Management of Alcohol and Drug Problems

Management of Alcohol and Drug Problems

Edited by

Gary Hulse
Jason White
Gavin Cape

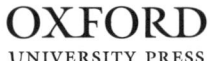
OXFORD

UNIVERSITY PRESS

OXFORD

UNIVERSITY PRESS

253 Normanby Road, South Melbourne, Victoria 3205, Australia

Oxford University Press is a department of the University of Oxford.
It furthers the University's objective of excellence in research, scholarship,
and education by publishing worldwide in

Oxford New York

Auckland Bangkok Buenos Aires Cape Town Chennai
Dar es Salaam Delhi Hong Kong Istanbul Karachi Kolkata
Kuala Lumpur Madrid Melbourne Mexico City Mumbai Nairobi
São Paulo Shanghai Taipei Tokyo Toronto

OXFORD is a trade mark of Oxford University Press
in the UK and in certain other countries

National Library of Australia

Cataloguing-in-Publication data:

Hulse, Gary.
Management of alcohol and drug problems.

Bibliography.
Includes index.
ISBN 0 19 551331 2.

1. Alcoholism. 2. Alcoholism—Treatment. 3. Drug abuse.
4. Drug abuse—Treatment. I. White, Jason M.
II. Cape, Gavin, 1958–. III. Title.

616.86

Edited by Elaine Cochrane
Text and cover designed by Racheal Stines
Typeset by Kerry Cooke
Printed through Bookpac Production Services, Singapore

Contents

List of Figures

List of Tables

Contributors

David Atkinson is Director of the Centre for Aboriginal Medical and Dental Health at the University of Western Australia. He has worked for many years as a medical practitioner in Aboriginal community controlled health services and in medical education. Recent projects include reports on health planning in the Kimberley, Aboriginal health-worker education, and collaboration on a review of injecting-drug use among Aboriginal people in Western Australia.

Maria Basso has worked for several years in the Unit for Research and Education in Drugs and Alcohol, School of Psychiatry & Clinical Neurosciences, Faculty of Medicine University of Western Australia. She has a history of involvement in facilitating medical management for migrants, and considerable experience working with and conducting research on dependent heroin use and affected persons.

Gavin Cape, MBChB, MRCPsych, is Medical Director of the Dunedin Alcohol and Drug Service, and a senior lecturer in the Department of Psychological Medicine, University of Otago, Dunedin, New Zealand. He has past experience working as a general adult psychiatrist within the alcohol and drug field in New Zealand and the United Kingdom. His current special interests include the evaluation of alcohol and other drug education and training for medical students, the influence of film media on drug use and outcome measures in methadone treatment programs.

Kate Conigrave Fafphm, PhD, MB BS (Hons) is a staff specialist in the Drug Health Services, Royal Prince Alfred Hospital, Sydney, and a co-joint associate professor in the School of Public Health and Departments of Psychological Medicine and Medicine at the University of Sydney. She is responsible for the coordination of drug and alcohol teaching within the medical program at the University of Sydney. Her research has focused on early detection and treatment of alcohol problems.

Jan Copeland, PhD, is a senior lecturer, National Drug and Alcohol Research Centre, University of New South Wales. Her research interests include: the treatment of cannabis dependence in adults and adolescents; women and substance use; substance-use intervention issues for young people in the juvenile justice system; and treatment evaluation and measurement of service utilisation and treatment outcome. She has been published in approximately 110 publications and has given 146 oral papers including keynote addresses at national and international conferences since 1990. She is an assistant editor of *Addiction* and the *Journal of Substance Abuse Treatment*.

Kennith Curry is the Medical Director of Canterbury Drug Health Services, staff specialist in Drug Health, Central Sydney Area Health Service and clinical lecturer, University of Sydney, Faculty of Medicine. His interests include: the management of pain in dependency; drug and alcohol education and cultural; and religious and spiritual relationships with drug use.

Daryl Deering, RCN, MHealSci has a joint appointment as lecturer in the Department of Psychological Medicine, Christchurch, New Zealand and is Director of Mental Health Nursing Practice, Christchurch. She has an extensive history of working as a clinician in the alcohol and drug services and youth mental health services. Her current research interests are in consumer outcome measurements and youth mental health.

Glenys Dore is a senior staff specialist psychiatrist and deputy medical superintendent at Macquarie Hospital, Sydney. She is also a clinical lecturer for the University of Sydney. She has worked for many years in drug and alcohol services, and general adult psychiatry. Her major interests include diagnosis and management of patients with dual diagnosis (substance misuse and mental health disorders); women and addiction; and management of opioid dependence. She is a co-editor of *The Long and the Short of Treatment for Alcohol and Drug Disorders* (1998), and an author in *Folding Back the Shadows: A Perspective on Women's Mental Health* (1998); *Affective Disorders* (1995); and *Foundations of Clinical Psychiatry* (2 nd Ed, 2001).

Mason Durie, (Rangitane, Ngati Raukawa, Ngati Kauwhata) is Professor and Head of School, Te Pūtahi a Toi, School of Māori Studies, Massey University, New Zealand. He has considerable research expertise interest and publications relating to the health and welfare of the Māori population. He was a foundation member of the New Zealand Alcohol Advisory Council

Gerald Feeney is a physician and Medical Director of the Alcohol and Drug Unit at the Princess Alexandra Hospital, Brisbane.

Rosemary Friend, MBBS, is a general practitioner working closely with the local needle exchange in Dunedin, New Zealand and works part-time as a clinical lecturer for the University of Otago, Dunedin with a special interest in the training of medical undergraduates and postgraduates in alcohol and other drug management. She also has interests in mentoring and works as a private psychotherapist.

Dennis Gray is an Associate Professor at the National Drug Research Institute, Curtin University of Technology, where he manages the Indigenous Australian Research Program. His interests focus on the political economy of alcohol and other drug use among indigenous peoples. With Sherry Saggers, he is co-author of a general text book on Aboriginal health *The Traditional and Contemporary Struggle for Better Health* (1991) and a book on indigenous alcohol use *Dealing with Alcohol: Indigenous Usage in Australia, New Zealand and Canada* (1998).

Margaret Hamilton, MSW, BA, Dip. Soc. Studs, is Professor/Director at Turning Point Alcohol & Drug Centre. She has worked for more than 25 years in the drug and alcohol area including clinical practice, education and research at the University of Melbourne. Her research includes: epidemiology; studying the specific needs of young people in relation to drugs; alcohol and women; examining the provision of treatment services to difficult-to-reach groups; patterns of alcohol consumption and related harms in the general population; the place of alcohol problems in remote rural mining towns; and an investigation into self-help. She has also been involved in policy advice and has sat on senior advisory bodies including the Australian National Council on Drugs, the National Expert Advisory Committee on Alcohol and NEACID (Illicit Drugs). Her publications include various articles, research monographs, reports and *Drug Use in Australia: A Harm Minimisation Approach* (Hamilton, M., Kellehear, A. and Rumbold, G.) (Oxford University Press, 1998).

Gary Hulse is an Associate Professor and Head of the Unit for Research and Education in Drugs and Alcohol, School of Psychiatry & Clinical Neuroscience, University of Western Australia {WA} Faculty of Medicine, Sir Charles Gairdner Hospital. He has worked in the area of problem alcohol and drug use for the past 21 years, initially for the first 11 years in clinical-based services. For the past 10 years he has held an academic appointment as coordinator of Alcohol and Drug Education and Training within the Faculty. His research activities are primarily directed at developing evidence-based information that will enhance clinical practice. He has a track record of public health advocacy, and has previously served on the Committee of Management for two community based alcohol & drug services and one hospital board. He is currently a board member of the WA Alcohol Advisory Council, and has a ministerial appointment under the WA Mental Health Act. He also chairs the Committee on Alcohol and Drug Education in Medical Schools (CADEMS) for the Committee of Deans (Australian Medical Schools).

Terry Huriwai (Te Arawa/Ngati Porou) BA, Dip. Health Sci, is currently working as a project manager, Ministry of Health, Wellington, New Zealand. His activities include the preparation of the National Methadone Guidelines of New Zealand. He has had experience as a clinician and researcher in the alcohol and drug field and has interests relating to the mental health of Māori peoples.

Eric Khong, MBBS, Grad Dip Primary Health Care, FRACGP, is a medical graduate of the University of Western Australia. He is medical education consultant at the Drug and Alcohol Office (West Australian Department of Health) and a general practitioner in Perth. His current teaching and writing interests lie in *Drug use in Medical Practitioners, Party Drugs* and *Drug Use in Adolescents*.

Henry Krum, MBBD PhD FRACP, is Head of Clinical Pharmacology at Monash University and Alfred Hospital, Melbourne. He has wide-ranging interests in clinical therapeutics of disease with a focus on drug interactions, cardiovascular pharmacology and adverse drug reactions among patients in hospitals. He teaches toxicology to undergraduate and post-graduate medical students.

Olga Lopatko, MD, PhD (Pharmacology), is a medical graduate of Tashkent Medical University. She has had a long-time interest in the clinical management of alcohol and other drug use, and joined the University of Adelaide, Department of Clinical and Experimental Pharmacology as a lecturer in 1999. Her current research interests include respiratory effects of tobacco and opioids and buprenorphine as a maintenance pharmacotherapy.

Noeline Latt, MBBS, MPhil, MRCP, is staff specialist at the Herbert Street Drug and Alcohol Clinic, Royal North Shore Hospital; consultant drug & alcohol physician, Northside Clinic, Greenwich; and clinical lecturer in Drug & Alcohol Medicine, University of Sydney. She has a background in clinical pharmacology and therapeutics and was a medical director in the Pharmaceutical Industry and medical director of the Ryde and Hornsby Drug & Alcohol Service. Her major interests include hepatitis C infection in pregnant injecting drug-users and their babies and the treatment of patients with alcohol and other drug related problems.

Simon Lenton, Bpsych, MPsych (Clin), is a senior research fellow at the National Drug Research Institute at Curtin University in Western Australia. He also works part time as a clinical psychologist in private practice. He has published numerous articles, reports and chapters on drug policy and drug-related harm. He is a deputy editor of the *Drug and Alcohol Review* and edits the *Harm Reduction Digest* that appears in each issue.

Jennifer Martin, MA (Oxon.), MBChB, FRACP is a clinical pharmacologist and physician at the Alfred Hospital, Melbourne. Her main interests include therapeutically and economically appropriate drug usage in medicine. She has taught medical students in Australia and New Zealand on drug and alcohol pharmacology, and also has an interest in alcohol and drug issues affecting doctors.

Stuart McLean, Mpharm, PhD, is Associate Professor of Pharmacology at the School of Pharmacy, University of Tasmania. He has worked in several universities in Europe and North America, as well as in Australia. His research focuses on how a better understanding of pharmacology can lead to the safer use of drugs and other chemicals. In the alcohol and drug field he has investigated the influence of tobacco advertising on primary school children and the relationship between licensed premises and drink-driving. He is currently coordinating the Tasmanian component of an Australian National Survey of Illicit Drug Usage.

Tuari Potiki (Ngai Tahu) is currently a manager with Ngai Tahu Development Corporation, Christchurch, New Zealand, a tribal organisation concerned with the economic and social development of the Ngai Tahu iwi. He has extensive experience as a clinician and coordinator of services within the alcohol and drug field. His special interests include the assessment and management of alcohol and other drug problems within the Māori population.

Robyn Richmond, BA, MA, PhD, DSc., is an Associate Professor in the School of Public Health and Community Medicine, at the University of New South Wales. Her current research is focussed on groups at high risk from cigarette related diseases: those with a mental illness, indigenous people, and inmates, and at evaluating pharmacotherapies (nicotine gum, patch and bupropion). For 19 years she has trained general practitioners and other health professionals (pharmacists and nurses) on how to assist people to stop smoking. For three years she was the chair elect of the Tobacco Prevention Section of the International Union Against Tuberculosis and Lung Disease (IUATLD), a non-government organisation based in Paris, and this was followed by three years as the deputy chair. Her main activities with the IUATLD were international tobacco control and prevention, particularly teaching medical students about tobacco globally. She has published more than 130 papers and books, mostly in the area of tobacco.

Paul Robertson (Ngai Tahu, Kati Mamoe, Waitaha) MA, DipClinPsy, MNZCCP is a lecturer/clinical psychologist at the National Centre for Treatment Development (Alcohol, Drugs & Addiction), Department of Psychological Medicine, Christchurch School of Medicine. He has a special interest in the assessment and treatment of Māori with alcohol and other drug problems, especially in increasing the relevance and quality of research in this area. He also has an active teaching and development role in several postgraduate papers on addiction taught at the Christchurch School of Medicine and short courses offered through NCTD, as well as being involved in the development of the medical curriculum in the area of Māori health.

Geoffrey Robinson, MBChB FRACP, is a full-time specialist physician in general medicine and in the alcohol and drug service in Wellington, New Zealand. He has written widely on alcohol and drug health issues for more than 20 years. His research interests include morbidity and blood borne viruses in the injecting drug user and pharmacological treatments and enzyme function in alcohol dependence. He is the author of the *Handbook on Alcohol and Drugs for Health Professionals* (1993) and has an on-going interest in the impaired practitioner and medical education at an undergraduate and postgraduate level.

Sherry Saggers is an Associate Professor in the School of International, Cultural and Community Studies, and program director in the Institute for the Service Professions. Her research includes work on indigenous health and society, women's work and childcare, and sustainable communities. With Dennis Gray she has published widely on indigenous health, including *Aboriginal Health and Society: The Traditional and Contemporary Struggle for Better Health* (1991) and *Dealing with Alcohol: Indigenous Usage in Australia, New Zealand and Canada* (1998).

John Saunders is the Professor of Alcohol and Drug Studies at the University of Queensland and Director of the Alcohol and Drug Services of the Prince Charles Hospital and Royal Brisbane Hospital Health Service Districts of Queensland Health. He qualified in science and then medicine from the University of Cambridge (UK) and specialised in acute general medicine, gastroenterology and addiction medicine. He has worked closely with the World Health Organization (WHO) for many years, being technical focal point (scientific director) for 10 years of WHO's collaborative studies on brief intervention. He is a member of the WHO Expert Advisory Panel on Mental Health and is the co-director of the WHO Collaborating Centre on Mental Health and Substance Abuse for Australia. From 1989 to 1993 he was a member of the Expert Advisory Panel on Alcohol and Drugs of the National Health and Medical Research Council. He has been editor of the *Drug and Alcohol Review* since 1984, and is a member of the Council of the Australian Professional Society on Alcohol and Drugs. Since 1995 he has been secretary of the International Society for Biomedical Research on Alcoholism. He has given guest lectures and workshops at international meetings on 40 occasions in the past five years, and has published two books and over 250 scientific papers and reviews.

Doug Sellman, MBChB, PhD, FRANZCP, FAChAM, is an Associate Professor in the Department of Psychological Medicine, Christchurch, New Zealand and Head of the National Centre for Treatment Development (Alcohol, Drugs & Addiction) in Christchurch. He has considerable research expertise and is actively involved in teaching and curriculum development with respect to alcohol and other drugs at an undergraduate and postgraduate level. He has developed university-based postgraduate courses leading to accredited qualifications in the addiction field in New Zealand. His current interests also include addiction issues relating to adolescents, pharmacotherapy of addiction, early interventions and treatment outcome.

Moira Sim, MBBS, Grad Dip Alcohol and Drug Abuse Studies, FRACGP, is senior medical officer for Practice Development in the Drug and Alcohol Office (West Australian Department of Health) and a general practitioner in Perth, Western Australia. She is also a clinical senior lecturer in the School of Psychiatry & Clinical Neuroscience, University of Western Australia, Faculty of Medicine. She has extensive experience in the provision of education at an undergraduate and post-graduate level for medical practitioners and other health professionals. Through her work with Divisions of General Practice at a local, state and national level, she has developed systems to support medical practitioners in caring for people with mental illness and alcohol and other drug problems.

Mary Surveyor, MBBS, has extensive experience as a general practitioner in Perth, Western Australia. She has had a long interest in education, having taught undergraduate medical students in her practice and has been a supervisor for the Royal Australian College of General Practitioners Family Medicine Training Program for several years. Since 2000, she has chaired the Prevocational Training and Accreditation Committee in Western Australia, which accredits all prevocational junior doctor positions and supervises junior doctor hospital training and experience. She has also been involved with the Australian National Prescribing Service since its inception, serving on the Prescriber Working Group. She was the foundation medical director of the Osborne Division of General Practice and chairperson of Quality Use of Medicine committees.

Stanley Theodorou, MBBS, DPH, MRCPsych, FRANZCP is Head of the Department of Drug Health Services at Concord Repatriation General Hospital, Sydney. He is currently the secretary of the section of Addiction Psychiatry of the Royal Australian and New Zealand College of Psychiatrists. He has wide clinical experience within the area of drug health, including pharmacotherapeutic interventions in opiate dependence, inpatient liaison services as well outpatient work. He is involved in both undergraduate and postgraduate medical teaching within the drug and alcohol field.

Fraser Todd, MBChB FRANZCP, is a senior lecturer, National Centre for Treatment Development (Alcohol, Drugs & Addiction), Dept Psychological Medicine, Christchurch School of Medicine, New Zealand. He has special interest in the development of effective treatments and service planning for co-existing disorders, cannabis and works as a psychiatrist for the alcohol and drug stream of the Youth Speciality Service, Christchurch.

Ross Young is a senior lecturer in Clinical Psychology at the Department of Psychiatry, University of Queensland and visiting senior clinical psychologist at the Alcohol and Drug Unit at the Princess Alexandra Hospital, Brisbane. His research involves the interface between genetic and psychological factors in the genesis and treatment of substance misuse as well as cognitive behavioural and pharmacotherapeutic treatments for nicotine, alcohol and opioid misuse. He has also served as national president of the Australian Association for Cognitive and Behaviour Therapy and is chair of the Early Intervention and Prevention Committee of the Queensland Cancer Fund.

Jason White, PhD, is Professor of Addiction Studies in the Department of Clinical and Experimental Pharmacology at the University of Adelaide and Head of the Maintenance Pharmacotherapies Unit, Drug and Alcohol Services Council. His research interests include the clinical pharmacology of opioid maintenance treatment and the adverse effects of substituted amphetamines. He has served on a number of national and international committees and is past-president of the Australian Professional Society on Alcohol and other Drugs.

Alex Wodak, MBBS, FRACP, FAFPHM, is the Director of the Alcohol and Drug Service, St Vincent's Hospital, Sydney. Major interests include the prevention of the spread of HIV and hepatitis C among injecting-drug users, brief interventions for problem drinkers, treatment of drug users in prison and drug policy. He is the president of the Australian Drug Law Reform Foundation and also president of the International Harm Reduction Association. He is a member of a number of state and national committees and has also often worked in developing countries, especially to assist efforts to control HIV infection among injecting drug users. He recently published, with Tim Moore, *Modernising Australia's Drug Policy*.

Preface

Problems associated with the use of alcohol and other drugs are of increasing concern today. One outcome has been an increased demand for accurate information on drugs, for appropriate and accessible treatment, and for programs for prevention of these problems. Together with other health professionals, medical practitioners are increasingly expected to provide appropriate information, assessment, and treatment. However, until recently, a major impediment to medical practitioners fulfilling these roles has been their limited education and training on drug and alcohol problems.

Since the late 1980s initiatives have been undertaken in Australia and New Zealand to improve undergraduate medical education in the drug and alcohol area. The continued maintenance of these programs and the setting of standards has developed under the auspices of the Committee for Alcohol and Drug Education in Medical Schools (CADEMS). The CADEMS group initially developed a core curriculum to be implemented across Australian and New Zealand medical schools. This book represents a further development by providing an appropriate alcohol and drug text. Most of the contributors have been or are involved in undergraduate drug and alcohol medical education.

The book is written for medical practitioners in training, but is also intended as an evidence-based reference text for doctors of all levels of experience, and for other professionals working in the area of alcohol and other drugs. The main goal of the book is to introduce the student or practitioner to the fundamentals of alcohol and drug misuse as applied to a clinical setting, complete with assessment, diagnostic and treatment strategies, and tools. While a clinical focus is maintained throughout the book, it is complemented with coverage of the research underlying practice.

The book is structured into three parts. Part 1 provides general introductory material that is largely common to the different drugs. This includes a historical perspective, an understanding of the biological and psychosocial bases of drug use and drug dependence, the types of problems that arise from drug use, and approaches to assessment, diagnosis and treatment. Part 2 covers specific drugs and drug classes. Although there are some differences, these chapters share a common structure. Part 3 is concerned mainly with sub-populations of drug users. These range from general groups within our society (adolescents, women, indigenous people) to those drug users with particular types of problems (for example, those with coexisting mental health disorders). There is also a final chapter on professional issues that covers important topics that should be considered by all medical practitioners.

This book is the product of the efforts of a number of people. We would like to thank the authors who contributed to the various chapters. It is very difficult for people to find the time within their busy schedules to take on additional commitments, and we are grateful for their valuable contributions. The collaborative nature of the book has meant that it required several meetings to plan the text, and to assemble and assimilate the material. We gratefully acknowledge the support of the Commonwealth Department of Health and Aged Care in Australia, and the Alcohol Advisory Council of New Zealand. We are also grateful to the Committee of Deans of Australian Medical Schools and especially to Professor Derek Frewin, the CADEMS spokesperson on this committee, who has been ever supportive throughout the development of this text.

PART 1

General Issues

The five chapters in part 1 provide a general introduction to alcohol and drug problems.

The first chapter begins with a historical overview. It then provides an outline of fundamental concepts relating to the use of drugs in society, including the response of the general population and policy makers. The role of medical practitioners and the broad health consequences of drug use are also considered.

Chapter 2 is concerned with why people use drugs, and importantly, why some people become dependent on them. As part of this examination the chapter considers the biological, psychological, and social bases of such dependence.

The next three chapters cover the practical issues of management of alcohol and drug problems in medical practice. The type of prevailing problems is considered first, followed by approaches to assessment and diagnosis, and finally general treatment options. These chapters provide a framework for the consideration of specific drugs in part 2.

1

History of Drug Use and Drug Policy Responses

Margaret Hamilton & Gavin Cape

Save for the occasional use of cocaine he had no vices, and he only turned to the drug as a protest against the monotony of existence …

Dr Watson's description of Sherlock Holmes, in Sir Arthur Conan Doyle 1893, 'The Yellow Face'.

From the quick-start cup of coffee to an ecstasy tablet at a dance party, from the celebratory glass of wine to the injecting of heroin or crushed morphine tablets, most people have some experience of psychoactive drug use. Drugs have attracted interest, symbolic meanings, desire, and fear throughout history. As Nietzsche said, 'the whole history of narcotica … is almost the history of culture'. Drug use is an integral part of human existence and is here to stay.

Understanding drugs is about understanding us, our histories and traditions, our make-up and our desires. It is also about an increasingly sophisticated scientific understanding of brain chemistry and behaviour. This area of study is rife with contradictions and paradox. Some substances that have been used by almost half of the population are illegal. At the same time, some legal drugs cost our community billions of dollars annually, and are promoted with sophisticated advertising while we, through our governments, derive substantial revenue from taxation associated with them. Some people use some drugs without apparent harm. Others develop severe problems and are harmed by their use.

This book provides a starting point for all students who wish to inform themselves adequately about a subject that most health practitioners are likely to encounter during their day-to-day practice.

WHAT IS A DRUG?

There are many definitions of a drug. For the purposes of this book the World Health Organisation (WHO) definition of a drug is used: 'a chemical entity used non-medically, self-administered for its psychoactive effect'. The psychoactive effect is an essential component of the definition and usually includes a change in mood, arousal and/or perception, cognition (thinking), and/or behaviour. The particular effect varies according to which drug is used, the amount used, the route of administration of the drug, the expectations the user has of the effects of the drug, the setting in which it is used, the previous experience of use of the drug and the possibility of tolerance, personal characteristics including gender, weight, and so on, as well as the mixture of drugs consumed at the same time.

> In the present context the term drug denotes a chemical entity, used non-medically, self-administered for its psychoactive effect.

A number of other terms may be used interchangeably with the word drug. 'Substance' and 'chemical' are often used when talking about the socially sanctioned drugs such as nicotine and alcohol. 'Addiction' is a general term that is slowly being replaced by the more narrowly defined 'dependence' (see later).

The definition of a drug can also be applied to a number of other chemicals or foodstuffs. Poppy seeds, nutmeg and even coffee can be misused, but are freely available. Some substances have managed to bypass the laws governing foodstuffs. For example, in New Zealand it is possible to buy kava (a powdered root used in Fijian ceremonies that has an intoxicating effect when consumed) from the local supermarket, while in other places it has been outlawed. Different cultures classify different drugs in different ways and the classification is not necessarily related to their potential for harm.

TYPES OF PSYCHOACTIVE DRUGS

Drugs are categorised in a variety of ways. A law textbook would divide them according to their current legal status. A users' guide might separate them according to availability, price, and uses. In the health area, we examine the mechanisms of action of the various drugs and their influence on physiology and behaviour, and how that ultimately impacts on the positive and negative consequences of their use. Many drugs have an important place in therapeutic medicine, but also have the potential to cause harm.

We are coming to a greater understanding of how drugs act on the human body. At a cellular or molecular level it is possible to pinpoint the actual sites of action and change in function of brain processes. With this knowledge it is possible to find pharmacological therapies to block or change specific actions of a drug, or provide less harmful substitutes for specific drugs, or to contribute to promising new drug treatments. An example of this was the discovery in 1973 of brain neurotransmitters that are very similar to morphine—endorphins (endogenous morphine). There are now drugs such as naltrexone that act to block this neural system and these are being tested for their potential therapeutic use (see chapter 6).

While it is possible to classify drugs by the effect they have on behaviour, this can be misleading. Our experience of a drug is influenced not only by the physiological effect of the drug on our body (usually the brain), but also by our expectations of the drug and the situation we use it in. The effects of a drug are thus not just the intrinsic property of the drug itself. Some drugs have several types of effects while others are unique in their properties. Some have a sedating effect on brain function but this might be experienced in mood and behaviour as stimulating or disinhibiting. For example, alcohol at low doses may have stimulatory effect while at high doses is a sedative. Other drugs can be included in more than one category: for example cannabis can have depressant effects on brain functioning but be experienced as stimulating, and it also can have a hallucinogenic effect.

A simple and commonly used framework classifies drugs according to their physiological effects. This gives rise to five broad categories: depressants, opioids, cannabinoids, stimulants, and hallucinogens.

Depressants include alcohol, which effectively lowers inhibitions. At higher doses it impairs perception including sight, as well as coordination and concentration, and it reduces the ability to make sound judgments and to respond to changes in the environment, such as a pedestrian stepping on to the road in front of a car. Other depressant drugs include inhalants (petrol or glue). Depressant drugs used to reduce anxiety or promote sleep include benzodiazepines such as diazepam (Valium) and the barbiturates.

Opioids, a category which includes morphine, heroin, codeine, and pethidine, are strong analgesics with euphoric properties and depressant action (impaired consciousness).

Cannabinoids have a mixture of mild hallucinogenic (altered perception of time and sound) and depressant (diminished physical coordination) properties.

Stimulants increase nervous energy and suppress sleep and appetite. This group of drugs includes the amphetamines (speed), cocaine, and ecstasy. These may cause anxiety and restlessness, and in large doses may provoke major psychiatric symptoms. Caffeine (contained in coffee, tea, cola drinks, and chocolate) and nicotine (tobacco) are also stimulants.

Hallucinogens such as LSD, psilocybin (magic mushrooms), and datura, powerfully distort perceptions of reality (time, sounds, and sight). Under the influence of these drugs, people experience things that do not exist or their experience of things that do exist is modified. Some anaesthetic agents (ketamine and phencyclidine) can also provoke visual hallucinations—seeing things that aren't there. Some other drugs including cannabis and ecstasy can produce mild perceptual distortions.

There are many other drugs which can be abused, or which can lead to harm, for example the steroids used in sport, betel nut, kava, and nitrous oxide.

> Drugs have an important place in therapeutic medicine. They can also cause harm.

DRUG TROUBLE AND DIAGNOSTIC CLASSIFICATIONS

Drugs are usually taken because they are enjoyed, or out of curiosity. They are seen to help the user relax or to ease a troubled mind, to make someone feel different, or to act as a social lubricant. Some drugs, such as alcohol, are ordinarily consumed in a controlled manner for these benefits. Many have potential to cause harm on a single occasion of excessive use (acute harm), as well as to cause harm as a result of a long period of consistent heavy use (chronic harm/problems). Certain patterns of use of any of these drugs can be hazardous.

> Drug use can cause harm in many ways to individuals, those around them, and the whole community. Harm can occur in an acute single episode of use and/or after sustained use.

The classification systems for dependence or addiction most widely used in Australia and New Zealand are the DSM-IV (Diagnostic Statistical Manual from the American Psychiatric Association) and the ICD-10 (International Classification of Diseases) from the WHO (see chapter 3). Both of these are based upon the dependence syndrome first described with regard to alcohol in 1976 by Edwards and Gross. This introduced the notion that dependence is at one end of a continuum of use from controlled use, and that there are many degrees of severity in between (see chapter 3).

THE CULTURE AND HISTORY OF DRUG USE

Over time and in all societies, human beings have identified and used naturally occurring psychoactive drugs. Over 4000 plants have been identified as having psychoactive properties, but only about 40 are used for human intoxication effects.

Drugs have been used since records began: 7000 years ago, Sumerians were aware of the effects of opium, and in 3500 BC the Egyptians knew how to brew alcohol on a large scale. As they recognised the power and potency of these substances, societies regulated access to the drugs and the appropriate manner of their use. Some examples of ways to understand drugs include appreciating their historic use in rituals and religion, and the recognition that, given their social potency, drugs are subject to changes in fashion. The use of many drugs has moved well beyond the traditions, rituals, and controls surrounding their geographic and social origins. They represent commodities, and as such have a place in international markets and, historically, in wars. They are ever-evolving as people seek new experiences or to enhance abilities and perceptions.

There have been many attempts to try to conceptualise the nature of drug use and drug dependence, including the moral and disease models.

Table 1.1 A brief history of drugs

Opium: first recorded reference on Sumerian tablets as 'plant of joy'	5000 BC
Alcohol: first recorded brewery	3500 BC
Cannabis: first recorded medicinal use	737 BC
Laudanum 'worthy of praise' (tincture of opium) introduced by Paracelsus	1525
Morphine first isolated from opium: 'cure for opium addicts'	1799
Tobacco smoking compulsory at Eton School (Thomas Hearne)	1721
Confessions of an English Opium Eater (Thomas De Quincey) published	1822
Opium wars start	1839
Le Club des Haschischins established, including Baudelaire and Alexandre Dumas as members	1844
Hypodermic syringe developed by Scottish surgeon Alexander Woodin	1853
Heroin isolated by Heinrich Dreser (inventor of aspirin)	1874
Cocaine prescribed by Freud (initially to treat himself)	1884
Coca-Cola (with cocaine) introduced by an Atlanta pharmacist as a tonic	1886
Heroin marketed by Bayer as cure for morphinomaniacs: 'a safe preparation free from addiction-forming properties'!	1894
Caffeine replaces cocaine in Coca-Cola	1903
MDMA (ecstasy) synthesised by Merk as an appetite suppressor	1912
Barbiturates: phenobarbitol introduced as Luminal	1912
Harrison Narcotics Act in US requires opiates and cocaine to be prescribed by a physician	1914
Prohibition amendment enacted in US—alcohol prohibited for 13 years	1920
Film *Reefer Madness* released	1936
LSD synthesised by Albert Hoffman and 5 years later he accidentally ingests a large amount	1938
Methadone synthesised and marketed as Dolphine ('pain ends')	1941
Benzodiazepines: chlordiazepoxide marketed as Librium	1959
THC isolated by Raphael Mechoulan	1964
League for Spiritual Discovery (LSD) started by Timothy Leary, and LSD made illegal in USA	1966
IOC (International Olympic Committee) ban amphetamines after a cyclist dies	1967
US President Bill Clinton states that he tried cannabis but did not inhale	1992

Moral model

The moral model was the prevailing addiction archetype up until the mid twentieth century, and it still has a wide following today. This model views the addicted user as weak-willed and morally bankrupt, someone who should be punished or sometimes pitied.

One outcome of the moral model was the Temperance Movement (misnamed as it advocated abstinence), whose members viewed alcohol consumption as something inherently evil, a poison that leads to social, moral and economic deterioration. The Temperance Movement started in the USA in the 1820s and contributed to the infamous years of Prohibition in the USA in the 1920s and 1930s. Under Prohibition, alcohol had a legal status akin to that of heroin today. Even though alcohol-related harm was reduced (but not eradicated) during this period, other negative consequences, such as a rise in organised crime and police corruption, became endemic. This, coupled with the general unpopularity of the Prohibition law, resulted in its eventual repeal in 1933.

Today this model tends to underpin the thinking of those who hold individuals entirely responsible for their drug use; assuming it to be an act of will whereby the individual's choice of behaviours, including drug use, is free and usually informed.

Disease model

The disease model represents a significant change of viewpoint from the moral model. It is a more humanistic response, advocating treatment rather than punishment. The disease model, coupled with a spiritual dimension, underpins the largest and most successful self-help organisation in the world, AA (Alcoholics Anonymous).

Although there had been some early writings on alcohol-induced diseases in the early nineteenth century, it was not until the 1960s that this model found favour within the academic establishment. A number of propositions underlie the disease model. These include the view that alcoholics (or other drug-dependent people) are different from the non-alcoholic drinkers, that abstinence is the only treatment goal, and that the alcoholic is not to blame for the disease. It is stressed that chemical addiction is a chronic, relapsing and progressive disorder.

Difficulties with this model include the idea that only certain people are vulnerable to chemical addiction, rather than anyone who uses drugs too much for too long. When the lives of people who are drug-dependent are followed, there is not always a progression down a slippery slope to death. Many do not escalate their use, and many stop or reduce alcohol or other drug use without formal treatment.

Genetic research has begun to reveal some specific vulnerability to dependence among some people, but the biological cause of dependence remains elusive. While there might be some physical predisposition, drug dependence has multiple origins, with a mix of pharmacological, psychological, social, and cultural determinants.

→ Drug dependence has multiple origins, with a mix of pharmacological, psychological, social, and cultural determinants.
→ Different models of drug use will lead to different prevention and treatment approaches.

The changing status of drugs

The status of particular drugs varies as cultures develop and change. Fashions and patterns emerge. Sometimes there can be a rapid rise in popularity and acceptability of a drug, followed by a rapid decline and vilification as unexpected consequences become evident. For example, phenacetin, a mild analgesic, was once used recreationally among the well-heeled in Scandinavian countries, and phenacetin-enhanced parties were very fashionable during the 1950s. Unfortunately this drug has very serious side-effects, including papillary necrosis (severe kidney damage). Once these side-effects became known, the drug-inspired parties soon ceased and so did the prescription of the drug. This same substance was a core ingredient of various patent medicines available over the counter through the middle of the twentieth century in Australia and New Zealand, and contributed to one of the highest rates of analgesic nephropathy in the world and a significant increase in the need for kidney transplants.

Since many drugs have both positive and potential negative consequences, it is not surprising to see warnings about caffeine from an earlier time. After the drinking of tea and coffee had become popular in Britain, a standard medical textbook written by a noted Cambridge physician and leading pharmacologist at the beginning of the twentieth century outlined in graphic detail the dangers of the humble cuppa:

> the sufferer is tremulous, and loses his self command; he is subject to fits of agitation and depression; he loses colour and has a haggard appearance. The appetite falls off, and symptoms of gastric catarrh may be manifested. The heart also suffers; it palpitates, or it intermits. As with other such agents, a renewed dose of the poison gives temporary relief, but at the cost of future misery. Tea produces a strange and extreme degree of physical depression … A grievous sinking may seize upon a sufferer … The speech may become vague and weak. By miseries such as these, the best years of life may be spoilt.

> Sir T. Clifford Allbutt & Humphrey Davy Rolleston (eds) 1909, *A System of Medicine*, vol. II, part I, Macmillan, London, pp. 986–7.

Alcohol has been and is viewed in many different ways by different societies and cultures. Current fashion (no doubt aided by expensive promotions in Western countries) contributes to the inclination of young people to drink certain alcoholic beverages, which are often spirit based, or promoted with youthful symbols such as vivid colours, sweet taste or by a suggested association with social popularity. Similarly, other products such as cigars, can become popular following high profile appearances in movies, for example in Wayne Wang's 1995 film *Smoke*. The use of party drugs, including ecstasy, represents a modern fashion.

Ritual and religion

Drug use has been associated with many human activities and has been incorporated in many celebrations and religious rituals. The Aztecs used a powerful hallucinogen—peyote—as a means of celebrating the rights of passage into adulthood. Peyote is still used in the Native American Church in the USA and Canada. Red wine plays a part in the communion of a mainstream Christian church, and the smoking of ganja, a potent form of cannabis, is used as a sacrament within the Rastafarian religion.

Ayahuasca tea is a brew of another powerful hallucinogen (dimethyltryptamine, DMT) used in many Christian churches in Brazil. The congregation, of all ages, imbibes this hallucinogen on a regular basis as part of their four- to six-hour church service. When this drug is used within these strict cultural boundaries there appears to be little risk to the user. One study reporting on the long-term use of this powerful hallucinogen within such congregations revealed that there were no significant differences between users and a matched population of non-users on a battery of neurological and psychological tests.

In these specific contexts there appears to be little harm in the regular use of powerful drugs.

War

Such is the power (or economic value) of some drugs that wars are fought over them. The Opium Wars from 1839 to 1842 and 1856 to 1858 were concerned with a clash of cultural values and claims to free (monopolistic) trade. The British insisted that the East India (Shipping) Company had the right to import opium into China, and, as a result of the wars, gained continued opium trade, Hong Kong, and a large sum of money. It was not until the People's Revolution in 1949 that opium use in China was virtually eradicated.

Drugs in sport

Drugs have become popular in sport as so-called performance enhancers. The degree of the deceit required to make detection difficult, and the risks involved, do not appear to discourage some athletes in continuing to use these drugs. The International Olympic Committee banned amphetamines in 1967 after a cyclist died of a heart attack related to their use. It is thought that amphetamines and other stimulants are responsible for more deaths than any other drug used in sport.

The use of androgenic anabolic steroids among sports people is often reported in the media, and is seen as giving users unfair advantage over their competitors. Studies of regular gym–goers have reported that up to 10% have used anabolic steroids. Steroid use is strongly associated with many physical problems and results in major mood disorders in up to a quarter of regular users, including so–called 'roid' rage.

TRENDS IN DRUG USE

Particular patterns of drug use and drug-related harm are a product of the social, cultural, and economic context of use, as well as of the pharmacological and toxicological properties of the drug itself.

In Australia and New Zealand large scale surveys on drug use are conducted every few years. These offer a guide to trends, although the information they provide may under-estimate some illicit drug use because of people's unwillingness to admit to such use.

Figure 1.1 Prevalence of drug use in Australia, 1998 National Drug Strategy Household Survey (Australian Institute of Health and Welfare 1999)

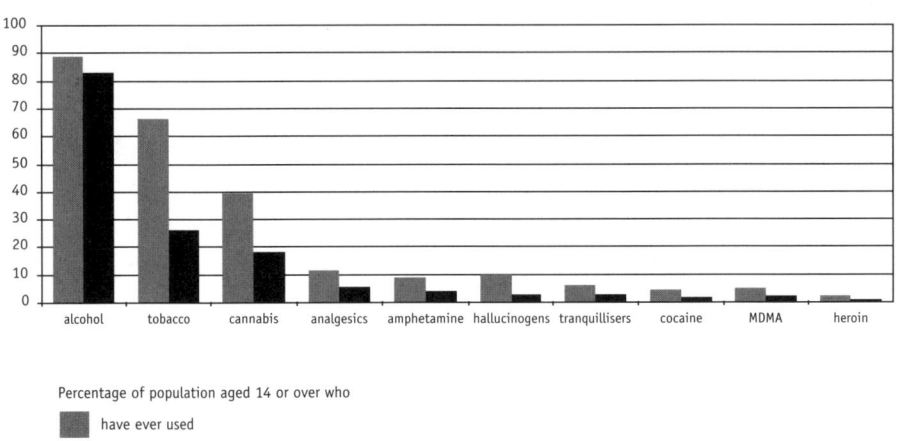

Percentage of population aged 14 or over who

☐ have ever used

■ have used in the last 12 months

Alcohol and tobacco use

Clearly the licit drugs—alcohol and tobacco—are the most widely used, as shown in figure 1.1. While the overall per capita consumption of alcohol in Australia and New Zealand has been gradually declining for some years, there is currently an increase in harmful (binge) patterns of use, especially by young people. Tobacco use has been declining, but the uptake of cigarettes among young people remains of concern (see chapters 7 and 15).

Illicit drug use

Illicit drug use among young people emerged in Australia and New Zealand in the 1960s. Since the start of the 1990s illicit drug use has increased, coupled with a lower age of initiation, paralleling a worldwide trend. The level of drug use in Australia and New Zealand is broadly comparable with the levels in Britain and the USA, albeit with some differences. New Zealand differs from Australia and most other developed countries by recording less use of cocaine, amphetamines and heroin, but more use of hallucinogens. Australia has higher drug use overall than New Zealand.

Drug use among indigenous Australians and New Zealanders is of increasing concern. With a backdrop of high rates of trouble with alcohol in these subgroups, there is increasing evidence of high rates of illicit drug use as well. These findings are consistent with other international work that has sought to analyse the complex broader environment of drug-related harm in communities with lower socioeconomic status. Other drug practices such as petrol sniffing are more common among indigenous Australians, especially among young people in remote communities (see chapters 17 and 18).

Cannabis is the most popular illicit drug and, although it has been tried at least once by a large proportion of the population, it is generally used infrequently. A small, but possibly growing, percentage of users report very frequent use, often associated with harmful consequences and dependence.

Use of amphetamines has been increasing in Australia and, to a lesser degree, in New Zealand. Amphetamine production is reported to be increasing internationally and the drugs that are available come from a mix of illegal importation and manufacture in clandestine laboratories. Use of amphetamines in Australia represents one of the highest rates in the world. Cocaine is less apparent, although in some locations, such as in Sydney, it appears to be more available.

The use of ecstasy (MDMA, see chapter 8) has been increasing, particularly among the late teen and early adult population, but is rarely used by people older than 35. Patterns of use of this drug might be changing to more frequent and longer sessions.

Hallucinogens have been tried by approximately one in ten Australians and New Zealanders. After a wave of popularity in the 1960s and 1970s this class of drug almost disappeared during the late 1980s and early 1990s. It has since resurfaced along with other drugs such as MDMA.

In New Zealand there is little heroin available but this is replaced by the manufacture of opioid alkaloids (including codeine, 'homebake', and morphine) through local laboratories, as well as the diversion of prescription drugs such as morphine tablets. A recent estimate indicates approximately 30 000 New Zealanders were opioid dependent. In Australia, recent research exploring a number of different methods of estimating the number of heroin users estimated that there were 74 000 dependent heroin users. The use of heroin appears to be increasing in Australia.

Many of the opioid-dependent users are also frequent users of other drugs and are often poly-drug dependent (see chapters 6 and 14).

POLICY RESPONSES TO DRUG USE

There are many ways a community or country can respond to drug use. One of the primary decisions is about the legal status of different drugs. Different drugs are made illegal in different countries. Some religious groups abhor alcohol for example, and some Muslim countries outlaw it, whereas in Australia and New Zealand alcohol is readily available to all except the young.

A number of international conventions provide some framework for international laws and potential international cooperation in policing them. Not all countries interpret them in the same way however, and some countries that are signatories of the UN conventions have contradictory policies and programs. The reasons for this are complex, relating to the sovereign rights of countries to decide their own laws and their various cultural, economic and social histories.

It is only since the 1980s that the focus has been on a public health approach on the whole population's use of these substances. This has increased interest in prevention and in ways of thinking about drugs that allow and require health, education, and community portfolios to come together with justice portfolios.

The dominant policy approach in many countries is prohibition for some drugs while legal products—tobacco and alcohol—are treated differently. The USA and Singapore are examples of countries where explicit policies focus on the illegal products and maximum resources go into policing. Policing of drugs includes interdiction (stopping their import at the borders), crop replacement programs in source countries, customs services, including the use of sniffer dogs, and support for special police in source countries or assistance with the supply of surveillance equipment. These environments tend to emphasise the dangers of the drugs themselves, and users of these products are punished and criminalised. Treatment is provided for users and the expected outcome of this treatment is abstinence.

Other countries (mainly in Europe) adopt a pragmatic stance towards drugs, and some of the more innovative responses have arisen here since the mid to late 1980s. The Netherlands is well recognised as having a more liberal and tolerant attitude to drug use. More recently, Switzerland has introduced the provision of prescribed heroin to heroin-dependent people, with considerable success in reducing drug use and crime, and increased involvement in work among those thus treated. Here, the focus is generally on the people who use drugs and the importance of managing public space to preserve safety and community life. There is less attention paid to prosecuting the drug users themselves.

Australia and New Zealand have adopted the principle of harm minimisation. This allows efforts to reduce and regulate the supply of drugs (the agent) and the demand for drugs or our appetite for psychoactive substances (the host) through education, information, and other preventative efforts at a community level, as well as treatment and harm reduction, including efforts to modify the environment of use to reduce harm (the context).

There are many reasons why this approach is the mainstay of drug policy in Australia and New Zealand. Methadone treatment and needle and syringe programs are examples of harm minimisation programs that became more prominent after the emergence of AIDS in the early 1980s. It is a pragmatic approach, and accepts that drug use is a common feature of human experience. It recognises that abstinence may be the ultimate goal, but accepts that this may not be achievable (or desirable), at least in the short-term.

Australia and New Zealand have a relatively low rate of HIV infection among injecting drug users. This is attributed to the early introduction of programs that make clean injecting equipment available to drug users to reduce the sharing of syringes with its concomitant risk of spreading blood-borne disease (see chapter 13).

Critics of the harm minimisation approach are concerned that the failure to be clear and tough about illicit drug use might send an implicit message that drugs are OK. While harm minimisation has provoked vehement criticism from many (in the USA for example, where it is equated with drug legalisation), it remains the central guiding principle for drug policy in Australia and New Zealand both for licit and illicit drugs.

THE ROLE OF THE MEDICAL PROFESSION

Patients with drug problems often present to the medical practitioners with multiple health and social issues that can seem overwhelming. It is tempting for doctors to turn a blind eye or to enter an agreement in which 'you do not mention drug use and nor will I'. However, when these issues are ignored or overlooked the intervention offered is at best inadequate or ineffective, and it might be inappropriate or even damaging. Many medical conditions have drug use as a significant or causative factor, a fact often ignored in health curricula. Likewise, alcohol and drug misuse often appear to go unrecognised in many clinical encounters (see also chapter 21).

Medical practitioners are in an ideal position to influence, assess, diagnose, and treat all people with health problems, including those whose alcohol and drug consumption contributes to their health problems. They are credible and highly regarded, and have expertise in the health field. Not only do they have a responsibility to explore, assess, and pursue health-harming drug use, the patient expects to be questioned and examined in this area. A medical practitioner can be seen as failing in his or her duty if an assessment of drug use is not carried out.

Another often-neglected area for practitioners is awareness of their own use of intoxicants. Doctors are particularly prone to the excesses of alcohol and drugs, and this is the commonest cause for disciplinary measures in the profession (see chapter 21). Doctors are also a major source of street and/or illicit prescription drugs that can be misused or be very lucrative for the drug-seeker/seller.

Drug use and health

We have known about the impact of tobacco on health for some fifty years and have sound knowledge about the effects of more than moderate doses of alcohol. The more recent concern about increased use of illicit drugs, especially among the young, heightens the need to understand their effects and to examine the role of doctors in responding to them.

It has been estimated that up to 25% of hospital medical admissions are directly due to the effects of excessive alcohol consumption through its cardiovascular, gastroenterological, and neurological consequences. It is estimated that 15 to 20% of all general practice attendees consume alcohol excessively and to such a degree that it will contribute to physical, psychological, and social harm. The WHO has estimated that alcohol-related diseases and injuries account for 3 to 4% of the annual global burden of disease and injury, and that tobacco smoking was responsible for 21 million deaths in developed countries in the 1990s.

Even when medical practitioners feel despondent about their impact on, for example, smoking among patients, it is important to recognise what a huge effect even a modest reduction in numbers of smokers can have in the community. If three

If you are a practising health professional you will be faced with patients or clients who have health problems that are either directly or indirectly due to alcohol and/or drug misuse.

Medical practitioners will:
- see many people who are using alcohol and other drugs harmfully
- have to treat the effects of harmful use of alcohol and/or other drugs
- be asked for help by the family and friends of those using drugs
- be seen as credible health experts, and have an opportunity for early identification of harmful drug use
- through their prescribing role be an important potential source for some drugs that may cause problems for some people.

Patients:
- with drug problems often have multiple health and social problems
- expect doctors to enquire and provide information about alcohol and other drugs. The failure to enquire and respond to this information could lead to professional malpractice in some situations.

In addition:
- some interventions available are simple, brief, and effective
- successful treatments are usually selective and targeted (although they might have to be repeated as with other chronic, relapsing conditions)
- new and promising treatments in this field require medical involvement.

out of every 100 patients quit smoking and this were spread across the whole community, it would mean a 3% reduction in smoking-related illness and could contribute to huge savings in people's life circumstances and in health care costs. It has been shown that even brief interventions offered as a part of a standard consultation can achieve this result.

CONCLUSION

The increasing ease of communication and trade, and the rapid expansion of markets through globalisation, means that illegal as well as legal products are increasingly available. It is in this context, when products are available in different groups, countries, or cultures to peoples without a tradition of beliefs, knowledge, experience, and social rules about the use of a particular drug, that these drugs are more likely to be used in ways or by people where there is an increased risk of harm.

In the near future we can expect a greater variety of new psychoactive drugs, both natural and manufactured, to be available in our community. Some of these might prove valuable in treating illness and alleviating suffering. Others will be used predominantly recreationally—some people will use them to enhance social discourse or for perceived pleasure. In this environment it is likely that some people will also develop problems associated with use of these drugs.

This book aims to provide you with fresh ideas, information, and ways of understanding drug use, as well as sources of further information and ways to develop knowledge and skills. Be ready for the patients you will see who will often present with explicit or implicit drug use problems: they will need your expertise, yet often not request it.

REFERENCES AND FURTHER READING

Australian Institute of Health and Welfare 1999, *1998 National Drug Strategy Household Survey: First Result*, Australian Institute of Health and Welfare cat no. PHE 15 (Drug Statistics Series), Canberra.

Edwards, G. & Gross, M. 1976, 'Alcohol dependence: provisional description of a clinical syndrome', *British Medical Journal*, vol. 5, pp. 1058–61.

Ghodse, H. 1998, *Drugs and Addictive Behaviour*, Macmillan, London.

Gossop, M. 2000, *Living with Drugs* (5th edn), Ashgate, Aldershot.

Hamilton, M., Kellehear, A. & Rumbold G. (eds) 1999, *Drug Use in Australia*, Oxford University Press, Melbourne.

McCrady, B. & Epstein, E. 1999, *Addictions—A Comprehensive Guidebook*, Oxford University Press, New York.

Why Do People Use Drugs?

Ross Young & Gerald Feeney

The reason behind human activity, as diverse as that activity might be, is always one: man's need to bring about events in the external world which, when reflected in his consciousness, will make him feel happiness.

M. Ageyev 1984, *Novel with Cocaine*, Dutton, New York.

Between two evils I always pick the one I never tried before.

Mae West, quoted in J. Sochen (1992), *Mae West: She Who Laughs, Lasts*, Harlan Davidson, Arlington Heights.

Substance use is influenced by a complex array of physiological, psychological, and sociocultural factors. There are no neat and all-encompassing explanations for drug use, and any scientific or theoretical dogmatism needs to be avoided.

It is clear from anthropological research that drug use is an ancient human activity, and it is probably ubiquitous, being found in all societies in some form. The earliest firm evidence of human use of psychoactive plants dates back to around 13 000 years ago. In the temperate rainforests of Monte Verde in southern Chile, archaeologists have found evidence of more than 20 medicinal plants being used, including two with hallucinogenic properties (*Drosera* sp. and *Peumus boldus*). Cocaine has been identified in hair samples in mummified remains from South America, and cocaine is still used to inhibit hunger and enhance work performance at high altitudes in the Andes.

Evidence of substance use for pleasure can be found further down the phylogenetic chain. For example, *Amanita muscaria* (fly-agaric mushroom) has been sought by animals partial to its stimulating and hallucinogenic properties. In Lapland this fungus has been traditionally eaten to induce hallucinosis during midwinter pagan ceremonies. The urine of humans who have consumed the mushroom contains isoxazole derivatives, which are intoxicating. Reindeer have been described fighting over urine-soaked snow in order to consume the excreted breakdown products of the fungus. The pagan Lapp myth of reindeer flight is attributed to the mushroom's hallucinogenic effects on humans combined with its motor agitation effects on the reindeer. The pagan image has been incorporated into the contemporary Western notion of Santa's flying sleigh.

The use of drugs by humans and other species may be broadly considered as the pleasurable alteration of state of consciousness. This can involve various sensation-seeking behaviours and, in many human cultures, is ritualised so that such alteration of consciousness does not interfere with the day-to-day responsibilities of life. For example, in some cultures (such as the Lapps described above and some indigenous Mexican peoples), hallucinogenic substances have been used by traditional healers and tribal elders to provide access to what is seen as a metaphysical reality of profound significance. Most individuals, whether in ancient or modern times, who consciously chose to alter their state of mind did so accepting the limitations imposed by ritual or self-restraint. Such individuals successfully balanced these activities with their physical, social, and resource needs.

In some circumstances there may be access to a diverse range of consciousness-altering experiences. In the contemporary Western world these experiences may include activities such as watching a horror movie, riding a rollercoaster, skiing, driving fast, climbing mountains, meditation, taking amyl nitrate to enhance orgasmic sensation, drinking a stubbie of beer, and taking a couple of snorts of intranasal cocaine. The majority of Australian youth today will have tried several pharmacological agents to alter sensation or perception before they reach adulthood. These agents include caffeine, alcohol, nicotine, and marijuana. A significant minority will also have experimented with stimulants and opioids.

Over the last few human generations, advances in pharmacology have considerably broadened the availability, range, and potency of drugs, with an attendant broadening of societal challenges. In the pursuit of civil stability and harmony there appears to have been a growing societal need to control human pleasure. A variety of social structures have developed to define the contexts of sanctioned drug use, to provide approval for or embargo access to drugs, and to attempt to effect control for what is often referred to as 'the common good'. It is only by trying to tease out the multiple strands of biological, cultural, social, and psychological factors, in diversity rather than adversity, that well-informed drug policy will emerge to face these challenges successfully.

THE PHYSIOLOGY OF NIRVANA

Understanding of the physiological basis of the pleasurable alteration of consciousness was advanced by the discovery in the 1950s of the primary brain circuits involved. Conditioning experiments involving stimulation of the medial forebrain bundle in the mesolimbic region identified the ventral tegmental area (VTA) and the nucleus accumbens as key areas in mediating what appeared to be extreme plea-sure in laboratory rats. These rodents would tolerate considerable discomfort to access environments in which VTA stimulation was provided, and would self-stimu-late with direct electrical stimulation in preference to other natural reinforcers such as food. Animals also developed a distinct place preference for the environment where the stimulation was administered. The phrase 'reward centre' was coined, proposing that the brain pathway involved was responsible for the positive subjec-tive experience related to natural reinforcers such as sexual activity and eating.

The neural circuits that underlie the experience of pleasure clearly have high evolutionary value, as there is powerful survival advantage in repeating adaptive behaviours associated with pleasure or the relief of suffering. Evolution has thus resulted in a brain neurophysiology that responds vividly and avidly to substances that essentially operate through the natural reward mechanisms. Therefore it is not surprising that throughout the ages people have displayed considerable ingenuity and enterprise in identifying substances or activities that can stimulate brain rein-forcement pathways. These activities, depending on complex social factors, may have been medicinal, religious, or recreational. It is ironic that key brain pathways associated with increased evolutionary fitness are also responsible for the addictive effects of potential substances of abuse.

There is now also a reasonably advanced body of work regarding the exquisite neurochemistry involved in pleasure, with dopamine the key neurotransmitter. Dopamine is released in anticipation of reinforcing activity, and it facilitates approach behaviour. Dopamine release, particularly stimulation of mesolimbic D1 and D2 postsynaptic receptors, is necessary for associative conditioning, essentially enabling emotionally tagged information to be acquired and retained efficiently. Dopamine thus has distinct motivational properties in signalling reinforcement and in incentive learning. In a fundamental sense the mesolimbic dopamine system may be a filter and gating system for sensory signals that have survival value. It is not active in humans alone. Dopamine precursors are released in molluscs when they are feeding, and in honeybees when they encounter nectar. The prairie vole (*Microtus ocrogaster*), a small North American rodent, forms a distinct pair bond which is regulated by dopamine release. The vole copulates continuously for up to 24 hours in the process of estab-lishing a mate. The copulation threshold needed to form a pair bond can be manipulated by the administration of dopamine agonists (less copulation is needed) or dopamine antagonists (where more copulation is needed).

The neurobiological mechanism for the positive-reinforcing effects of drugs of abuse (other than benzodiazepines) similarly resides in the mesocorticolimbic dopamine system and connections in the basal forebrain. The cell bodies arise in the midbrain and from the VTA project to the nucleus accumbens, the amygdaloid nucleus, hippocampus, olfactory bulb, and parts of the prefrontal cortex. Microdialysis, electrophysiological and brain imaging techniques have shown that dependence-inducing drugs, including opioids, nicotine, amphetamines, ethanol, and cocaine, substantially increase the release of dopamine in the VTA and nucleus accumbens.

Other rewarding repetitive activities, such as playing computer games, similarly result in dopamine release as demonstrated by PET scan studies. Watching pornographic videotapes also has a similar effect on mesolimbic activity.

Surgical interruption to mesolimbic dopaminergic pathways in animals impairs approach behaviour to reinforcing activities, including drug-seeking behaviours. For example, under normal circumstances rats will lick their mouths and paws in pleasure after eating sugary foods, and they will rapidly acquire responses that are reinforced with sugary snacks. Following establishment of the conditioned response, rats will release dopamine in the brain reward centre in anticipation of the food. Microsurgical ablation of the VTA, or the administration of dopamine antagonist drugs, inhibits rats' seeking out the sweet food, but it does not disrupt their expression of pleasure when they are force fed. This has prompted speculation that dopamine reward pathways may be more strongly related to wanting rather than liking.

Anticipatory release of dopamine may assume an attentional role and be the biological substrate of drug-related desire or craving. This effect is evident in the presentation of drug-related cues that have been conditioned to ingestion (such as drug-use implements) to drug users. This increases cerebral blood flow to the amygdala despite no drug being administered. However, it is also clear that dopaminergic activity influences liking, as in animal studies drugs of abuse lower the threshold of electrical stimulation required to provide reinforcement. Drugs of abuse can be thought of as reward synergists that operate via either increasing presynaptic dopamine release or inhibiting postsynaptic dopamine reuptake. For example, cocaine operates via inhibition of dopamine uptake, amphetamine increases dopamine release, and opioids indirectly release dopamine through the removal of GABA-ergic interneurone tonic inhibition in the VTA. Furthermore, given projections to the amygdala and hippocampus, which are key memory structures, dopamine release following initial drug intake may help to form strong memories associated with the pleasure derived from substance use.

The influence of drugs on brain function is not all due to dopamine. Dopamine in turn modulates the presynaptic release of glutamate (the major excitatory neurotransmitter) and gamma-aminobutyric acid (GABA, the major inhibitory neurotransmitter), both of which have been implicated in drug reward. Generally speaking, the more efficiently a substance alters neurochemical function the stronger its potential reinforcing value. The reverse corollary has important implications for diminishing a drug's rewarding potential. With opioids, for example, use of a partial agonist (such as buprenorphine) or an antagonist (such as naltrexone) that produce opioid receptor blockade can diminish reinforcement, and this can confer potential benefits in treatment.

Each drug of abuse has its own reinforcing properties through its impact on specific combinations of neurotransmitter systems. Thus NMDA, GABA, glutamate, serotonin (5-HT) and endogenous opioid peptides all contribute to ethanol's positive reinforcing properties. For example, the action of long-term potentiation (repeated stimulation) on NMDA receptors in the hippocampus leads to the formation of multisensory memories. The NMDA receptor is sensitive to high doses of alcohol, and this in part accounts for alcohol's amnesic effects. The powerful conditioning effects due to dopamine release at low doses, and the higher dose amnesic effects due to the disruption of NMDA receptor dysfunction, contribute to the maintenance of problematic drinking in the absence of sustained powerful rewards.

Brain homeostatic processes subsequently alter the CNS response to repeated drug administration. The complexities of subsequent alteration in neurotransmitter activity on brain function are incompletely understood. Chronic alcohol, cocaine, or amphetamine intake diminishes the number of postsynaptic D2 dopamine receptors and there is also a reduction in general dopamine availability. Alcohol withdrawal states are more severe among those individuals with less active CNS dopaminergic systems. Noradrenaline, a product of dopamine metabolism, is also reduced in response to chronic ethanol ingestion. When a physiological system reaches a steady state due to the administration of a drug that involves reduction of activity, drug cessation typically has an opposing or rebound effect. The increased rebound noradrenergic activity in the alcohol withdrawal state is thought to be responsible for tachycardia, hallucinosis and delirium tremens. Chronic exposure to alcohol also leads to a decreased density of GABA-A receptors and upregulation of NMDA receptors. Furthermore, specific neurotransmitter enzyme disruption is possible with chronic drug use. For example, an as yet unidentified non-nicotine component of cigarette smoke suppresses the mitochondrial enzyme monoamine oxidase B (MAO-B). Smoking is thus not only pleasurable because of dopamine release but also because of the increased availability of dopamine due to impaired breakdown.

The collective impact of drugs of abuse is that neurotransmitter release is occurring as a result of direct stimulation of brain pathways, as opposed to their stimulation by sensory input. The ease, reliability, intensity, and rapidity of such effects go a large way towards explaining the potential of such drugs to lead to abuse.

GENETIC VULNERABILITY

The underlying brain structures and processes responsible for drug-related reinforcement are at least partially under genetic control. Animal models have been instrumental in understanding the neurobiological basis of addiction. Even animals with an alcohol preference do not spontaneously self-administer alcohol as humans do, however, so there are limitations in the generalisability of this research. Rodents (and most other animals) have a natural aversion to alcohol, but selective breeding has resulted in strains of rodents who consume alcohol more readily than their wild counterparts. Neurochemical, neuroanatomical, and behavioural studies confirm that innate differences exist between the high-alcohol-consuming and low-alcohol-consuming rodents. These differences are manifested in limbic structures, anxiety, and acute response to alcohol when administered intraperitoneally. This animal research collectively indicates that the genetic propensity to use substances, or to develop problems, is complex and is influenced by a wide array of genes. It is not the product of a single gene locus and simple Mendelian genetics.

Alcohol remains one of the most commonly misused substances, and is the best studied in terms of genetic susceptibility. In humans, family, twin, half-sibling, and adoption studies of alcoholic subjects suggest that the heritability of liability to alcoholism is at least 50%. The concordance rate for alcoholism is 55% in monozygotic twins, but only 28% in dizygotic twins. There is almost a 50% lifetime risk of alcoholism among sons and brothers of alcoholic fathers, and an even higher risk in siblings with an alcoholic mother. Adopted sons of alcoholic men show a rate of alcoholism closer to their biological fathers than that of their adoptive fathers

This genetic risk is probably common for many addictive substances. The specific substances abused may be more related to availability, social and cultural factors than underlying genetic risk. For example, those with alcohol dependence are frequently also nicotine dependent, abusing both these legal and readily available dopamine agonist substances. One male twin–pair study estimated the heritability of nicotine dependence as 60.3% and that of alcohol as 55.1%, and concluded that a common genetic vulnerability to both agents existed. Intergenerational data supports this common underlying risk model. Parents of current cannabis or stimulant abusers are much more likely to be, or have been, alcohol abusers than are the parents of non-stimulant abusers. This pattern contrasts markedly with that predicted by gateway drug hypotheses, where abuse of drugs like cannabis was seen as a causal factor in the abuse of drugs like amphetamines. It seems more likely that those individuals with the propensity to become addicted in general will become addicted to whatever substances are readily available.

Recent advances in molecular biological techniques have given rise to increased interest in identifying specific genes or sets of genes which may contribute to the effects of potential substances of abuse. Initially this work focused on individual differences in alcohol metabolism, in particular the influence of acetaldehyde accumulation and its alcohol deterrence capacity in some Asian populations.

In the major pathway for alcohol metabolism, ethanol is metabolised to acetaldehyde, mainly by alcohol dehydrogenase (ADH). ADH is then catalysed, mainly by aldehyde dehydrogenase (ALDH), to acetic acid. Less than 10% of ingested ethanol is metabolised by a microsomal ethanol oxidising system (MEOS) involving cytochrome P450 oxygenase (CYP2E1). Genetic polymorphisms of ADH, ALDH and CYP2E1 occur, resulting in multiple isoenzymes with differing relative activity. People with ADH2*2 and ADH3*1 alleles generate acetaldehyde more rapidly than those with ADH2*1, ADH2*3, and ADH3*2 alleles, and among Chinese samples these people are consequently at a lower risk of developing alcohol dependence. These alleles do not themselves confer any direct protection amongst Caucasians, but they may interact with adjacent DNA regulatory sequences. Deficiency of the ALDH2 isoenzyme (ALDH2*2) also results in higher acetaldehyde levels after ethanol consumption due to slower clearance of acetaldehyde, and it is responsible for the aversive flushing syndrome noted in Asian groups. A low proportion of ALDH2 deficiency (ALDH2*2 allele frequency) is found in Asian alcoholics compared with healthy Asian controls. However, this genetic protective factor is also influenced by other social factors. With the adoption of more liberal attitudes towards alcohol, Japanese drinkers and Japanese Americans in Hawaii who are heterozygous for the ALDH2*2 allele have increased alcohol consumption despite its aversive effects. A more complete protection appears to be offered amongst those homozygous for the ALDH2*2 allele. The ALDH2*2 allele is not found in Caucasians, but some less effective variants of the ALDH1 gene occur. Despite impaired clearance of acetaldehyde and associated facial flushing in such drinkers these genetic variations confer no protection against alcohol abuse, again indicating the power of sociocultural factors or the influence of other genes.

Similar enzyme research has been conducted in smokers. In humans, 60–68% of smoked nicotine is metabolised to cotinine by the genetically polymorphic enzyme CYP2A6. Three alleles have been identified: a wild-type (CYP2A6*1), and two inactive (null) alleles (CYP2A6*2 and CYP2A6*3). Smokers who are heterozygous for CYP2A6-null alleles smoke significantly fewer cigarettes per week than smokers with two CYP2A6 active alleles. Impaired nicotine metabolism thus gives a smoker some protection against becoming dependent, and is a determinant of the number of cigarettes smoked by a dependent smoker. Carriers of the CYP2A6-null alleles may also have decreased risk of developing cancers, not only because of their decreased risk of becoming a smoker or smoking less if they become dependent, but also because the nitrosamines in tobacco smoke can be activated to carcinogens by CYP2A6.

Genetic influences on brain neurotransmitter function may have a greater effect on the reinforcing potential of psychotropic substances than the metabolic breakdown of the substances themselves. Given the key role of central dopaminergic systems in drug-related reinforcement, considerable interest has focused on polymorphisms of dopamine receptor and transporter genes, particularly those related to D2 and D4 activity. A significant association between the Taq1A polymorphism (A1 allele) of the D2 dopamine receptor gene (*DRD2*) and severe alcoholism was reported in 1990. Subsequent studies of both association and linkage analysis have been variable, but this polymorphism has consistently been associated with the more severe forms of alcoholism and other drug dependence. The A1 allele (either homozygous A1/A1 or heterozygous A1/A2) has been associated with severe alcohol, nicotine, opioid and stimulant dependence, and with obesity related to a preference for high carbohydrate food. Quantitative trait loci techniques have also identified the A1 allele in alcohol-preferring mice on mouse chromosome 9. Humans with the A1 allele have lower numbers of postsynaptic D2 receptors, and this appears to be reflected as a hypodopaminergic state. It is hypothesised that this state increases the likelihood that dopamine agonist substances will be highly reinforcing. Phenotypic characteristics associated with the A1 allele include poorer visuospatial functioning, a longer EEG P300 latency (indicating impaired attentional capacity), an impulsive personality style, biologically influenced craving, and a rapid onset of substance problems. It is likely that the Taq1A polymorphism is in linkage disequilibrium with a mutation of the promoter or regulatory gene element that affects expression of the dopamine D2 receptor.

The dopamine D4 receptor 7 repeat allele has also been associated with alcohol dependence, opioid dependence, heavy cigarette use, and the personality trait of novelty seeking. These effects are less significant than those due to A1 *DRD2* status, and they show a greater variability across studies. A handful of studies has noted an association between D1 dopamine receptor gene status and D3 dopamine receptor gene status and substance use risk. A variant of the *MAO-A* gene has also been associated with early-onset substance use, and there is some evidence that certain variants of the DAT1 human dopamine transporter gene may be associated with more severe alcohol withdrawal. This work collectively indicates that genes associated with dopaminergic function are related to patterns of substance use.

Similar work has been conducted examining 5–HT transporters. Some alcohol dependent individuals have lowered central 5–HT neurotransmission, and there is an extensive literature on the role of 5–HT neurotransmission in obsessionality, compulsiveness, depression, suicidal behaviour, and eating disorders. Studies of the $5\text{-}HT_{1B}$ receptor gene show promise in identifying a subtype of alcohol-dependent individual with antisocial features and aggression. These individuals show an early onset of problems and are more typically identified in the criminal justice system than in clinical settings. Initial research also associates the human 5–HT transporter gene as a marker for severe dependence. There is evidence that endogenous opioids are involved in alcohol consumption, and blockade of this system (for example, by administration of naltrexone) reduces alcohol consumption. Some opioid μ receptor gene (*OPRMI*) variants are modestly associated with substance dependence, and research on the delta opioid receptor gene shows some promise.

GABA appears to play a major role in the negatively reinforcing effects of alcohol, that is, those effects that are reinforcing because they terminate an aversive event or sensation, such as anxiety. Genetic variation in GABA receptors is emerging. For example, the GABA α 6 receptor gene Pro/ser genotype is associated with a muted acute response to alcohol. *GABA-A* β *3* subunit non-G1 alleles (there are 11 in all) have been associated with increased risk for developing severe alcohol dependence, and these alleles add unique variance to this prediction over that associated with the A1 allele of the D2 dopamine gene. Polygenic impact is likely to be a focus of future research into patterns of substance use.

PSYCHOSOCIAL INFLUENCES ON SUBSTANCE USE RISK

The studies of Japanese and Japanese Hawaiians mentioned earlier indicate the potential influence of social factors over the partial genetic protection offered by heterozygous ALDH2*2 status. These illustrate that information about genotype is only pertinent if it is considered under the specified environmental conditions that influence gene function or expression. There are a myriad psychosocial influences, and the body of research on their nature is vast and difficult to integrate. The key psychosocial influences on drug use patterns are summarised in table 2.1.

Table 2.1   Identified psychosocial risk factors for heavy adolescent substance use

---

Social environmental factors

Low socioeconomic status
Liberal, cultural, or subcultural norms towards use
High population density
Low population mobility
High crime
High unemployment
Alienation
Drug availability

Family factors

Parental substance abuse
Positive family attitudes towards use
Family disruption
Parental anti-social behaviour
Inconsistent, negative parenting
Poor attachment
Low involvement
Poor parental monitoring

Peer factors

Heavy substance use among peers
Positive peer attitudes to use
Greater attachment to peers than to parents
Delinquent peer group

Individual factors

Positive expectations of use
Poor coping skills
Interpersonal difficulties
Psychological trauma
Conduct disorder (a precursor of adult ASPD)
Impulsiveness
Tolerance of deviance
Low self-esteem
Anxiety
Depression
Poor academic performance
Sensation-seeking personality

At the start of the nineteenth century, real incomes per head in the world's richest and poorest countries were in a ratio of three to one. By 1900 it was 10 to one and by 2000 it has risen to 60 to one. During the latter half of the twentieth century there has also been a considerable redistribution of wealth within many countries, with considerable inequity between rich and poor. Affluence has an impact on the extent and pattern of drug use. Across many large-scale data sets from the developed world the relationship between socioeconomic status and drug use is a robust one. Higher drug consumption is associated with lower socioeconomic status, and the effects of poverty are often compounded by social and political disempowerment, a sense of hopelessness, and low perceptions of control. Frequently the consumption pattern amongst these groups is bimodal, for example in surveys of alcohol use among Aboriginal Australians there is an increased likelihood of both abstention and hazardous alcohol consumption than among non-Aboriginal Australians. Similar patterns have been documented amongst disempowered subgroups within a single community, such as gay men. Additionally, communities with low socioeconomic status are more likely to be exposed to a broad range of stressors such as crime and poor living conditions. These contribute additional risk of problematic substance use and may also be related to transient changes in substance use patterns in response to acutely stressful events. Similar effects have been demonstrated in alcohol-preferring rodent colonies. Rodents reared in a crowded environment with limited resources or in one where there are unpredictable stressors are at significantly higher risk of consuming drugs than are those reared under more ideal conditions.

Within a given community, the drugs of choice are influenced by cultural and subcultural norms. For example, in a comparison between Francophone and indigenous high school students in Quebec, the lifetime prevalence figures indicated that the use of stimulants and inhalants was significantly higher among indigenous students, with the consumption of alcohol more important to the Francophone students. Some drugs are highly specific to particular groups, largely related to availability, and cultural norms with traditions and etiquette have developed around their use. Kava (derived from a plant belonging to the pepper family, Piperaceae) has been used ritually among Pacific Islander peoples, predominantly by males, for over 3000 years. It has mild euphoric and sedative properties. This has prompted some Pacific Island authorities to support its use in preference to alcohol, as alcohol is a more recent arrival that has been associated with major psychosocial problems.

Within a given community the shared expectations of what is appropriate in terms of drug use clearly interact with genetic risk. A longitudinal study of alcohol use in Massachusetts showed that cultural group was the most powerful predictor of drinking status over time, with those from an Irish background showing most risk and those from a Chinese or Jewish background the lowest risk. Irish-Americans reported more positive cultural beliefs about intoxication, whereas low risk groups, while not against the use of alcohol, had strong and negative cultural proscriptions against excessive consumption. These normative beliefs can vary widely within subcultural or cultural groups over time.

Independent of the nature of the community an individual is born into or the collective cultural beliefs of the individual's family, it is clear that the stability of early life experience influence the disposition to use psychotrophic substances. Secure attachment to a caregiver is a protective factor for a whole raft of psychological problems. The nature of this attachment is also associated with later patterns of substance use. The experience of parental divorce in childhood, frequent childhood relocation, and a variety of adverse childhood experiences (including sexual abuse) are associated with increased likelihood of misusing psychotrophic substances.

The influences of the family on later drug use are fundamental and complex. Substance use patterns are familial, which means that, in addition to the genetic factors already noted, social learning factors such as parental modelling of use are involved. These are not independent events. Factors that correlate with adolescent drug use include ineffective parental management (lack of, or inconsistent, discipline), negative communication patterns (blame or criticism), and poor family relationships. Parental modelling effects include the use of poor coping strategies, anti-social behaviour, positive parental attitudes towards drug use, and parental drug use itself. Consistent with this is the finding that drug dependence is present in at least half the families who come to the attention of child welfare authorities for child abuse or neglect, indicative of the high level of family stress and chaos accompanying drug dependence. These factors can also contribute to future patterns of pathological family interaction and substance misuse continuing into successive generations.

Prospective studies indicate that stable and secure attachment is reflected in early adolescent personality attributes of greater responsibility, less rebelliousness, and intolerance of deviance. These non drug-prone personality and behavioural attitudes, in turn, insulate the young adult from affiliating with drug-using peers, and these attitudes are related to less drug use in adulthood. In a rejecting and punitive family with a lack of closeness to parents, a precocious and strong orientation towards peers adds further risk to the progression to more severe drug use. Many of these youngsters are inadequately supervised by parents, and this allows unsupervised early experimentation with drugs. Poor parental vigilance also adds independently to the prediction of drug problems.

Adolescence is a time of clarifying a sense of self, of learning to plan beyond the immediate, and of improving control over emotion when confronting the challenges of life. This period of risk-taking in the process of developing independence and individual identity can be a volatile time. Adolescents often harbour a sense of invulnerability and have underdeveloped powers of introspection. Constitutional impatience and impulsiveness can compromise decision-making processes further.

For most adolescents, experimentation with substances is part of natural curiosity, associated with little harm, and represents healthy psychosocial adjustment. Peer-group influences contribute to drug initiation in young people as they enter adolescence and are more receptive to influences outside the family. After controlling for family and cultural factors, drug use by peers and delinquent participation strongly differentiate drug users from non-drug users. Generally young people involved in early onset or protracted drug use are alienated from two of the most important institutions in their lives: school, displaying poor attendance, and family, with strong orientation away from parents and towards peers. For those who develop drug abuse or dependence in adolescence there is inevitably significant psychological distress or biological vulnerability present. Premorbid depression and some anxiety disorders are associated with additional risk, and drug use possibly reflects an attempt to adapt to or cope with this underlying psychopathology. This reliance on drugs to cope, and affiliation with dysfunctional peers, diminishes the likelihood of the vulnerable adolescent developing autonomous coping skills.

Adolescent misuse of drugs can be viewed as just one aspect of problematic functioning. These multiproblem deficits are likely to be reflected in such ways as poor school performance, impaired family relationships, greater psychological symptoms, delinquency, more active involvement with their peers, and selection of social environments where the use of drugs by other adolescents and adults is the norm. Delinquency and the extent of perceived drug use consistently increase with the extent of misuse. Adolescents using amphetamines or opioids exhibit a particularly poor level of psychosocial functioning. Over time, as drug use itself creates more difficulties, it becomes very difficult to tease out the causal relationships between drug use and other psychosocial problems.

Despite adolescence being the time when the actual risks associated with drug use itself are manifested, the beliefs about substance use are likely to have been developing for some time. For commonly available drugs, such as alcohol, children at five years of age are beginning to form concepts about the effects of alcohol on mood, behaviour, and cognition. These beliefs, frequently referred to as alcohol expectancies, develop maximally between the ages of five and ten years primarily on the basis of parental modelling and media influences. The nature of these beliefs prior to the onset of alcohol being consumed predicts the style of subsequent drinking behaviour. Those who view alcohol as able to transform negative emotional or cognitive states (such as depression, anxiety, or worry) are at the highest risk of problematic use. While these beliefs about alcohol are further refined by actual drinking experience, they represent a significant premorbid risk. Those who view alcohol as a prosocial drug and who have a strong repertoire of coping skills, as opposed to those who view drinking as a means of solving problems, are most likely to drink without problems.

Expectations about drug use are important, as they represent a common pathway through which genetic and psychosocial risks operate: that of learning. Drug users are not born dependent. Drugs are reinforcing either through the generation of positive psychological states (positive reinforcement) or through the elimination of aversive states (negative reinforcement). This is essentially an operant conditioning paradigm, and behaviours which are operantly maintained by intermittent reinforcement are particularly resistant to extinction. Substance use and gambling are good examples of intermittent reinforcement, and this explains why many substance abusers persist with behaviours that do not generate powerful reward on every occasion: episodically powerful reinforcement is enough to maintain use. The parameters which influence whether drug use will be reinforcing on any given administration are typically a combination of the drug (potency, dose, route of administration), the user's cognitive set (attitudes, expectations, beliefs), and the setting (both external, such as social setting, and internal, such as mood state). Furthermore, operant theory specifies the conditions under which the reinforcement of any behaviour will be most powerful. Two parameters particularly relevant to substance use relate to the potency of immediate reinforcement and the ineffective impact of delayed consequences. Drugs of abuse generally have a fairly rapid onset and thus have high reinforcing potential. As dependence develops, the user is more likely to use more direct routes of administration that offer a more immediate reward, for example the move from intranasal to intravenous use of amphetamines. As our behaviour is more powerfully influenced by immediate than by distant consequences, the delayed punishments, such as a hangover the next day or the possibility of carcinoma of the lung in 30 years time, have little influence over the decision to use a substance.

Classical conditioning processes are responsible for the powerful reactions elicited by previously neutral environmental cues (so for example a smoker may crave a cigarette after dinner). The reaction to cues associated with drug administration can be strong even in non-dependent users. In those who are dependent and have undertaken thousands of conditioning trials through repeated self-administration, these reactions can be extremely intense. Classically conditioned responses are thought to be the psychological basis of craving. Intravenous drug users will even inject inert solutions when in a craving state to elicit a conditioned 'rush'. These classically conditioned effects can be manifested as low self-efficacy (situational confidence) in resisting drugs under particular environmental conditions, such as when with drug-using friends, when depressed, when seeing a syringe, or on benefit payment day. Both operant and classical conditioning processes are likely to influence the likelihood of drug use together, with operant processes being more related to the acquisition of drug use and classical conditioning being more related to the maintenance of drug use in those who are dependent. Both processes are likely to involve dopamine and NMDA in the limbic system as previously noted.

GENE–ENVIRONMENT INTERACTIONS

Given that the influence of genes is not static and can be expressed differently in the presence of different environmental conditions, there are valuable insights to be gained by examining gene–environmental interactions. A powerful example of the combined role of genes and environment can be found in the study of children or adolescents prior to the establishment of their drinking careers, at a stage when the potential impact of drug use on behaviour is not a confounding factor. In adolescents who have not commenced substance use, the A1 allele of the *DRD2* receptor gene interacts with family stress to produce the characteristic decrements in EEG P 300 response and visuospatial functioning associated with the A1 phenotype. The genetic effect is not a pure one, but reflects a gene–environment interaction.

While neuropsychological risk is important, most research to date has embraced the notion of personality, which clearly has both genetic and environmental components. The notion of an addictive personality achieved widespread currency in the 1950s. Although useful in highlighting to patients in treatment their vulnerability to transfer from one drug of dependence to another, research using psychological rating instruments has failed to find a consistent collection of personality features in all problematic drug users.

Many of the risks associated with dysfunctional use (chaotic families, poor early attachment, impaired psychosocial functioning) are expressed in terms of personality disorder. It has long been recognised that there are individuals who have psychiatric problems that represent extensions of the usual range of variation in character or temperament. These refer to a range of personality attributes that are sufficiently problematic to result in distinct and enduring impairments in social functioning and personal relationships. Characteristics such as being difficult to comfort or being oppositional may have been present since birth. There is a problem in diagnosis in separating the behaviours inherent in the activity of drug misuse from the diagnosis itself. This is especially true with anti-social personality disorder (ASPD), where criminal activity may reflect the cost of maintaining drug supply. In studies, predominantly of opiate users (in treatment settings), almost two-thirds fulfil diagnostic criteria for ASPD. Other less frequent diagnoses include avoidant, borderline, and paranoid personality disorders. Increased psychiatric distress, poorer social functioning, increased criminality, poorer treatment retention, increased HIV-risk behaviours, and increased hepatitis C or HIV infection rates have been noted in this group. The personality pattern is formed by adolescence and is associated with impaired interpersonal, social, and occupational functioning. In these circumstances it can be difficult to resist the allure of psychotrophic substances affording fleeting mood elevation, secondary gain or transient repose. Identification of personality subtypes on the basis of gene–environment interactions with genes such as the $5\text{-}HT_{1B}$ receptor gene shows future promise.

CONCLUSION

Drug use is universal, and for the majority of users it is functional and is associated with pleasure and improved adaptation. A myriad of interacting factors impact on the nature of drug use, and the influence of these factors is not static. A growing body of scientific knowledge has established key biological, cultural, and psychosocial risks associated with misuse; however this work also indicates that the cumulative and interactive nature of risk operates at both an individual and a community level. Protective factors, particularly in the presence of risk, are not well understood. To add to this complexity it is clear that there are multiple paths to problematic and non-problematic use, and subgroups of individuals characterised by specific parameters of risk and protection require identification.

Generally speaking, those groups who are most disenfranchised, whether through early life adversities or through social and cultural dislocation, show the most problematic use. It comes as no surprise that those facing considerable difficulties with little inherent material or other reward should be at the highest risk for substance abuse, and it is a sad irony that their substance use, although providing short-term relief, typically complicates underlying problems further. Human adaptation under these circumstances, in simplistic terms, is to short-circuit the brain mechanisms that respond to natural rewards. It remains an enormous scientific, humanitarian, and ethical challenge to provide a more rewarding and nurturing environment to prevent or treat substance misuse that acknowledges the richness of influences involved.

REFERENCES AND FURTHER READING

Drummer, O. 2001, *The Forensic Pharmacology of Drugs of Abuse*, Edward Arnold, London.

Higgins, S.T. 1997, 'Applying learning and conditioning theory to the treatment of alcohol and cocaine abuse', in Johnson, B.A. & Roache, J.D. (eds) *Drug Addiction and its Treatment: Nexus of Neuroscience and Behavior*, Lippincott-Raven, Philadephia, pp. 367–85.

Koob, G.P. & Le Moal, M. 2001, 'Drug addiction, dysregulation of reward and allostasis', *Neuropsychopharmacology*, vol. 24, pp. 97–129.

Nutt, D.J. 1996, 'Addiction: Brain mechanisms and their treatment implications', *Lancet*, vol. 347, pp. 31–6.

3

Medical and Psychosocial Problems

John Saunders & Ross Young

THE CORE DIAGNOSES

Alcohol and drug use is not an all-or-nothing phenomenon. It exists as a spectrum that extends from abstinence, through intermittent non-hazardous (and sometimes beneficial) use, risky or hazardous use, and harmful use, to dependence (see figure 3.1). Medical, psychological, and social problems may occur due to occasional, high-level (binge) use, repeated harmful but non-dependent use, or dependence.

In general, the greater the frequency of use and the greater the amount of alcohol or drug taken per occasion, the more severe the dependence, and the more severe and disabling the medical and psychosocial consequences.

There are four core diagnoses: hazardous (or risky) use, harmful use, substance abuse, and dependence.

Hazardous use

Hazardous substance use is defined as a repetitive pattern of use that confers a risk of harmful physical and psychological consequences. As such it is significant in public health terms, although it is not included in the World Health Organisation (WHO) *International Classification of Diseases*, 10th edn (ICD-10) (World Health

Figure 3.1   The spectrum of disorder

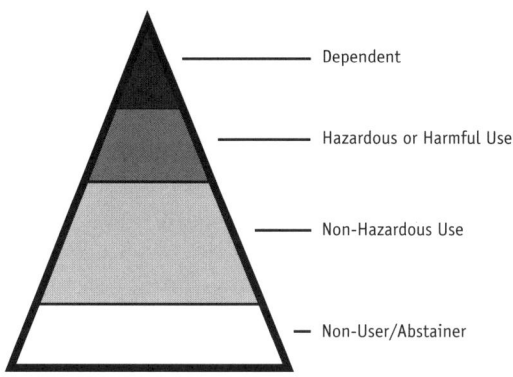

Organisation 1993). The WHO and some national authorities, for example the National Health and Medical Research Council (NHMRC) in Australia, define hazardous or risky alcohol consumption as a regular daily intake of more than 40 grams for men or more than 20 grams for women. Hazardous substance use is also definable in terms of at-risk behaviours, such as sharing intravenous needles, bingeing to severe intoxication, and using substances in unsafe settings such as while driving or operating machinery. This diagnosis identifies people at increased risk of experiencing substance-related social and medical problems, and of progressing to harmful use, abuse, or dependence.

Brief interventions that provide information and advice are effective in reducing many forms of hazardous use.

Harmful use

Harmful use is defined in ICD-10 as a pattern of substance use that is actually causing physical or psychological harm to the individual. No specific level or pattern of substance use is inferred. The Australian (NHMRC) and New Zealand definition of harmful alcohol use emphasises high-risk levels of consumption (over 60 grams for men and 40 grams for women per day in Australia and per session in New Zealand) rather than the specific consequences.

Substance abuse

Alcohol and drug abuse are diagnostic terms in the *Diagnostic and Statistical Manual* of the American Psychiatric Association, 4th rev. (DSM-IV) (American Psychiatric Association 2000). The DSM-IV definition focuses on social and interpersonal consequences of substance abuse, such as failure in role obligations, and recurrent legal, social, or interpersonal problems. Substance abuse can thus be defined as the use of drugs or alcohol in a way that disrupts prevailing social norms. These norms vary with culture, gender, and generation.

Dependence

One of the paradoxes of many patient presentations of substance use is the persistent use of a substance despite negative consequences. Some of these negative consequences may contradict the original motives for substance use in the first place, for example an alcohol-dependent patient may recount the early use of alcohol to relieve anxiety yet now maintain dependent use despite increased worry due to a failed marriage, unemployment, and episodic gastritis, all directly related to alcohol. Sometimes the individual may consider that the remaining reinforcing effects of use outweigh the potentially punishing consequences of use: immediate reinforcement is a more powerful influence on behaviour than more distant punishers, so the patient may also minimise the negative consequences.

Dependence is a psychobiological syndrome that explains this seemingly paradoxical behaviour. It arises from repeated and excessive alcohol or other drug use, and in turn acts as a driving force for continued substance use. It is defined as a core syndrome (Saunders, Young & Dore 2000), and exists as a continuum of severity. Essentially, it consists of a number of behavioural, cognitive, and physiological disturbances that tend to cluster together in time. The central features are impaired control over the use of a psychoactive substance, a strong desire or craving to take it, a high priority given to substance use over other activities, a stereotyped or predictable pattern of use, tolerance, withdrawal symptoms (in some cases), and continued use despite harm. The trajectory in the recurrence of the syndrome when substance use resumes following a period of abstinence is shorter than the trajectory when dependent use first developed. This is called rapid reinstatement. The physiological components of the syndrome represent a state of neuroadaptation resulting from repeated exposure of the brain to a psychoactive substance, and is referred to as physical dependence. Rapid reinstatement suggests some CNS sensation which persists even when the user is abstinent.

A diagnosis of dependence is made if three or more of the above criteria occur together repeatedly over 12 months (American Psychiatric Association 2000). It is not defined by a particular level or pattern of substance use, but specifically by these behaviours and physiological changes. It is noted that tolerance and withdrawal (physical dependence) are not necessary for a diagnosis of dependence to be made.

> ➡ The dependence syndrome exists on a continuum. Severe dependence is typically associated with drug withdrawal upon cessation of use.

Withdrawal state

A withdrawal state (or withdrawal syndrome) occurs in a physically dependent individual when substance use ceases or is markedly reduced. The symptoms of withdrawal are usually the opposite of the drug's effect in intoxication. For example,

CNS depressants such as alcohol and sedative–hypnotics have a withdrawal syndrome characterised by tremor, agitation, hallucinations, and seizures, while withdrawal from psychostimulants is typified by lethargy and inertia. Withdrawal is often accompanied by psychological symptoms such as anxiety, depression, and sleep disturbance. The dependent person may use the substance or a related one to avoid or alleviate withdrawal. Some succeed in alleviating withdrawal by maintaining continuous high blood levels of the substance.

The onset and duration of withdrawal is related to duration of action of the substance. With short-acting substances such as alcohol or heroin, withdrawal usually starts within 48 hours and settles within a week. With longer duration drugs such as diazepam or methadone, the withdrawal state may be delayed for several days and continue for six to eight weeks.

MEDICAL SEQUELAE

Substance misuse may have both immediate and long-term adverse effects. These may be due to direct toxicity (such as alcohol-induced liver disease), the route of administration (such as hepatitis C or B infection acquired through sharing contaminated injecting equipment), or be secondary consequences (such as Wernicke's encephalopathy due to malnutrition, or loss of income or depression related to family separation). Many adverse effects occur in non-dependent users or in those with mild dependence. The number and severity of physical and psychosocial problems typically increases with severity of dependence. Major complications associated with alcohol and other drug use are discussed below. More detailed information is available in the chapters on the respective individual drugs.

Complications of alcohol use

Alcohol is unique among psychoactive substances in having the capacity to cause widespread tissue damage. Of all drugs of abuse, alcohol is associated with the greatest variety of presenting problems. Physical sequelae may also be due to concomitant nutritional deficiency, to trauma sustained while intoxicated, or to infections as a result of reduced immune function. Alcohol is a risk factor for HIV infection and other sexually acquired disorders, because of its disinhibiting effects on behaviour.

The risk of physical sequelae is correlated with the average level of consumption and the frequency of binge drinking. The risk of chronic diseases such as cirrhosis, pancreatitis, and cardiomyopathy increases above a mean daily intake of 40 grams (four standard drinks) for men and 20 grams (two standard drinks) for women. Certain complications, such as gastritis, acute pancreatitis, and trauma, are also related to heavy sessional drinking.

The gastrointestinal tract and associated organs bear much of the brunt of alcohol-induced injury. Alcoholic liver disease is one of the commonest causes of morbidity and mortality in the developed world. It exists in three main forms: fatty liver, alcoholic hepatitis, and cirrhosis. Fatty liver is a predictable metabolic response to alcohol and in most individuals is of little consequence. Often it is asymptomatic and is detected only by abnormal liver function tests, but it may cause pain in the right abdomen, dyspepsia, nausea, and vomiting. Alcoholic hepatitis presents typically with jaundice, fever, and right abdominal pain. Cirrhosis can present with non-specific gastrointestinal symptoms, or signs of hepatic decompensation such as ascites, encephalopathy, or variceal haemorrhage. Both alcoholic hepatitis and cirrhosis can be asymptomatic, being detected only on routine medical examination or abnormal liver function test results. The threshold of use associated with significant liver disease varies widely across individuals. The factors responsible for these individual differences are not yet known.

Alcohol misuse may also lead to alcoholic pancreatitis. Acute pancreatitis typically presents with mid-abdominal pain of variable degree, accompanied by nausea, vomiting, and, in severe cases, hypotension and renal failure. The chronic form is characterised by chronic upper abdominal pain and weight loss, and may be accompanied by exocrine deficiency (for example steatorrhoea) and endocrine deficiency (diabetes mellitus).

Gastritis and peptic ulcer are associated with alcohol misuse, in part because alcohol enhances back diffusion of hydrochloric acid through oesophageal and gastric mucosa. An alcoholic binge may lead to acute gastritis, with mucosal erosions and bleeding. Alcohol is a risk factor for peptic ulcer, and complications of peptic ulcer such as perforation and haemorrhage are more common in alcohol-dependent persons. Oropharyngeal and oesophageal cancers are strongly associated with alcohol consumption, particularly if it is combined with nicotine dependence. Colon and rectal cancers share a weak but significant relationship with alcohol consumption.

The effects of alcohol consumption on the cardiovascular system are both injurious and protective. Alcoholic cardiomyopathy is a form of dilated cardiomyopathy that typically presents with heart failure. Alcohol misuse is now established as a risk factor for systemic hypertension, with 20 to 30% of cases of essential hypertension being attributed to it. On the other hand, moderate levels of consumption reduce the risk of coronary heart disease by up to 40%. Peak protection is obtained at an intake of approximately 20 grams (two standard drinks) per day for men and 10 grams (one standard drink) per day for women.

Alcohol consumption also has a considerable impact on the central nervous system. Both haemorrhagic and thrombotic stroke are more common in hazardous, harmful and dependent drinkers. Chronic diffuse brain damage occurs due to the toxic effects of alcohol and thiamine (vitamin B_1) deficiency. The Wernicke–Korsakoff syndrome, which is related to thiamine deficiency, is characterised by defective short-term memory but better preserved immediate recall and remote memory. Frontal lobe syndrome causes defects in conceptualisation, planning, and organisation. Cerebellar atrophy mainly affects the vermis and causes ataxia of stance and gait; it is thought to be due to a combination of alcohol toxicity and thiamine deficiency. Peripheral neuropathy results in sensorimotor disturbance manifested by numbness, dysaesthesiae, and paraesthesiae in a glove-and-stocking distribution, and sometimes weakness of proximal or distal muscle groups.

Foetal alcohol syndrome is now recognised as one of the two commonest causes of intellectual disability in many developed countries. The mean IQ of affected children is 70, and there is no improvement in intellectual function with time. Affected children have distinct facial characteristics, with a depressed bridge of the nose, thinning of the upper lip and absent philtrum, and low-set ears. Cardiac abnormalities are frequent.

➡ Of all drugs of abuse, alcohol is associated with the greatest variety of presenting problems.

Complications of nicotine dependence

Although nicotine is a highly toxic substance, acute presentations of nicotine toxicity are rare. Toxicity is associated with gastrointestinal distress, delirium, seizure, and coma. Fatal respiratory failure may also result. Death due to oral ingestion of tobacco is uncommon, as vomiting is usually stimulated rapidly. It is more likely that patients will present with more chronic problems, such as coronary heart disease or chronic obstructive pulmonary disease (COPD). Smoking also acts synergistically with other risks for cardiovascular illness, in particular hypertension, raised fibrinogen, and a high lipid fraction. Atherosclerotic lesions are exacerbated by cigarette smoke, probably via the actions of nicotine on platelet adhesiveness and blood pressure in addition to hypoxia. This may result in myocardial infarct. Ischaemia may result from the increased oxygen demand that occurs as a result of enhanced catecholamine release, but this is in the context of reduced oxygen delivery due to elevated carbon monoxide. Efficient lung function and gas exchange may also be further compromised by COPD. Presentation of myocardial infarct, angina or ischaemia can be directly as a result of smoking. Damage to peripheral vessels, or their occlusion, can result in necrosis. These patients may present with claudication on exertion. In extreme cases this requires amputation of the affected limb, often when the patient also has a diagnosis of diabetes mellitus. Ischaemic cerebrovascular accident is also related to smoking, and subarachnoid haemorrhage in women is twenty times more likely in women who smoke and are using the oral contraceptive pill than those with neither risk factor.

Cigarette smoke contains numerous potential carcinogens. Substances such as tar are complete carcinogens, both initiating and promoting malignant change. Other highly reactive compounds in the smoke, such as aromatic hydrocarbons, also have considerable carcinogenic potential. Carcinoma of the lung, oropharynx, breast, liver, genitals, pancreas, kidney, bladder, and the alveolar space are all associated with smoking. Response to chemotherapy or postoperative healing following surgical intervention is poorer in continuing smokers with cancer.

Male erectile dysfunction is associated with smoking. Fertility can be impaired by nicotine, and menstrual problems are well documented. Maternal smoking is also associated with spontaneous abortion, ectopic pregnancy, premature birth, poor neonatal health, and early delayed development in the infant. Childhood asthma, pneumonia and bronchitis are also associated with parental smoking.

Smoking increases basal metabolic rate and may suppress appetite, leading to smokers being significantly underweight. Poor wound healing, the delayed subsidence of bruising, and slowed postoperative recovery are common. Skin elasticity is compromised by exposure to cigarette smoke. Other dermatological problems can be secondary to burn. Burns can indicate a likelihood of concurrent alcohol abuse, with the patient falling asleep while holding a lit cigarette. Smoking in bed poses a particularly high risk.

> ⇒ Nicotine use is associated with significant cardiac, respiratory, endocrine, and dermatological complications.

Complications of sedative–hypnotic use

Sedative–hypnotics have little intrinsic tissue toxicity. Morbidity and mortality are usually related to intentional overdose, often in combination with alcohol or other CNS depressants. Overdose resembles alcohol intoxication, with confusion, disorientation, memory impairment, reduced consciousness, and abnormal vital signs.

In lower doses benzodiazepines lead to memory impairment, anterograde amnesia, impaired psychomotor performance, and ataxia with postural unsteadiness. Benzodiazepines may cause paradoxical disinhibition, particularly when combined with alcohol, manifesting as irritability, hostility, or inappropriate behaviour. Several drugs, including midazolam, flunitrazepam and gamma-hydroxybutyrate, have been termed date rape drugs because of their disinhibiting effects, especially when they are mixed with alcohol.

The withdrawal syndrome resembles an anxiety state, but may be accompanied by distorted or intensified perceptions, seizures and delirium. Withdrawal delirium is characterised by confusion, hallucinations, delusions and autonomic hyperactivity, and is more likely when there is an abrupt cessation in use.

Complications of cannabis use

The major health risks of acute cannabis use are psychosis, which generally abates within five days, and psychomotor impairment. Long-term use may produce subtle changes in the higher cognitive functions of memory, attention, and integration of complex information; the longer cannabis is used, the more pronounced the impairment. While subtle, these changes may affect everyday functioning, particularly in adolescents with marginal educational aptitude and in adults whose occupations require high levels of cognitive functioning. Adverse physical effects include respiratory disease associated with smoking, such as wheezy bronchitis and chronic airflow obstruction. Carcinoma of the bronchus is not definitely associated with cannabis use.

Complications of psychostimulant use

Complications of psychostimulant use arise from both CNS effects and sympath-omimetic actions. After both acute and chronic use, psychosis, a hyperactive (hypomania-like) state, seizures and, less commonly, delirium may occur. Psycho-stimulants are well-recognised causes of acute myocardial infarction and ventricular arrhythmias in young people with no underlying cardiac disease. Complications of cocaine use, in particular, include dilated cardiomyopathy, myocarditis, non-cardiogenic pulmonary oedema, subarachnoid haemorrhage, rupture of the aorta, bowel infarction, rhabdomyolysis, and acute renal failure. Sniffing cocaine may result in ulceration and perforation of the nasal septum.

Complications of hallucinogen use

The presentation following the ingestion of a hallucinogen is almost exclusively psychiatric. It may be a hyperadrenergic state related to panic, or be more similar to psychosis with flight of ideas and hallucinosis. Injury may be related to the ingestion of a hallucinogen, particularly if the circumstances surrounding the trauma are unusual, and related to poor or bizarre decision-making. These cases are rare and may involve, for example, a paranoid patient under the influence of LSD trying to stop traffic on a freeway being subsequently hit by a car, or someone under the influence of PCP jumping out of a second-floor window because he or she thinks that he/she has powers of flight.

Complications of opioid use

Opioids such as heroin have little toxic potential per se. They may, however, cause anoxia due to overdose because of the variable quality of street drugs and co-use with other drugs acting as central nervous system depressants. Neuropsychological damage can result from anoxic episodes and subsequent necrosis of brain tissue. Ancillary problems may occur from, for example, cigarette burns due to smoking while in a drowsy drug-induced state, anorexia or nausea leading to poor nutrition, or reproductive system impairment, for example menstrual irregularities. The greater part of the associated morbidity is related to injecting drug use.

> ⇒ Of the illicit drugs, opioid use is commonly associated with accidental overdose. Cannabis, hallucinogen, alcohol and psychostimulant use can all be associated with acute psychological disturbance. High-level cannabis use may be associated with chronic respiratory disease. Cardiovascular abnormalities are often observed following acute psychostimulant-related presentations.

Complications of injecting drug use

Sharing injecting equipment results in rapid transmission of communicable diseases, particularly hepatitis B and C, and human immunodeficiency virus (HIV). Drug use also leads to disinhibited and high-risk behaviour such as unprotected sexual contact, further increasing the likelihood of contracting these diseases. Insoluble additives to the drug, such as talc and starch, may cause granulomas and thromboembolism in the lung. Bacterial and fungal infections may be local or systemic. The injecting site is a portal for entry of these micro-organisms, and is often the site of an abscess, from which thrombophlebitis, septicaemia and endocarditis may develop. The most common bacterial infection is with *Staphylococcus aureus*. In many countries, including Australia and New Zealand, sterile syringes and needles are provided to reduce the spread of communicable diseases among injecting drug users.

Hepatitis C is currently the most widespread viral infection in injecting drug users. It presents insidiously, with non-specific symptoms such as fatigue. Hepatic pain is unusual. Jaundice is a sign of advanced disease, often heralding other features of hepatic decompensation. Hepatitis C infection responds to combination antiviral treatment in approximately half the cases. However, the dosing schedules are demanding, and only a minority of injecting drug users are in treatment. Patients on maintenance programs are better candidates because of their greater residential and occupational stability.

> ⇒ Much of the harm associated with injectable drugs relates to the manner of use of injecting equipment.

PSYCHOLOGICAL AND SOCIAL PROBLEMS

It is often difficult to ascertain whether psychosocial problems are a cause or an effect of drug misuse. Those with the most significant problems are more likely to report significant psychopathology or substance misuse in their family of origin. They are likely to have had an early onset of drug misuse, and to display sensation-seeking and antisocial personality features. Sadly, these early dysfunctional patterns may be repeated in the patient's own life with significant psychological, emotional or cognitive deficits resulting in impaired adult adjustment and poor coping. Those with a drug dependence are also more likely to form relationships with other drug-dependent individuals, and those relationships are likely to be highly unstable. Poor, inconsistent parenting is associated with an increased likelihood of behaviour problems emerging in their children.

The deterioration in psychosocial functioning evident as drug use becomes more central to the person's life is typically associated with multiple loss. This loss may include relationships, employment, financial security, material wealth, and self-esteem. In extreme cases significant poverty and homelessness can result in considerable impairments in psychological and physical health. Among individuals with intact intimate relationships and social support there may be significant resentment from a spouse who has undertaken more responsibility in an attempt to compensate for the drug user's diminished activity. Repeated promises of change not supported by action can also result in impaired trust. The stigma of drug use and pessimism regarding change can also create a significant psychological burden for the drug user.

> Presenting psychosocial problems which are indicative of underlying drug use reflect a combination of chronic and acute difficulties. In those with severe dependence repeated losses are common.

Comorbid psychiatric issues are often difficult to ascertain as they may be wrongly attributed to the substance use, may be masked by the intoxication or withdrawal, or may unfold gradually following abstinence. There may be an active delirium or residual amnestic disorder or intellectual impairment. Mood disorder may be evident.

It can be very difficult, even for a medical specialist, to discern which is the primary disorder and which is the complicating condition. Of the anxiety disorders, social phobia is more likely to precede the onset of substance misuse, and panic disorder to follow. Post-traumatic stress disorder (PTSD), although less common, may be a result of poor decision-making while intoxicated that leads to enhanced risk of trauma, with the drug use contributing to impaired processing of traumatic memories. Increased alcohol or drug use is common during a hypomanic episode in a person with bipolar disorder. Chronic alcohol and drug use is associated with dysthymia or depression, and it is often impossible to tell which is the primary disorder. Despite the compulsive nature of drug use, obsessive compulsive disorder is rare among substance misusers. Other diagnoses, including psychosis, problem gambling, eating disorders, sexual dysfunction and personality disorder (particularly borderline and antisocial), need to be screened for.

Medical practitioners need to be wary of the over-diagnosis of comorbid disorders, as substance misuse can present in a manner similar to any psychiatric disorder. For example, antisocial personality disorder may be erroneously diagnosed on the basis of crime committed to get money to buy drugs. Many users experience considerable guilt and self-loathing because of their criminal activity or prostitution. It is crucial to examine the psychological impact of these behaviours; they should not be taken at face value.

The assessment and management of substance use and psychiatric comorbidity is discussed in chapter 20.

Table 3.1 Negative psychosocial consequences of substance use that may be evident on initial presentation

---

Acute psychological problems

Anxiety states
Social phobia
Panic disorder
Traumatic reaction
Depression or dysthymia
Amnesic episodes
Delusional psychosis
Low self-esteem
Poor coping
Suicidal ideation
Suicidal attempt
Guilt
Sense of hopelessness

Domestic and allied problems

Poor relationship satisfaction
Loss of friends
Deterioration in marital and other significant relationships
Separation
Divorce
Domestic violence

Occupational difficulties

Failure to gain promotion
Demotion
Dismissal
Unemployment

Financial problems or problems related to obtaining money to buy drugs

---

Homelessness
Loss of regular income from employment
Hardship from money spent on drugs
Gambling and other debts
Victim of fraud
Prostitution
Theft

---

continued

Table 3.1   Negative psychosocial consequences of substance use that may be evident on initial presentation

---

Legal problems

Drug dealing or possession
Property crime
Assault or domestic violence
Homicide
Neglect or abuse of children

Legal problems are also common. Some problems are directly related to the illegal nature of much drug use, and users may sell drugs in order to take a cut of the drugs or to obtain sufficient money to sustain a habit. Alcohol use may be associated with intoxicated aggression and domestic violence or assault. In rare cases homicidal ideation may be acted upon when intoxicated. A summary of the psychosocial problems associated with drug use is presented in table 3.1.

→ Alcohol and drug use is a spectrum from abstinence, through intermittent non-hazardous and sometimes beneficial use, risky or hazardous use, and harmful use, to dependence.

→ The greater the frequency of use and amount of alcohol or drug taken per occasion, the more severe the dependence, and the more severe and disabling the medical and psychosocial consequences.

→ The dependence syndrome's central features are impaired control over substance use, a strong desire or craving to use, priority given to substance use over other activities, a stereotyped or predictable pattern of use, tolerance, withdrawal symptoms, and continued use despite harm.

→ A diagnosis of dependence syndrome is made if three or more of the above criteria occur together over a 12-month period.

→ A withdrawal syndrome occurs in a physically dependent individual when substance use ceases or is markedly reduced.

→ The symptoms of withdrawal are usually the opposite of the drug's intoxication effects, with the onset and duration related to duration of action of the drug.

→ Substance misuse may have both immediate and long-term adverse effects, due to either direct toxicity, the route of administration, or secondary physical or psychosocial events.

→ Those with the most significant substance use commonly have the most significant physical and psychosocial problems.

→ Psychiatric morbidities are common amongst those with significant substance use, but are often wrongly attributed to the substance use.

REFERENCES AND FURTHER READING

American Psychiatric Association 2000, *Diagnostic and Statistical Manual of Mental Disorders* (4th edn, text revision), American Psychiatric Association, Washington, DC.

Saunders, J.B., Young, R. & Dore, B. 2001, 'Substance misuse', in Bloch, S. & Singh, B.S. (eds) *Clinical Foundations in Psychiatry*, Melbourne University Press, Melbourne.

World Health Organisation 1993, *The ICD-10 Classification of Mental and Behavioural Disorders: Diagnostic Criteria for Research*, World Health Organisation, Geneva.

4

Assessment and Diagnosis

John Saunders & Ross Young

Alcohol and drug misuse is so common throughout society that it must be considered as a possibility in nearly every patient seen in medical practice. The conditions with which it is associated are extremely varied, encompassing not only the purely medical but also psychological disorders and an array of social, occupational, and legal problems. Alcohol and drugs follow a range of patterns of misuse: it may be sporadic and binge-type, or regular but low-level, or regular, frequent, and high level such that the person exhibits features of dependence. The nature of the complications typically reflects these patterns. For example, sporadic use of cannabis may not result in many discernible ill-effects but high-level use on a single occasion may cause an acute psychosis, regular daily use may result in recurrent episodes of bronchitis, and daily high-level dependent use may result in the person's life being so dominated by the drug that work, friends, and family are progressively abandoned and the user's health is seriously compromised.

Because of the wide variety of substances available and the range of possible use, the alcohol and drug history must be elicited carefully, with at least the same attention paid as to the past medical and medication history. In everyday medical practice, alcohol and drug misuse is, however, commonly missed. Reasons for this include the non-specific nature of substance-induced symptoms, the reluctance of many patients to report alcohol and drug use due to concern about the implications of doing so, embarrassment or lack of insight, and a low index of suspicion on the part of the clinician. In addition, disorders related to substance misuse typically mimic other conditions. This results in there being a wide differential diagnosis and the understandable assumption that the presenting condition is unrelated to substance misuse.

Given the widespread misuse of psychoactive substances and community expectations that doctors will be at the forefront of providing advice and help for substance-related conditions, it is ethically unacceptable to ignore a patient's use of alcohol and drugs. This must be considered in all clinical presentations and a history of substance use properly blended into the medical history. An effective diagnostician must be aware that alcohol and drug-related conditions occur in all areas of medical practice, and be ever alert for them.

The purpose of eliciting information about substance use is to make diagnoses so that an appropriate management strategy can be developed and implemented. In this chapter we identify how to elicit this information, and consider a number of methods that can be used to enhance the accuracy of the solicited information.

PRESENTATION AND ASSESSMENT

Presentation and symptoms

As was noted in chapter 3, the disorders that result from (or are associated with) alcohol and drug misuse span the entire medical spectrum.

Acute presentations include intoxication and withdrawal states, multiple fractures from motor vehicle accidents, convulsions and delirium, acute abdominal pain (for example from an acute alcoholic pancreatitis), and bacterial endocarditis (consequent on injecting drug use).

In a general medical clinic, patients will be seen with common medical conditions like hypertension, obesity, hyperlipidaemia, and gout, all of which may be due to alcohol misuse, or with recurrent pulmonary disease related to cigarette smoking or cannabis use. A general practitioner will often see a patient with a cluster of problems that embrace medical conditions (such as dyspepsia), psychological distress (for example recurrent depression), and social difficulties (such as constantly running out of money).

In psychiatric practice, acute intoxication and withdrawal from psychoactive substances may present as delirium, psychosis, sleep disturbance, anxiety, depression, or agitation. Chronic substance use disorders may present as depression, dementia, phobias, paranoid states, and psychosis.

When patients present to specialist services for people with alcohol and drug problems, the existence of an alcohol or drug problem is usually self-evident. Even in these services, however, an aspect of the person's substance use may not be revealed, and the complete picture may be obtained only after careful and repeated enquiry.

In medical settings, substance misuse may be suspected first because of unexplained social or occupational malfunctioning, a previously successful businessperson failing in business, or an elderly person who appears physically healthy having recurrent falls at home.

Diagnosis of problems related to substance misuse may be difficult if the presentation mimics other conditions, but missing the diagnosis can have serious consequences. Consider, for example, a patient presenting with right-sided abdominal pain, nausea and vomiting, jaundice, and intolerance of fatty food. These are the symptoms of an acute viral hepatitis (hepatitis A), but could also be caused by an acute alcoholic hepatitis. If alcoholic hepatitis is the cause, the patient may become progressively more anxious and agitated because of undiagnosed alcohol withdrawal, and may progress to generalised seizures.

Hidden substance misuse must also be considered during follow-up, even if there is no apparent problem when the patient is initially interviewed. It is a common cause of unexplained treatment failure. A typical scenario is prompt improvement in a person's condition after admission to hospital, but equally sharp deterioration (often repeatedly) after discharge from in-patient care.

The context of assessment

The process of assessment will be influenced by the nature of the presentation and its setting. Patients in an emergency department are likely to be distressed due to pain, recent trauma, and the rapidity with which they have fallen ill, or because family members have also been admitted with illness or trauma. In this setting the emphasis should be placed on obtaining the key information on alcohol and drug use necessary for their immediate management. For example, it is highly important to assess whether their alcohol, sedative, or opioid use is so high that a withdrawal state may soon develop. A history of opioid use is also important in gauging a patient's requirement for analgesia: the usual doses of morphine will be inadequate if there is a history of heroin dependence. A history of injecting drug use will indicate a potential infectious risk. The subtleties of more minor forms of substance use and their overall contribution to the clinical picture and the history of social and occupational problems may have to wait until the patient is stabilised and recovering from the acute illness.

Patients in a medical, surgical, or psychiatric ward may present with a disorder that is clearly related to substance use, but they are more likely to have a condition not obviously caused by it. Nonetheless, their substance use is highly important, for it may result in an unexpected withdrawal syndrome, and this may interfere with accuracy of diagnosis or efficacy of analgesic treatment, or predispose the patient to pulmonary complications (for example from tobacco or cannabis use), post-operative infections (due to immunosuppression by alcohol or injecting drug use) or delayed wound healing (from malnutrition due to alcohol, amphetamine, or injecting opiate use). The emphasis is again on identifying patterns of alcohol and drug use that have immediate implications for the patient's management. However, following control of the acute illness and after ensuring that potential withdrawal states are being monitored appropriately, attention should be paid to amplifying the alcohol and drug history to obtain a full account.

The hospital setting provides an opportunity for intervention. If substance use is at the hazardous or risky level, intervention may entail brief advice on reducing or ceasing use of a particular substance. Where there is a more damaging pattern (such as recurrent binge use, use with harmful consequences, or clear-cut dependence), the opportunity should be taken for referral to an alcohol and drugs consultation service, a community alcohol and drug service, to the patient's own general practitioner, or to a specialist in drug and alcohol medicine. Such treatment, as will be described in a later chapter, may involve pharmacotherapy, counselling, a rehabilitation program, attendance at a self-help group, or, where no fundamental change in substance use is expected, harm-reduction approaches such as advice on safer injecting practices, and vitamin and nutritional supplementation.

The accuracy of assessment

There is a common view that the alcohol and drug history will invariably be inaccurate. This is untrue. The accuracy of the history depends much on the skills of the interviewer and the context in which the history is obtained. Patients often feel guilty, ambivalent, or embarrassed about their substance use. It is important not to interpret this automatically as denial.

People may not perceive their substance misuse as a problem in situations where their level of use, although hazardous, is similar to that of their peers. Lack of awareness of the negative physical, social, and psychological effects contributes to their under-reporting. Under-reporting also occurs where excess consumption is socially unacceptable (for example, of alcohol in women) or punishment is likely (such as heroin use in prisoners). Sensitivity to these issues when taking a history will result in more accurate and meaningful assessment. Some patients do strongly deny substance use or minimise the severity of their problems, but they are in the minority.

The history also needs to be considered in the light of the treatment environment (for example a hospital versus a probation and parole service). In clinical settings, accurate reporting on substance use will enhance the efficiency of diagnosis and the adequacy of treatment. There are, or should be, no negative implications. On the other hand, revealing a history of continuing substance use to a probation officer is highly likely to have negative implications for the individual. It is important for the medical practitioner to stress the confidentiality of all information. Time should be taken to reinforce that, while other professionals might be preoccupied by the illegality of the patient's activities, you are only interested to the extent that they negatively affect the patient's psychosocial or physical well-being.

Other factors influencing the accuracy of the history include personality factors, neuropsychological impairment, state of intoxication or withdrawal, and staff attitudes and behaviours towards the patient. In those who self-refer, the self-report is generally valid, but intoxication or cognitive impairment related to chronic use may limit this.

The validity of clinical information provided by the patient is enhanced by the clinician:

- establishing the legitimacy of enquiring about substance use (explaining that this information is necessary to make a diagnosis, to ensure that treatment is appropriate, and to avert hazardous interactions between drugs that are prescribed and those the patient may have been taking)
- providing reasons why information on specific drugs is being obtained (for example that the clinician needs to know of any heroin use to gauge whether the patient is likely to be tolerant to opioids)
- outlining the professional, legal, and ethical responsibility of the doctor to provide optimal patient care.

Taking the history

Assessment includes taking a history of substance use (see tables 4.1 and 4.2). The validity of the self-report is improved by obtaining corroborative information, as well as the medical practitioner's use of appropriate organisational, presentation, and verbal skills

Organisational and presentation skills

The issue of substance use is approached in a friendly, non–judgmental manner. Sometimes it is useful to introduce the topic of alcohol and drug use as an unremarkable behaviour, so that the patient's substance use is seen as falling within the spectrum of normal human activities. Asking questions about the use of alcohol and cigarettes is less confronting (because they are legal substances) than enquiring immediately about injecting drug use. Beginning by assessing the frequency and quantity of licit substance use will help to legitimise subsequent questioning on illicit use, make the patient more comfortable, and ultimately increase the accuracy of the information obtained.

For example, for alcohol, it is important to establish the quantity and frequency of consumption, and the beverage type. The average weekly or daily level of consumption can be calculated from this information. It may be useful to show a standard drink chart. Questions can then be posed about possible physical and psychosocial sequelae, and dependence (table 4.1). A convenient screening tool for alcohol use is the Alcohol Use Disorders Identification Test (AUDIT), which explores all of these domains (figure 4.1).

The clinician may then ask about the use of tobacco, prescription drugs, and then illicit substances (table 4.2). With regard to tobacco, the two most useful questions are:

- How many cigarettes do you smoke each day?
- Do you smoke within half an hour of waking up in the morning?

Figure 4.1 The alcohol use disorders identification test (AUDIT)

The AUDIT is a 10-item questionnaire designed to screen for excessive drinking in primary care settings. It takes the patient two minutes to complete and the clinician can identify in one minute which category the patient is in.

AUDIT

Please place a mark in the box next to your answer.

---

1 How often do you have a drink containing alcohol?

❑ Never ❑ Monthly or less ❑ Once a week ❑ 2 to 4 times a week ❑ 5 or more times a week

---

2 How many standard drinks do you have on a typical day when you are drinking?

❑ 1 ❑ 2 ❑ 3 or 4 ❑ 5 or 6 ❑ 7 or more

---

3 How often do you have six or more drinks on one occasion?

❑ Never ❑ Less than monthly ❑ Monthly ❑ Weekly ❑ Daily or almost daily

---

4 How often during the last year have you found that you were not able to stop drinking once you had tried?

❑ Never ❑ Less than monthly ❑ Monthly ❑ Weekly ❑ Daily or almost daily

---

5 How often during the last year have you failed to do what was normally expected from you because of drinking?

❑ Never ❑ Less than monthly ❑ Monthly ❑ Weekly ❑ Daily or almost daily

---

6 How often during the last year have you needed a drink in the morning to get yourself going after a heavy drinking session?

❑ Never ❑ Less than monthly ❑ Monthly ❑ Weekly ❑ Daily or almost daily

---

7 How often during the last year have you had a feeling of guilt or remorse after drinking?

❑ Never ❑ Less than monthly ❑ Monthly ❑ Weekly ❑ Daily or almost daily

---

8 How often during the last year have you been unable to remember what happened the night before because you had been drinking?

❑ Never ❑ Less than monthly ❑ Monthly ❑ Weekly ❑ Daily or almost daily

---

9 Have you or someone else been injured as a result of your drinking?

❑ No ❑ Yes, but not in the last year ❑ Yes, during the last year

---

Continued

Figure 4.1   The alcohol use disorders identification test (AUDIT)

10 Has a relative, a friend, a doctor, or other health worker been concerned about your drinking or suggested you cut down?

❏ No   ❏ Yes, but not in the last year   ❏ Yes, during the last year

For the first eight questions, each response is scored 0, 1, 2, 3 or 4 from left to right; questions 9 and 10 are scored 0, 2 or 4.

AUDIT scores are interpreted as follows:

Women		Men
0	Abstainer	0
1–5	Non-hazardous safe drinking	1–6
6–12	Hazardous or harmful alcohol use	7–14
13+	Alcohol dependence	15+

The first answer quantifies the risk of dependence and of pulmonary and other malignant complications (typically by calculating the 'pack-years' of smoking). The second question is the most efficient way of determining whether the person is physically dependent on nicotine (a 'yes' response indicating that physical dependence is highly likely).

Information on prescription drugs centres on the quantity of the medication taken (in number of tablets and in mg or gram amounts), the duration of use, whether the drug has been taken only under medical prescription, or whether some at least has been obtained through subterfuge or illegally, and whether the stated dose is within the therapeutic range or in supra-therapeutic amounts.

The medical, psychiatric, and social history provides useful information on the presence, severity, and course of any neuropsychiatric, physical, or social complications. These disorders may often be the only pointers to the presence of substance misuse.

Corroborative information

Corroborative history can be obtained from relatives, friends, other treating professionals like the local general practitioner, and from past records. Understatement of substance use by collateral sources may occur due to fear of retribution or of negative social or legal consequences. Overstatement by relatives may result from false assumptions based on previous behaviour or hearsay, or from a wish for retribution.

Other techniques to enhance history taking

While problems in establishing the quantity and frequency of low-level alcohol and other drug use are not common, difficulties can be encountered when patient consumption patterns are more significant (to the levels of harm, substance abuse, or

Table 4.1   The alcohol history

Approaching the topic

In many consultations it will be appropriate to elicit the drinking history as soon as an alcohol problem is suspected. Alternatively, it is often convenient, and acceptable to patients, if the inquiry about drinking is introduced with other lifestyle issues such as smoking, diet and exercise. One method of broaching the subject is to say, 'We often find that people's eating, smoking, and drinking habits have a significant effect on their health or how they feel about themselves. I'd like to ask you some questions in these areas.'

Introduce drinking as a normal, everyday experience

Assume that your patients will be regular or occasional users of alcohol. You can begin your questions with statements like, 'Most of us like to have a drink on a regular basis. How often would you have a drink during the week and at the weekends?'

Suggest high levels of drinking to the patient

When inquiring about the number of drinks taken during a drinking session, it is useful to suggest a quantity towards the extreme range of the scale such as 'A bottle of gin a day?', 'Two dozen beers at a sitting?', and so on. The person is more likely to admit to a high intake of alcohol if several quantities at the high end of the range are suggested. Suggesting a high figure allows the patient to correct you downwards. The amount you suggest should depend on the sex and socioeconomic background of the patient, and any knowledge you may already have about the person's alcohol consumption.

Do not allow personal attitudes to affect the assessment

Under-diagnosis of alcohol problems may sometimes be related to the doctor's own denial mechanisms. Sometimes this is based on an unjustified pessimism about the outcome of intervention, sometimes on the doctor's own problems with alcohol. On the other hand, judgmental attitudes can creep in if the doctor believes that any drinking is inappropriate.

Avoid labels

It is best to avoid using terms like alcoholic unless the patient him- or herself feels comfortable using that term. Patients who feel they are being accused of being an alcoholic may become defensive, and so may be frightened away from treatment. It is often more appropriate to talk about 'problems related to alcohol' or 'a drinking problem'. Thus it may be more appropriate to say 'I wouldn't say you are an alcoholic, but from what you've told me, there do seem to be a number of problems related to your drinking.'

Home-poured drinks

People tend to underestimate greatly the size of home-poured drinks. Try to estimate the specific amount of alcohol consumed, such as half a bottle of wine rather than four glassfuls, as the size of glasses can be hard to quantify.

Table 4.2   The drug history

Name of each drug ever used

Establish which drugs the patient has ever used.

Current use

For each of these drugs, establish the current pattern of use. This should include information on:
- quantity: the amount of the drug used each time
- frequency: how often this amount of drug is used
- duration: how long this pattern of use has been occurring
- route of use: oral, intravenous, intranasal, inhaled, smoked
- last use: when the drug was last used
- cost: how much per day or per week
- source: how the client is obtaining drugs and the money for drugs (doctor shopping, prostitution, or crime to pay for street drugs, and so on).

In addition:
- assess for substance-related problems
- assess for substance dependence.

Past use

For each drug ever used, establish:
- first ever use: age or year when the patient first ever used the drug
- heaviest period of use: assess quantity, frequency, duration, route of use, cost, source, substance-related problems, symptoms of dependence at that time.

Drug(s) of choice

Establish the drug(s) most used, most preferred.

Most problematic drug

Establish the drug(s) causing most problems.

Purpose and meaning of the substance use for the client

Establish:
- reasons for substance use: why does the client use the substance?
- precipitants: identify situations that trigger substance use for the client
- effects: what effect on mood and behaviour does the client experience when the drug is taken?
- consequences: what are the consequences of using the substance, both positive and negative?

Continued

Table 4.2   The drug history

Family history

Ask if any other members of the family have had any problems with alcohol or other drug use.

Treatment history

Ask about any past or current treatment the patient has had, including counselling, self-help groups (Alcoholics Anonymous, Narcotics Anonymous), residential programs, detoxification, medication.

Assess risk–taking behaviour

Assess the risk of hepatitis C, hepatitis B and HIV infection by asking about:
- injecting drugs: how often does the client inject drugs? how often does he/she share needles with other users? how often and how effectively does he/she clean the needles before reusing them?
- sexual behaviour: how many sexual partners has your client had in the past month? does he/she use condoms when having sexual intercourse?

Assess motivation for change

To assess your patient's stage of change, simply ask him/her some direct questions about change. For example:
- how interested are you in changing your (*substance*) use now?
- do you feel that you *need* to stop using (*substance*)?
- do you really *want to* stop using (*substance*)?
- what do you feel you could do to get on top of your use of (*substance*)?
- how confident are you that you could achieve this?

---

dependence syndrome). The accuracy of the alcohol and drug history in these people can, however, be enhanced by methods that are non-threatening and non-judgmental, but that at the same time encourage the patient to reveal the truth about their substance use without allowing an escape from the line of questioning (see tables 4.1 and 4.2).

The clinician should pay close attention to the subject's facial expression and body language during this part of the interview. The patient frequently gives a fleeting look of recognition or adopts a defensive body posture when the correct intake is mentioned. This level is often higher than the one the patient is prepared to admit to verbally. If no acknowledgment—verbal or otherwise—is forthcoming for a particular level of consumption, progressively lower intakes should be suggested in a stepwise manner. When there is acknowledgment of a certain level of consumption, the clinician should probe further to establish a consistent response. The clinician adopting this technique should pay proper attention to the patient's reaction to the style of questioning because, if used in an unsophisticated way, it can backfire badly. History-taking must not deteriorate into harassment. A similar approach can be used to elicit quantitative information about dependence and problems related to drinking.

Examination

Examination of the patient's physical and mental state may reveal evidence of recent substance use (for example the smell of alcohol or signs of use of intravenous needles), intoxication or withdrawal, or the physical complications. Substance misuse commonly leads to decline in global functioning, evidenced by poor general appearance, personal hygiene, overall health, and nutrition. Neuropsychiatric testing may reveal patterns of abnormality consistent with the effects of substance misuse, such as alcohol-related brain damage.

A physical assessment to identify evidence of alcohol and drug use and its complications should include the following:
- general appearance—evidence of agitation (due to a withdrawal state or stimulant use), malnutrition (for example, giving rise to a gaunt appearance), premature ageing, Cushingoid facies (in alcohol-dependent persons), covering up the arms by wearing long-sleeved garments in warm weather (to hide injection marks)
- signs of intoxication—garrulousness, unclear thinking, ataxia, smell of alcohol on the breath
- signs of withdrawal—tremor and sweating of hands, tremor of face and tongue
- cutaneous stigmata of alcohol and drug use, such as injection sites (in the ante-cubital fossae or the back of the hand, for example), injection of the conjunctivae (recent heavy alcohol consumption or cannabis use), facial telangiectasia (alcohol), rhinophyma (alcohol), inflammation of the nasal septum and alae (cocaine), periorbital wrinkling (tobacco smoking), thinning of skin (alcohol, heroin), Dupuytren's contractures (alcohol), bruises, especially of different ages (alcohol, sedative–hypnotics, opioids), and scars unrelated to surgery (alcohol, opioids, psychostimulants)
- cutaneous stigmata of liver disease such as spider naevi and/or palmar erythema
- pulse rate and blood pressure
- evidence of cardiac disease (especially of valvular heart disease, endocarditis, cardiac enlargement or failure)
- abdominal examination to assess size and consistency of liver, presence of splenic enlargement, or ascites
- evidence of head injury
- on cranial nerve examination, the presence of nystagmus or ophthalmoplegia
- ataxia, especially of stance and gait
- signs of peripheral neuropathy
  In the mental state examination, particular attention should be paid to:
- clouding of consciousness
- abnormalities of perception, especially visual and auditory hallucinations
- abnormalities of thought, especially paranoid ideation

- affect, anxiety, dysphoria, depression, blunting, lability
- suicidal ideation
- cognition, including awareness of current events, immediate recall, short-term and long-term memory, abstraction, conceptualisation, and planning

Formal cognitive function testing should await the resolution of any clouding of consciousness. The Short Mental Status Examination questionnaire is used by some as a simple screening instrument for alcohol-related brain damage. More sensitive screening procedures make use of a short battery of tests, usually under the direction of a clinical neuropsychologist. Among those commonly employed are the New Adult Reading Test, to assess pre-morbid IQ, Visual Reproduction Test from the Wechsler Memory Scale, the Rey Auditory Verbal Learning Test, the Rey-Osterrieth Complex Figure Test (executive function), and the Reitan Trailmaking Test B (also executive function).

Laboratory tests

Laboratory tests may provide evidence of substance misuse.

Most substances are detectable by urine or serum tests, or (in the case of alcohol) breath tests. However, drug testing should never replace history taking, and should be undertaken only when there is a concern about underlying substance use and the information is clinically relevant. For example, drug testing is particularly valuable when the patient is unable to give a clear account of any substance use because of psychosis or delirium. Unnecessary or inappropriate use of drug testing can significantly impair the development of a therapeutic relationship between patient and doctor.

Alcohol misuse is best detected by the physiological markers of consumption, such as mean corpuscular volume (MCV) and gamma glutamyltransferase (GGT). However, abnormal values are found in only 20 to 50% of those with recent alcohol misuse. Carbohydrate deficient transferrin (CDT) is a more sensitive marker of excessive alcohol consumption than conventional laboratory markers (being abnormal in 40–60% of patients), but the test is expensive.

There are several commercial assays that allow for simultaneous testing of 200 or more psychoactive substances. The most accurate technique is gas chromatography–mass spectroscopy, though the availability of this is limited by its cost. A number of personal identification kits are also becoming available; however, these commonly have high false positive and false negative rates.

In practice, urine drug testing is often less useful than one might suppose. There are frequently delays in the results being available to the clinician who requests the test, and drug testing provides information only on the absence or presence of the substance or its metabolites. Unlike history taking, it provides no information on frequency of use or quantity consumed on which the clinician may assess, for example, the likelihood of physical dependence, onset of withdrawal, or likely presence of a dependence syndrome. As most substances are cleared rapidly from the body, tests will be negative if there has been no recent use. Exceptions are cannabis (THC), which is detectable in urine and serum for several weeks after cessation of use, and long-acting benzodiazepines such as diazepam, for which metabolites may be detectable for several days.

Collateral history and ethical issues

Obtaining a collateral history is important from a number of perspectives. It serves as a reliability check, it affords a somewhat independent perspective that may be less influenced by a patient's acute intoxication or neuropsychological impairment, and it provides an opportunity to assess the impact of substance use and the ability of a spouse or partner to cope. However, it is crucial that such information not be gathered in a punitive sense, that it is obtained with the patient's permission, and that any limitations or concerns about ethical issues are addressed (such as divulging information to the parents of an adolescent).

Collateral information

A history of the patient's substance use, dependence, and problems obtained from the spouse, another relative, or a friend may be pivotal in making a diagnosis. As already noted, consent should always be sought from the patient first, unless the need to make a prompt diagnosis outweighs privacy concerns. Exceptions might include, for example, the adolescent who is admitted with severe psychotic symptoms, or in the case of accidental overdose. Collateral information is also especially valuable in patients who exhibit strong denial of their substance-use disorder. In this instance, however, extreme care needs to be taken to ensure that the patient is not alienated by the solicitation of this information. Important information can also be obtained from the hospital medical record or that of the general practitioner. Such sources are neglected to a surprising degree.

Direct observation

Sometimes it is possible to observe the effects of a person's substance use by the smell of alcohol on the breath, by the unsteady gait of an intoxicated individual, or by a chance meeting outside the clinical setting.

Drug-seeking behaviour

Some patients seek a prescription for psychoactive drugs as the main (or only) goal of the medical consultation. They are especially likely to be dependent on sedative–hypnotic drugs such as benzodiazepines, or opioids, and regard the doctor as the most convenient, and often the cheapest, source of supply. When the request is for sedative–hypnotics, patients are likely to present with complaints of anxiety, tension, or insomnia, and it can be very difficult to identify whether the complaint is genuine or not. When the request is for opioid drugs, the typical complaint is of acute or chronic pain. Renal colic, migraine and chronic back pain are common complaints in this context. Frequently the patient claims to be an interstate visitor, and may come with discharge summaries and X-rays. In nearly all cases the patient knows the desired medication by name, prefers short-duration and rapidly acting drugs in preference to sustained-action preparations, and may become abusive when a prescription is denied (see chapter 21).

FROM ASSESSMENT TO DIAGNOSIS

As already noted, the purpose of eliciting information about substance use is to make diagnoses that can form the basis for a management plan. On the basis of the history, supplemented where relevant by the examination and collateral and laboratory information, the clinician should determine, for each drug category, whether:

- a diagnosis of risky or hazardous use can be made
- there is evidence of physical or psychological harm related to substance use (making a diagnosis of harmful use)
- there is recurrent maladaptive use causing social complications (making a diagnosis of substance abuse), or
- there is evidence of a cluster of psychological, behavioural and physiological features that amount to dependence.

The information obtained should be analysed against the diagnostic criteria for the core conditions. Following this, the presence of physical, neuropsychiatric, psychological, and social complications related to these core conditions should be examined.

After assessment is completed, the core diagnoses related to substance misuse are recorded (for example alcohol dependence and withdrawal, amphetamine abuse), followed by the chief physical and psychosocial complications. A definitive statement about the relationship of concurrent physical and psychiatric conditions to substance misuse may have to await special investigations or longitudinal observations.

Clear record-keeping is very important. In most cases patients have access to their records, and the more detailed the information recorded, the more likely the doctor will be able to justify a particular course of action.

REFERENCES AND FURTHER READING

Krabman, P.B. & Saunders, J.B. 1996, 'Diagnostic criteria for substance misuse and dependence', in Rommelspacher, H. & Shuckit, M.A. (eds), *Drugs of Abuse: Bailliere's Clinical Psychiatry*, vol. 2, Bailliere Tindall, London, pp. 375–404.
Saunders, J.B., Sitharthan, T. & Krabman, P.B. 2001, 'An overview of substance use disorders and their management', in Henn, F., Sartorius, N., Helmchen, H. & Layter, H. (eds), *Contemporary Psychiatry*, vol 3 part 2, Springer, Berlin, pp. 253–71.

5

Identifying Treatment Options

Gary Hulse, Jason White & Katherine Conigrave

Greek mythology tells us that Damastes (also known as Procrustes, 'the stretcher') was a brigand of ancient Attica who lived in the area of Eleusis, beside the road to Athens. He would entice travellers to lie down on his iron bedstead. Those who were short were stretched until they were of the correct length. Taller victims received amputations to make them meet the bed's specifications. While Damastes clearly identified the means to accommodate differences in presentation, his use of available resources was poor and the final human outcome less than optimal.

Chapter 4, 'Assessment and Diagnosis', tells us that people with problem drug use can present with distinctly different clinical scenarios and have a variety of needs and characteristics. It follows that these different presentations may require different types or combinations of interventions to achieve an optimal outcome. A range of therapeutic options is available for dealing with problem drug use. These differ for those who are identified early compared with those with longstanding and more entrenched drug-use problems. In this chapter we identify commonly used management tools and the patients for whom these are best suited.

INTERACTING WITH THE PATIENT

Many patients with alcohol or other drug problems do not present seeking help for these problems. The vast majority of patients in primary health care and generalist health care settings who have an alcohol and/or drug problem will be attending for other reasons. In some cases the presentation may be related to the drug use (for example the patient with hypertension who drinks excessively), while in other cases it may be unrelated.

Whether the presenting problem is related to alcohol or drug use or not, the patient may be reluctant to divulge the alcohol or drug use. This is because there is a general disapproval of alcohol and drug problems in our society, and because medical practitioners are frequently seen as judgmental, even though they may also be regarded as an important source of information and help regarding alcohol and drug problems. This has two major implications. First, one of the roles of the medical practitioner is to identify people with alcohol and drug problems. As discussed in chapter 4, a skilled practitioner should be able to recognise someone with a drug problem based on their presentation and medical history, and should approach assessment in a non-threatening, non-judgmental manner. Second, it cannot be assumed that the patient will want to change his or her behaviour or to engage in treatment in order to effect such change. Many patients do not see their drug use as a problem and so do not recognise any need to change.

The medical practitioner therefore needs to be skilled in helping patients recognise the true consequences of the drug use. This can be done in two main ways. One is a confrontational approach; that is, the patient is presented with evidence of the drug use and the damage it is causing, and then, if the patient denies such evidence, argument is used to try to change his or her views and a treatment goal is prescribed. This type of approach was common in the past and is still widely practised. However, confrontation may produce defensive behaviour in the patient, including minimising the problem or denying its existence. It should generally be used only when a less confrontational approach has failed. An alternative to confrontation is known as motivational interviewing, or motivational enhancement therapy.

Motivational interviewing

The goal of motivational interviewing is to encourage the patient to recognise both the problems and benefits associated with the drug use, and so to determine if the harms outweigh the benefits and from this assess whether action might be needed. Instead of the medical practitioner (or other health professional) confronting the patient, the patient is encouraged to discuss the drug use in an open manner.

The first step is to ask the patient to list the benefits he or she gets from the drug use and the costs it incurs. Patients are often surprised by a medical practitioner asking them to list benefits, and this can help counter the perception of doctors as judgmental. If you are familiar with the typical effects that a drug produces you can often assist patient in listing benefits, asking, for example, whether the patient feels less anxiety when drinking alcohol, or whether the patient finds it easier to go to sleep after smoking cannabis. Some help may also be provided if the patient finds it difficult to list the problems associated with the drug use. As a medical practitioner, you may be able to show a link between drug use and medical problems that the patient may not have recognised. For example, the patient presenting with hypertension may not understand that there is a link between alcohol consumption and hypertension, and you may have to explain this.

After listing the various problems and benefits there should be some discussion of any concerns raised by the patient. Instead of confrontation between doctor and patient, the conflict should be within the patient as he or she considers the costs and benefits of his/her actions. Only after the patient has recognised that the costs are considerable and outweigh the benefits should you move on to consider behaviour change.

For some patients, an initial discussion of drug problems may not proceed beyond consideration of the problems and benefits. It may be appropriate to suggest the patient go away and think a little bit more about the issues before returning for a follow-up appointment. Some patients will change their views about their drug use when allowed time to consider the costs and benefits.

A number of techniques can make motivational interviewing more effective. These include:

- using summary statements from time to time, trying to pull together the views of the patient into a coherent statement
- responding to resistance by reframing the patient's statement, for example 'So you don't think there are any negative aspects to your amphetamine use?'
- encouraging and supporting the patient whenever he or she makes statements about actively choosing or changing his/her behaviour.

The technique of motivational interviewing can be extended to many other types of behaviour change that may be sought in medical practice. Compliance with medication schedules, dietary changes, exercise, and so on are all issues about which patients are likely to be ambivalent, with associated costs and benefits. In any of these situations motivational interviewing can be a useful approach.

Establishing a treatment goal

For the non-dependent user whose drug use problems have been identified prior to the development of major physical and psychosocial consequences, controlled drug use may be more acceptable than complete abstinence. For example, a 25-year-old binge drinker who has experienced only minor adverse consequences of his drinking is unlikely to be ready to accept a goal of a lifetime of abstinence from alcohol. However, if the goal is more realistic, then it is likely to be accepted and hence to be associated with positive treatment outcomes. In contrast, for the highly dependent drug user the best outcomes are associated with treatments that have the ultimate goal of abstinence.

A good social support network and positive employment history, coupled with early identification of problem drug use and absence of dependence, are factors that make controlled drug use a more appropriate and feasible treatment goal than abstinence. Absence of social support and poor employment prospects, despite early identification, may indicate that abstinence, at least for the initial treatment period, is a more appropriate goal. Another key factor in identifying an appropriate treatment goal is the individual's desire to become a more moderate user or to abstain.

NON-DEPENDENT PROBLEM USE

People with early-stage problem drug use commonly present to general practitioners and community health services for reasons that are not drug-related. Acute trauma presentations, such as accident, injury, and overdose, are common consequences of drug use. The identification of these people before the development of more significant drug use, dependence, and associated physical and/or psychosocial problems, is one of the important areas covered in chapter 4.

Those who have early problem drug use but are not dependent, or who have a dependence which is mild to moderate and who have good and stable psychosocial support networks, are more likely to be suitable for a goal of moderation of drug use. The most widely accepted method of achieving a moderation in drug use is by use of a brief intervention.

This is generally used as part of a general consultation in a primary care setting, such as general practice or a community health service. Some brief interventions may be instigated at a 'teachable moment' such as in general hospital emergency, medical or surgical departments, when patients may be highly motivated to change their behaviour.

Use of brief intervention has been shown to reduce the level of hazardous or harmful licit (especially alcohol and tobacco), illicit, and poly-drug use, and the harm associated with this use. Efficacy has been demonstrated with diverse groups, including college students, women, the elderly, adolescents and war veterans.

While the exact composition of a brief intervention may vary, a number of common elements can be identified. A typical brief intervention consists of a structured therapy of short duration (5–30 minutes) that is offered to help the individual to cease or reduce drug taking, and it commonly includes motivational interviewing, information, and counselling on problem-solving strategies.

The components of brief intervention have been summarised using the acronym FLAGS:
- Feedback on risk or impairments due to drug use
- Listen to the patient's concerns
- Advise patients about the consequences of continued drug use
- Goals of treatment should be defined, for example to reduce or cease drug consumption
- Strategies for treatment should be discussed and implemented, for example identify triggers to drug use and strategies to overcome them, and offer a follow-up appointment.

More detailed information on the FLAGS model is provided in chapter 10, 'Alcohol'.

Importantly, this type of approach with early-stage problem drug use provides outcomes comparable to long-term conventional inpatient treatment. Given the considerable cost involved in providing conventional inpatient treatment, there is therefore good economic argument for brief intervention.

MANAGING PHYSICAL DEPENDENCE AND WITHDRAWAL

Repeated and frequent drug use leads to the development of tolerance to and physical dependence on the drug. The development of a withdrawal syndrome following cessation or marked reduction in drug use is commonly used to define physical dependence. People presenting with physical dependence therefore have a history of regular and significant levels of drug use, often with frequent episodes of intoxication. However, although frequent intoxication is common in drug dependence, it is not a necessary component. For example, the elderly woman who regularly consumes several nips of sherry or repeatedly uses night-time sedative–hypnotics may not exhibit signs of intoxication, but may nonetheless develop withdrawal symptoms when the drug use is significantly reduced or ceased.

The symptoms of withdrawal are usually opposite to a drug's effect. For example, the withdrawal syndrome associated with CNS stimulants is characterised by features of CNS depression such as lethargy and inertia, while for CNS depressants such as alcohol and sedative–hypnotics the withdrawal syndrome is characterised by symptoms of CNS stimulation, such as restlessness, tremors, agitation, hallucinations, and seizures. Withdrawal is often accompanied by symptoms such as anxiety, depression, and sleep disturbances.

The onset and duration of withdrawal is related to the duration of action of the drug to which physical dependence has developed. For drugs with a short half-life, such as alcohol or heroin, withdrawal usually starts within 48 hours, with major symptoms absent by the end of seven days. For drugs with a longer half-life, such as diazepam or methadone, the withdrawal state may be delayed and not observed for several days, and then may continue for several weeks. The severity of withdrawal is determined by several factors, including duration of use, poly-drug use, the general health of the person, and the withdrawal setting.

Managing withdrawal

Withdrawal management refers to a structured procedure for assisting the physically dependent person to reduce his or her drug use, while minimising withdrawal symptoms. It may be delivered on an inpatient, outpatient, or home basis. Within these broad frameworks, the process may be medicated, with pharmacotherapies employed to control withdrawal symptoms, or non-medicated. Each of these broad withdrawal management systems is described below and the suitability of each for different patient presentations is described.

Withdrawal management is often confused with comprehensive treatment. However, although assistance to withdraw from drug use is commonly an important component of a treatment strategy, especially where the degree of physical dependence is significant, the benefit of withdrawal management commonly lies in it creating an opportunity for entry into a longer-term management strategy that provides for systematic life change. This may involve pharmacotherapy, psychotherapy, a therapeutic community, or other treatment options.

Even where entry into long-term management does not eventuate, if withdrawal management significantly reduces levels of drug use post-withdrawal it provides positive outcomes in health promotion and disease prevention, although these may be short lived.

Non-pharmacological treatment

Non-pharmacological treatment of withdrawal involves withdrawing from drug use without assistance of prescribed medications. This approach is appropriate for persons who are likely to experience mild to moderate withdrawal symptoms and who have no coexisting medical problems.

Mild to moderate withdrawal symptoms, for example anxiety and agitation, can be significantly reduced by providing support and counselling in a non-stimulating and safe environment. There are a number of ingredients that can help to reduce patient distress and anxiety and improve treatment outcomes. Importantly, those overseeing the withdrawal should provide reassurance and comfort to the patient. This is particularly important in alcohol and benzodiazepine withdrawal, where the patient is in an overstimulated, anxious state and where, in more severe cases, orientation and perception may be affected. During the withdrawal process, confrontation and argument should be avoided as far as possible. Stimulation should be kept to a minimum, and loud noise and bright lights avoided. Withdrawal should be undertaken in an environment familiar to the patient, or with familiar items present, to reduce patient distress and the likelihood of perceptual confusion.

Pharmacotherapies

The pharmacological treatment of alcohol and drug withdrawal involves relief of symptoms and prevention of escalation of withdrawal severity. This is most important when the withdrawal syndrome can be both severe and dangerous, as in the case of alcohol or barbiturate withdrawal. Several major pharmacological strategies are used to alleviate withdrawal severity.

One approach is the administration of the drug on which the patient is dependent or another drug from the same pharmacological class. Controlled administration of an agonist drug in this way can be used to alleviate withdrawal. The dose is gradually reduced over time so that there is little re-emergence of withdrawal symptoms. This approach is used for benzodiazepine and opioid withdrawal.

A related approach is the administration of a drug with similar pharmacological actions. An agonist drug that does not belong to the same pharmacological class as the drug on which the patient is dependent, but which has a similar action, may be used to alleviate withdrawal. The best example is the use of benzodiazepines in the treatment of alcohol withdrawal. There is cross-tolerance between alcohol and benzo-diazepines, so benzodiazepines can be used effectively to alleviate the symptoms of alcohol withdrawal.

Some withdrawal syndromes cannot be adequately treated with agonist drugs or there may be reasons to avoid these drugs, for example if medication is to be given on an outpatient basis and there is significant potential for its abuse. Symptomatic medications may be used to relieve specific withdrawal symptoms. An example is the use of a cocktail of medications to relieve the various symptoms of opiate with-drawal. The presence and severity of current and past withdrawal symptoms are considered in deciding which if any medications to administer.

A controversial approach is the precipitation of withdrawal by an antagonist in order to reduce the duration of the syndrome. It has been used only for opioid withdrawal, and is used in combination with symptomatic medication. On one hand it offers the potential advantage of a greater completion rate for the with-drawal process, but on the other hand the risks of the withdrawal process may be increased. Precipitated withdrawal will be discussed further in chapter 6.

Withdrawal setting

Where a person is assessed as having only mild to moderate withdrawal, is not in need of sedation and no medical or psychiatric complications are anticipated, then outpatient withdrawal or withdrawal at home is appropriate. Ideally, there should be a reliable person available to monitor withdrawal and, if necessary, to oversee the timely provision of pharmaceutical agents. This is particularly important for alcohol and benzodiazepine withdrawal.

Inpatient withdrawal is indicated where severe withdrawal is expected, such as in the case of recent high-level alcohol use of long duration, in poly-drug users, in patients with poor general health, and in those with a history of present or past major medical or psychiatric complications. Inpatient withdrawal may also be advis-able in less severe withdrawals where there is no friend or relative to assist with home withdrawal, or there is a lack of an alternative community support framework or suitably structured outpatient services to assist with home withdrawal.

The best conditions for inpatient withdrawal are provided by special-purpose withdrawal units rather than acute medical wards. These specialist-built facilities are created to provide a quiet, non-stimulating, and safe environment, and so maximise a patient's ability to tolerate the withdrawal state. Staff are trained to monitor patients and to be ready to detect and respond to more significant prob-lems. The staff also become highly experienced in managing patients with an altered cognitive state, making use of appropriate techniques including testing the patient's reality base, repeated orientation, reacquaintance of patients with their environment, dealing with the nature of illusions and hallucinations, and providing clear directions and appropriate calm response when a patient is endangering themselves or others.

LONG-TERM MANAGEMENT OF DEPENDENCE

The term dependence is used to describe the cluster of physiological and behavioural changes that arise through repeated high-level drug use (see chapter 3). People who are dependent often exhibit physical withdrawal signs and symptoms when they stop using drugs, but this is not a prerequisite for the diagnosis. Severe drug-related health, social, and financial problems are common in drug dependence.

Psychosocial complications include truncated education and training, frequent job changes or unemployment, disruption of relationships with partners, parents, and their own children, and unstable accommodation, including homelessness, debt, and incarceration. Mental health problems are common, and compound these issues. It is often difficult to decide whether the mental health problems are the cause or the result of drug use, but improvement often follows cessation or reduction in drug use.

Presentation

Dependent drug users may present at specialist drug treatment services, or at hospital emergency medical or surgical units following admission for morbidity associated with drug use or the associated lifestyle. They also present at mental health services and social welfare, police or correctional services, or services that deal with poverty and homelessness.

People presenting with a long history of drug dependence, although commonly distressed by their current life circumstances, are frequently considered by doctors to be unmotivated to resolve their problems. This assessment may occur because of the vast disparity between what the drug dependent person feels they can do to address their drug use and what the doctor believes should be undertaken. Unrealistic expectations of what the patient can achieve can lead to frustration for both the doctor and patient.

Goal

While noting the desirability of long-term change for the dependent individual, it may be prudent for the doctor to negotiate short-term treatment goals in the first instance—goals that focus on partial or short-term resolution of drug use problems and small improvements in psychosocial and physical status. In this way the patient can see an achievable goal, rather than the seemingly insurmountable obstacle of life-long abstinence with its complete transformation of lifestyle.

With each successful step, growing motivation is provided to both patient and doctor to continue the process. Gradual steps may, for example, be a safe and controlled withdrawal followed by a short period of abstinence, for example two to three weeks, followed by a review and planning for the next step. In some cases the patient may not be willing to cease drug use, even in the short-term, and in these circumstances it may be possible to negotiate restricting drug use to certain times of the week, such as weekends. In other cases the patient may wish to cease drug use immediately, with no intention to return. Abstinence may also be necessitated by the form of treatment being used, for example maintenance antagonist therapy.

Long-term maintenance medications

A range of pharmacotherapies have been developed for use in the long-term treatment of drug dependence. These can be broadly characterised as follows.

Agonist drugs

The substitution of an agonist drug with similar effects to the drug of dependence can be used in long-term treatment. The best known example is methadone for the treatment of heroin dependence. As discussed in chapter 6, methadone has typical opioid properties and will itself produce dependence. Nevertheless, given in controlled doses and administered orally once a day, it is a very effective treatment for heroin dependence. The goal of this type of treatment is to suppress withdrawal symptoms and to provide stability while the patient addresses lifestyle changes. Nicotine replacement therapy is an example of maintenance therapy with an agonist where the change is not in the drug itself but the form in which it is administered.

Acamprosate for the treatment of alcohol dependence (see chapter 10) and bupropion for the treatment of nicotine dependence (see chapter 7) act on receptors that are influenced, directly or indirectly, by alcohol and nicotine respectively. They do not belong to the same pharmacological classes as those drugs as they have different actions and effects. Nevertheless, they can, to some degree, be considered as substitutes.

Antagonists

Drugs that block all or part of the effects of the drug of dependence may be used in long-term treatment. The goal is for the patient to continue taking the antagonist drug so that if they relapse there will be little or no effect of the drug administered. The best example is naltrexone for the treatment of opioid dependence (see chapter 6). Naltrexone is able to block the effects of heroin completely so that administering heroin has no effect. This drug is also used for the treatment of alcohol dependence, but the mechanism is somewhat different (see chapter 10). Here naltrexone is blocking only one effect of alcohol, the increase in endogenous opioid action.

Aversive therapy

Disulfiram is used in the treatment of alcohol dependence as it can produce an unpleasant reaction if the person relapses to drinking (see chapter 10). While this and other medications have been used to produce aversive reactions in an attempt to dissuade people from continued drug consumption, these are no longer widely used because of limitations of patient compliance and the risks of a severe reaction to alcohol.

Development of medications

While we have a range of maintenance medications for some classes of drug (for example the opioids), there are no pharmacotherapies of proven efficacy available for other drug classes (such as cannabis and stimulants). In some cases the development of such medications awaits a clearer understanding of the pharmacology of the drugs of dependence. In the case of cannabis, the pharmacology is beginning to be understood and we can look forward to the prospect of having agonists and antagonists available in the future. In other cases the pharmacology is well understood, but we simply do not have effective treatments (as with the stimulants).

Psychosocial interventions

Psychosocial interventions are primarily aimed at achieving one or more of four major interconnected outcomes to achieve behavioural change. The first is to reduce drug use to non-problem levels; this often means abstinence. The second is to prevent relapse following reductions in drug use. The third is to assist the patient to cope with current lifestyle predicaments while making appropriate lifestyle changes that promote safer, reduced drug use or abstinence. The fourth outcome is to improve the psychosocial status of the patient with the goal of integration back into the fabric of society.

Psychosocial interventions can be employed as treatment in their own right, but there is also increasing evidence that the outcomes associated with a pharmacotherapy are more likely to be successful if they are supported by psychosocial therapy. The approach discussed below is based on the principles of cognitive behavioural therapy (CBT). Although other therapeutic approaches are sometimes adopted, CBT is the most widely used approach for management of drug dependence.

It is sometimes assumed that changing an unhealthy behaviour requires nothing more than informing the patient of the need for change. This fails to recognise that the patient is deriving benefits from the drug use, even though these benefits may be difficult for others (including the practitioner) to recognise and understand. In the treatment of drug problems we are seeking to produce a long-lasting change in behaviour, and not simply short-term improvements that are lost in weeks or months. This requires a program to be developed with the patient that is carried out over a number of months with repeated follow-up appointments. The approach below sets out a simple step-by-step method that can be used for a variety of alcohol and drug problems. The behavioural program may be used in isolation or together with pharmacotherapy treatment (such as nicotine replacement therapy for tobacco use, naltrexone for alcohol problems).

Measurement

It is useful for the patient to measure and monitor his or her drug use behaviour. Patients are sometimes unaware of the exact amount of drugs that they use. This is more likely with a drug such as alcohol, where consumption occurs in social situations with other activities occurring simultaneously. By itself the act of measuring behaviour typically produces a decrease in drug consumption as patients become aware of their own use patterns.

It is important to discuss with the patient the units they should use (these will depend on the drug), and how they should go about monitoring their drug use. It is sometimes useful for them to use a diary in which they record the time and date of drug use, the location, the amount and type of drug consumed, and the form in which it is used on that occasion. For a more in-depth analysis, diaries can also include other information, such as the psychological state of the individual before and after use and the events leading up to drug use. The diary can then be brought to the next session to review the pattern of drug use and the information used in discussing drug use behaviour.

A second purpose of a diary or record of drug use is for the patient to be able to recognise changes when they occur. If the decrease in drug use is gradual, the patient often does not recognise how much he or she has achieved. It is important to be able to reflect back on, for example, the amount of alcohol he or she used to consume or the number of cigarettes he or she used to smoke.

Treatment goals

The goal of treatment needs to be determined and agreed upon. There are two major types of goals: abstinence from the drug, and controlled use. The choice will depend on a number of factors. In general, if there is a significant level of dependence a period of abstinence is usually necessary. For people with little or no dependence, but a pattern of excessive or problematic use, controlled use may be more appropriate. Consideration needs also to be given to the safety of the drug and the route of administration.

Once the goal is established, some decision needs to be made about how this is going to be reached. Is this to be done in one step, or as a serious of sub-goals with the eventual major goal to be reached some time in the future? If consumption is to be ceased in one step, then consideration needs to be given to the management of any withdrawal syndrome. Sub-goals need to be achievable so that the patient receives positive feedback as he or she reaches each sub-goal and progresses towards the major goal.

Reward

In order for long-lasting behaviour change to occur, the patient needs to derive some positive benefit from the change. If drug use is more rewarding than living without the drug, then the person will relapse. It is important, therefore, to help the patient recognise the benefits received from reduced drug use.

In earlier interaction with the patient, the benefits and costs of drug use will have been discussed. Some of the reward from reduced drug use will be obtained in the form of a reduction in those costs initially highlighted. The medical practitioner can highlight any improvement in the patient's health. It is helpful if concrete evidence can be given to patients of changes that have occurred, such as improvements in liver function tests. Such feedback can have a considerable impact on the patient's future drug-use behaviour. By understanding the typical adverse effects of drugs, you can prompt the patient to recognise positive changes that may have occurred in his or her life. For example, the patient who has been using amphetamine may have decreased paranoia or improved sleep as a result of a reduction in drug use. Decreased drug use is frequently accompanied by improved relationships with both relatives and friends. Patients may be encouraged to recognise the money that they are saving due to decreased spending on the drug.

High-risk situations

Once behaviour change has commenced it is important that the patient recognise those situations in which relapse is most likely. Typically, these will be situations in which drug use has occurred frequently in the past or in which the rate of drug use has increased. Sometimes drug use may be associated with a particular physical location or time of day (for example the cannabis user who only smoked after 8 p.m. or the drinker who mainly consumed alcohol at a particular hotel). A high-risk situation may arise when the person finds him- or herself in the company of other drug users, on payday, or in a particular psychological state (anxiety, joy). By discussing the situations in which drug use has occurred in the past you can determine the individual's high-risk situations.

Once the high-risk situations are identified, strategies can be developed to deal with these. One is avoidance: if at all possible, high-risk situations are best avoided rather than confronted, particularly in the early stages of changing drug use. If they cannot be avoided, then alternative ways of coping need to be developed. The exact approach will depend on the nature of the high-risk situation. For example, if it is the presence of certain people, then drug refusal skills may have to be considered. If it is a particular psychological state, the person needs to consider other ways of dealing with that mood or experience or may have to be considered for treatment of a recurring disorder such as depression or anxiety.

Re-establishing social activities

A common feature of drug dependence is that previously important social activities will have disappeared as drug use has grown. A reduction in current drug use that does not address this deficit can create a lifestyle which seems empty, devoid of pleasure, and ultimately less attractive than the drug-use lifestyle. It is therefore essential to reinstate old activities and develop new interests to fill any void created by reductions in drug use.

Follow-up

Changing drug use behaviour is a complex and often lengthy process. During this process it is essential to include patients in decision making and encourage their active participation. Simply prescribing ways of changing drug-use behaviour is unlikely to be effective. It also needs to be recognised that relapses are common, with long-term management of the dependent drug user often involving patient movement in and out of treatment initiatives (either the same or different) over an extended period. This is an important realisation for both the patient and doctor, and recognising this will assist the patient not to be viewed by the practitioner or him or herself as a failure.

Given that relapse to drug use is common, the practitioner's role should be to plan for possible relapse, and if it occurs to encourage the patient to re-enter treatment. Optimally, re-entry to treatment should be initiated before drug use patterns have escalated back to dependent levels. Failure to act quickly will mean that ground is lost, and the patient will be likely to require withdrawal management before treatment can be initiated again. Impediments to the patient returning for assistance should be minimised. It is also helpful to have frank discussions with the patient on the likelihood of relapse and on what to do should relapse occur. Even though relapse to drug use is common, improvements are usually observed with each remission and subsequent entry into treatment.

Additional therapeutic tools

A number of behavioural and social interventions have been shown to be effective in assisting patients to achieve and maintain behavioural change. These are identified below.

Cognitive behavioural therapy for associated problems

Cognitive behavioural therapy teaches patients to moderate their responses to their environment by improving social coping and problem-solving skills. For example, improved treatment outcomes have been noted with social skills training, where persons are trained to manage social situations previously perceived as difficult, such as interpersonal communication and conflict. It can also be used to assist patients to manage situations where they may be tempted to use drugs.

Comorbid anxiety and depression are commonly associated with dependent drug use, and CBT has been noted to improve treatment outcomes in these patients. The use of CBT as an adjunct to treatment of comorbid presentations is important, since these patients usually have a poor prognosis, with depressive episodes and anxiety both associated with relapse back to drug use. CBT can be delivered to either a group or an individual.

Significant others

The involvement of significant others, often family members or partners, in the treatment process may help to engage initially unmotivated patients in treatment. Clearly, this outcome is more likely if the patient consents to the initial involvement of the significant other. Compliance with pharmacotherapy treatment is also commonly improved when a significant other is involved.

Mutual-help groups

A variety of mutual-help groups are available to individuals in treatment and to affected family and other significant people. These groups are commonly run by community-based not-for-profit organisations. Some mutual-help groups, such as Alcoholics Anonymous or Narcotics Anonymous, are worldwide institutions with a clear documented philosophy for recovery and support, but other groups may be less structured.

The common objective shared by these groups is to support those who are in the early stages of recovery from dependent drug use and to assist them to maintain their non-dependent status. While the efficacy of many of these services has not been formally evaluated, many people who attend report that they have been significant in assisting them to refrain from dependent drug use.

Affected family and friends also commonly report positively on attendance at mutual-help groups, where they have had the opportunity to discuss issues with others who are dealing with the often traumatic consequences of problem drug use.

Residential treatment and support

The approaches described above can all be used on an outpatient basis. However, some people benefit from treatment in a setting apart from their normal social environment. This is particularly the case where there are very strong social pressures in their normal environment to use drugs, or where the patient requires more intensive therapy than can be provided via outpatient appointments.

Therapeutic communities

Therapeutic communities are commonly provided for those who have experienced problem alcohol, opiate or poly-drug use, although occasionally users of other illicit drugs also become involved. Communities commonly require abstinence, so patients may require assistance to withdraw as preparation for entry. They have strict rules regarding the rights and responsibilities of community participants, with well-defined structures giving higher status to those who have attended longer and who have demonstrated a level of psychosocial stability. These people often act as lay therapists and counsellors and work in association with trained health professionals.

The objectives of the therapeutic community are to provide interpersonal, vocational and coping skills through community collaboration in a structured environment, and to discourage relapse. To facilitate these objectives, contact with the outside community is commonly restricted until a level of stability has been achieved.

Attrition is high, with many people leaving after only one or two weeks. The major obstacle for the majority of those who enter a therapeutic community is assimilation from the drug-using culture into one with strict rules and consequences.

Supported accommodation

Drug users with long-term dependence commonly lack stable residential accommodation, and are dislocated from previous social support networks and from the normal fabric of society. Involvement in mutual-help groups or in therapeutic communities may not be possible for this most socially disadvantaged group of drug users. General counselling, CBT, and other forms of psychosocial therapy also may offer little assistance. Providing a level of psychosocial stability is the initial goal of management. This is commonly achieved by the provision of supported care in a structured abstinent environment.

Places providing supported community accommodation, frequently referred to as half-way houses, are located in general community settings and can provide medium- to long-term residential accommodation to the significantly drug-dependent person who otherwise lacks accommodation and social support. They provide an environment that is conducive to abstinence and that allows the significantly impaired drug user to re-establish personal self-esteem and skills slowly, with a long-term goal of return to the general community. They may provide the opportunity for personal and lifestyle changes, such as retraining with the goal of eventual employment, identification of recreational activities, the development of new social networks, and the rekindling of links with salient others and family.

For those long-term drug users with more significant mental health morbidity and cognitive impairment, a more structured and supervised residential environment is required, often within a mental health facility. While these services, like half-way houses, provide supported care in a structured abstinent environment, full return to mainstream community life is not a common goal. Nevertheless, some level of integration back into the community is often achievable.

OVERDOSE TREATMENTS

Overdose amongst drug users can be accidental or intentional, and can occur in those who are non-dependent as well as in those who are dependent. Overdose is treated by supportive measures and, in some cases, by use of specific antagonists. The most widely used is the opioid antagonist naloxone for the treatment of heroin or other opioid overdose. It effectively reverses the effects of opioids, particularly respiratory depression, which can be fatal. The benzodiazepine antagonist flumazenil has also been used for overdose treatment of that class of drugs, but is used uncommonly, and with great caution, because of the risk of precipitating seizures. For most other classes of drugs there are no effective antagonists available. In such cases treatment is supportive, sometimes with use of symptomatic medications.

➡ Brief intervention or advice is appropriate to the primary care setting, including general practice, community health services, and the general hospital environment.

➡ The less dependent problem drug user is more likely to benefit from brief intervention and advice and to achieve controlled drug use.

➡ The more dependent drug user who commonly lacks social support and/or stable psychosocial profiles is more likely to benefit from a treatment where abstinence is the goal.

➡ Where abstinence is the goal, this may need to be worked towards by achievable short-term steps, for example withdrawal and then a two to three week abstinence with a review.

➡ Although an important part of a treatment strategy for the physically dependent drug user, withdrawal is not a treatment in its own right.

➡ In most instances outpatient withdrawal is as effective as inpatient withdrawal.

➡ Home withdrawal can often be initiated where suitable support for observation and pharmaceutical supervision is available within the outpatient context.

➡ Inpatient withdrawal is recommended for people where significant withdrawal symptoms are anticipated based on history of drug use and past withdrawals, for those involved in polypharmacy, or where major physical or psychiatric comorbidity is present.

➡ Pharmacotherapies are effective treatment components in the long-term management of significant problem drug users.

➡ The use of psychotherapies conjoint with pharmacotherapies is associated with better outcomes, and improves pharmacotherapy compliance.

➡ Given that relapse to drug use is common, the practitioner should plan for possible relapse and, if it occurs, encourage the patient to re-enter treatment.

➡ Cognitive behaviour therapy is associated with improved treatment outcomes, both in its own right and as an adjunct to the pharmacotherapy.

➡ Involvement of salient others may prove helpful in encouraging problem drug users to engage in treatment.

➡ While the efficacy of self-help groups has rarely been formally evaluated, many people report that they have been significant in assisting them to refrain from drug use.

➥ Some patients, particularly those with more severe dependence and social dysfunction, may benefit from residential treatment.

REFERENCES AND FURTHER READING

Finney, J.W. & Moos, R.H. 1998, 'Psychosocial treatments for alcohol use disorders', in Nathan, P.E. & Gorman, J.M. (eds) *A Guide to Treatment that Works*, Oxford University Press, New York.

Miller, W.R. & Rollnick, S. 1991, *Motivational Interviewing: Preparing People to Change Addictive Behavior*, Guildford Press, New York.

O'Brien, C.P. & McKay, J.R. 1998, 'Psychopharmacological treatments of substance use disorders', in Nathan, P.E. & Gorman, J.M. (eds) *A Guide to Treatment that Works*, Oxford University Press, New York.

Poikolainen, K. 1999, 'Effectiveness of brief interventions to reduce alcohol intake in primary health care populations: A meta-analysis', *Preventive Medicine*, vol. 28, pp. 503–9.

Specific Substances

Part 2 is concerned with different drugs and drug classes. While not all of the drugs that are used non-medically are considered, most of the major recreational drugs and drugs of dependence are included. In order to provide some comparability, there is a similar structure across chapters. In addition, where possible, the same authors have been responsible for equivalent sections across the different chapters. For each chapter, the first-named author has taken primary responsibility for collating the material.

Part 2 should be read after consideration of the general issues raised in part 1.

6

Opioids

Ross Young, John Saunders, Gary Hulse, Stuart McLean,
Jenny Martin & Geoff Robinson

*What an upheaving, from the lowest depths, of the inner spirit! What an apocalypse of
the world within me! That my pains had vanished was now a trifle in my eyes … here
was the secret of happiness, about which philosophers had disputed for so many ages, at
once discovered: happiness could be bought for a penny, and carried in the waistcoat
pocket: portable ecstasies might be had corked up in a pint bottle: and peace of mind
could be sent down in gallons by the mail coach.*

Thomas De Quincey 1822, *Confessions of an English Opium Eater.*

The word 'opium' is the Greek word for juice, referring to the juice of the opium
poppy, *Papaver somniferum*. Opioids have been used since at least 4000 BC by the
Sumerians, and from 2000 BC by the Egyptians. Opium was probably introduced to
post–Roman empire Europe by the returning crusaders. Heroin (diacetylmorphine)
is now the most commonly abused opioid in the Western world. It was produced
commercially in 1898 by the same Bayer pharmaceutical team that developed
aspirin commercially. At that time heroin was viewed as a less effective analgesic
than morphine, but it was thought to hold great promise as a cough suppressant.

PHARMACODYNAMICS AND PHARMACOKINETICS

Morphine, an alkaloid, is the major active constituent of the opium poppy. Both
morphine and codeine are derived from opium, the milky juice or dried exudate of
the poppy. The opioids as a class are substances with morphine-like effects that can
be reversed by the specific antagonist naloxone. Some opioids are semisynthetic
chemical derivatives of morphine (such as heroin). Others, which are fully synthetic
(such as pethidine and methadone), share a common core structure that allows them
to interact with opioid receptors.

Heroin (smack, H) is prepared by acetylation of morphine extracted from opium. In Australia the prepared heroin is likely to come from South-East Asia; in New Zealand acetylation of prescription opioids to produce domestic 'homebake' is more common. The purity of both of these forms of street opioids varies widely, and their appearance may range from tan granules to a white powder. Adulterants are routinely added to illicit opioids to dilute the opioid (see chapter 13). Pharmaceutical opioids, such as methadone and slow-release oral morphine may also be used by dependent and recreational opioid users.

Figure 6.1   The appearance of street heroin varies and can range from tan granules to a white powder.

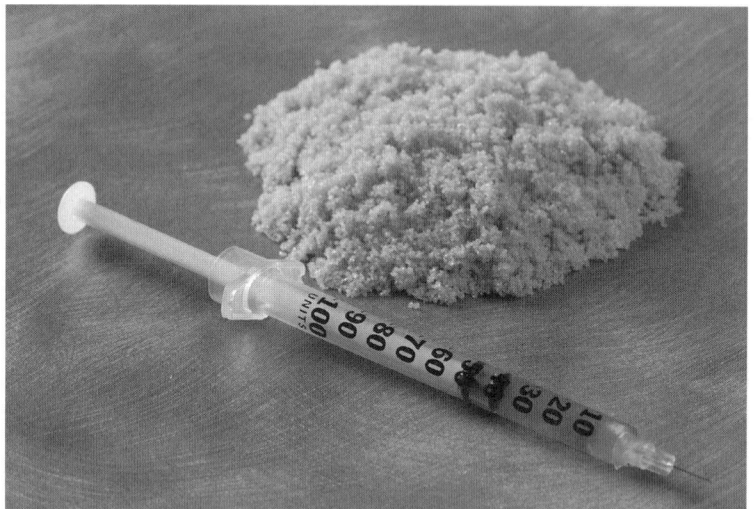

Artwork reproduced with permission of the Prevention Branch, Drug and Alcohol Office (Department of Health, Western Australia)

Pharmacodynamics

The opioid system in the central nervous system (CNS) and periphery includes three main types of opioid receptor, μ, κ and δ. There are thought to be subtypes of each, although the exact number and characteristics have yet to be determined. Four groups of endogenous opioid peptides (enkephalins, endorphins, dynorphins and endomorphins) are produced by peptidases that cleave inactive precursor peptides (for example, pro-opiomelanocortin to β-endorphin). Opioid receptors act via G-proteins and are inhibitory. They inhibit adenylate cyclase, open potassium channels, and block voltage-gated calcium channels, thus reducing the release of a variety of neurotransmitters including 5-HT, acetylcholine, glutamate, and GABA.

The opioid peptides and their receptors are widely distributed in the brain and spinal cord and in many non-neuronal tissues, including the gastrointestinal tract. The endogenous opioid system is activated by stress, and is involved in the modulation of pain perception and mood and the regulation of physiological systems such as respiration. Opioids also have a role in regulating immune function.

The principal effects of morphine are drowsiness and mood change, typically contentment or euphoria, analgesia, and respiratory depression. The analgesic response, rather than removing pain, completely alters the perception of pain, making it no longer aversive. Cognition is impaired, but consciousness and coordination are generally intact at low doses. Respiration is depressed partly through the inhibition of the brainstem response to carbon dioxide, and this can be fatal in overdose. Cough is suppressed, and nausea and vomiting arise from stimulation of the chemoreceptor trigger zone in the medulla. Gastrointestinal motility is depressed and constipation is common. Miosis occurs via increasing parasympathetic tone to the pupil. Urethral and bladder tone are also increased, leading to urinary retention. At high doses there is an increase in the tone of large trunk and intercostal muscles, which can impair breathing.

Morphine activates μ receptors in the mesolimbic reward pathway, increasing dopamine release by inhibiting GABA interneurones. The increase in dopamine release may contribute to the dependence potential of these drugs (see chapter 2). Tolerance, discussed below, starts to develop after the first dose and involves both down-regulation (a decrease in the number of receptors) and desensitisation (a diminished response to receptor activation).

> Opioid drugs stimulate opioid receptors, producing drowsiness, reduced pain perception and euphoria. The latter effect is highly reinforcing.

The consequences of binding to opioid receptors vary with the nature of the ligand. Strong agonists, such as morphine and methadone, activate opioid receptors in the manner already described. Partial agonists, such as buprenorphine, are unable to elicit this full response, even after high doses. Antagonists, such as naloxone, occupy but do not activate the receptor, and so block the effects of agonists.

Both agonists and antagonists can show selectivity for specific receptor subtypes. Buprenorphine is a partial μ agonist and is therefore useful in blocking some of the reinforcing effects of full μ agonists. Pentazocine is a mixed κ agonist and μ antagonist and, because of the κ action, tends to produce dysphoria instead of euphoria. As a mixed agonist–antagonist drug, it may precipitate a withdrawal syndrome if administered to a patient who is currently opioid dependent.

Pharmacokinetics

As would be expected from the great variety of chemical structures in the opioid class, there are important differences in their pharmacokinetics. Most are metabolised by oxidation, but morphine and buprenorphine are conjugated with glucuronic acid in the liver. Morphine is rapidly metabolised after oral administration so that only a small fraction of an oral dose reaches the systemic circulation (that is, it has low bioavailability). Despite this, oral morphine is a common therapy for chronic severe pain, given as a slow-release formulation. Morphine is also given parenterally for acute pain. Morphine-6-glucuronide is an active metabolite that contributes to the opioid effects of morphine, and it can accumulate in the patient with renal failure.

Heroin (diacetylmorphine) is more lipophilic than morphine, and therefore enters the CNS more rapidly, leading to intense euphoria. It is hydrolysed to monoacetyl-morphine and then morphine. Codeine is also converted to morphine, its active form, via demethylation by the enzyme CYP2D6. This enzyme is absent in about 8 to 10% of Caucasians and about 2% of South-East Asians. In such individuals codeine has no analgesic effect.

Methadone is an orally active strong analgesic with a long duration of action. l-α-acetylmethadol (LAAM) is even longer acting because it produces two active metabolites with very long half-lives. The actions of pethidine are complicated by conversion into a metabolite, norpethidine, which is a CNS stimulant. Fentanyl is a potent agonist that can be absorbed transdermally.

TOLERANCE, PHYSICAL DEPENDENCE, AND TOXICITY

Tolerance

Tolerance to opioids is characterised by a shortened duration and reduced intensity of the analgesic, euphorigenic, and sedative effects. Postulated mechanisms for this include receptor adaptation to the recurrent agonist binding (a decrease in receptor numbers), adaptive changes in second messenger systems, and a negative feedback process influencing production of the endogenous ligand.

Binding of opioids to μ receptors results in the activation of Gi (an inhibitory G-protein coupled receptor system), and subsequent inhibition of adenylate cyclase, the effector enzyme. Long-term administration of morphine causes a compensatory increase in adenylate cyclase activity, and resultant increase in second messengers like cAMP (which phosphorylates protein kinases). This results in rebound excitability of neurons during opioid withdrawal. Negative feedback due to higher concentrations of exogenous opioids also reduces the synthesis of endogenous opioids in the CNS.

There is marked variation between individuals in the development of tolerance. This is likely to be due to genotypic variations in receptor characteristics and second messenger systems. Other substance use and environmental influences are also important. Tolerance does not develop equally or at the same rate to the various effects of opioids. Even chronic users experience respiratory depression and miosis. Clinically, higher concentrations of opioids can be required to achieve a given analgesic effect among those with high genetic tolerance. While important in all patients, it is particularly crucial in those with high tolerance to reduce the opioid dose slowly at the end of treatment to allow neuroadaptation to reverse, and thus reduce the likelihood of withdrawal. Opioid analgesia in chronic opioid drug users also poses significant challenges due to the heightened tolerance they have acquired through previous drug exposure.

Withdrawal

The opioid withdrawal syndrome is well documented. The withdrawal state, although unpleasant, is not life threatening, except in the neonate. Rather than life-threatening features, it is the subjective sensations of withdrawal and discomfort from psychological changes that require treatment. Withdrawal symptoms include insomnia, irritability, restlessness, malaise, pain, fatigue, and gastrointestinal hypermotility. Most patients will develop some withdrawal symptoms, even with a gradual reduction in dosage. One form of treatment involves a reducing dose of methadone, which, as noted, is a μ agonist with pharmacodynamic properties similar to morphine. Methadone suppresses withdrawal symptoms, including craving. The partial agonist buprenorphine has a similar effect, but with less likelihood of withdrawal reaction from the treatment itself. Clonidine (a centrally acting α_2 agonist) can reduce some of the autonomic symptoms, but not the craving or anxiety. Despite the effectiveness of methadone, some illicit drug users find the withdrawal state experienced from methadone more aversive than that of heroin as it is more protracted.

As noted above, binding to μ receptors causes enhanced dopamine release from the nucleus accumbens. On withdrawing from morphine there is severe inhibition of dopamine release from the nucleus accumbens, and a consequent dopamine deficiency.

Toxicity

The acutely toxic effects of opioids are numerous and involve many systems. Briefly, from mild to severe, they include pruritus, constipation, nausea, vomiting, confusion with possible delirium, stupor, miosis, urinary retention, hypothermia, non-cardiogenic pulmonary oedema, hypotension, coma, and death from respiratory depression.

There is no evidence of long-term direct toxic effects on the CNS. In fact, good health and productive work are not incompatible with the regular use of opioids. Many of the long-term health-related complications are a product of antisocial behaviour, poor general self-care, imprisonment, drug impurities or contaminants, and blood-borne disease. However, some recent evidence suggests that repeated non-fatal overdoses may result in brain damage as a result of the hypoxia.

> ⇒ The opioid withdrawal state is unpleasant but not life threatening.
> ⇒ The main risks related to drug use are acute toxicity.
> ⇒ The long-term effects of opioids themselves are relatively benign, however adulterants and use-related behaviour are associated with harm.

83

ASSESSMENT

Of the possible laboratory analyses related to opioid use, assays to determine the presence or concentration of opioid in the urine are used most frequently. A determination of the presence or absence of drugs may be part of an initial screen. While only small amounts of most opioids are excreted directly, metabolic breakdown products are detected readily. Urine analysis is preferred to blood analysis because the collection is less invasive, multiple samples can be collected easily, urine samples are more stable over time, and, due to the concentrating actions of the kidneys, the urine concentrations of drugs and metabolites are relatively high. To avoid the possibility of substitution, urine samples in drug clinics may be taken under direct observation. Shorter-acting opioids such as fentanyl may be detected for up to seven or eight hours; longer-acting drugs such as methadone for up to 72 hours.

Estimating the precise amounts of street drugs used can be challenging because of the contaminants present, and consequently the amount spent per day by a dependent user of illicit drugs may be a more reliable index. Street heroin typically contains an average of 50% drug, but this is highly variable. Use can also be approximated by determining the frequency of administration: daily administration is commonly considered the threshold for dependent use, while those with a strong dependence typically administer heroin three times daily. Contrary to community stereotypes of heroin use, many and perhaps most heroin users are episodic recreational users who are not dependent. Furthermore, there are also users who show fluctuating use that is related to their current life situation. Having the patient estimate the number of hours intoxicated per day can also be informative.

Opioids can be administered by inhalation (smoking is colloquially called 'chasing the dragon'), orally (this is rare today), intranasally, and, most popularly, intravenously. Smoking produces less efficient absorption than intravenous injection because vapour is lost in the atmosphere. Prescription opioid abuse is generally oral, although multiple presentations to medical professionals seeking intramuscular opioid analgesia for a migraine or back pain are relatively commonplace.

As with any drug-related assessment, consideration needs to be given to the stigma associated with abuse of opioids: a non-threatening, empathic interviewing style is more likely to elicit an accurate history than a judgmental approach. However, there is a high representation of personality disorder amongst those who are dependent on illicit opioids and among those with chronic pain disorders associated with vague physical pathology. The self-report of such individuals is often unreliable and, in the case of drug-seeking patients, typically represents a significant distortion of the truth. Government inspectors who monitor the use of restricted schedule drugs can provide accurate data regarding prescribing patterns. This is also of potential legal importance as the prescription of opioids to opioid-dependent individuals is restricted (see chapter 21). The self-report of the patient who is in withdrawal or who is acutely intoxicated is also likely to be compromised. It is also vital that patients be routinely asked regarding prescription of naltrexone, as recent use will negate the use of opioid analgesia. Information from a spouse, partner, or family member is often very useful in establishing the validity of the patient's self report.

> ➡ While the patient should be dealt with in a non-judgmental way, the history should not be taken at face value. Chronic opioid users may present a distorted picture because of personality issues, abnormal behaviour as part of illness, or drug seeking. Collateral information is highly valuable.

Physical examination

Clinical observation for signs of intoxication or withdrawal is vital. In acute intoxication, sedation, constricted pupils, impaired respiration, and euphoria may be present. In patients with compromised lung activity, respiratory depression can significantly impair function even at relatively low opioid doses. Acute withdrawal symptoms vary according to the time since the last opioid dose. The first signs emerge as soon as four hours after a dose, and are manifested as a marked drive to use the drug. At 8–12 hours the signs include lacrimation, rhinorrhoea, yawning, and sweating, followed by dilated pupils, anorexia, irritability, tremor, and gooseflesh/piloerection. Restlessness begins at about 12–14 hours. In most medical settings the level of dependence and severity of the withdrawal state are unlikely to be assessed using standardised paper and pencil instruments, but in specialist clinics use of measures such as the Severity of Opiate Dependence Scale and the Short Opioid Withdrawal Scale are common. In all settings, provision of information about possible withdrawal symptoms is beneficial and results in less distress, particularly in the novice.

> Assessment and information about likely withdrawal symptoms and their sequence is crucial.

As previously noted, the chronic physical and medical problems associated with the use of pure opioids are not severe. Most of the significant problems are related to mode of administration or to the presence of contaminants. Physical examination also needs to include inspection of limbs for increased pigmentation over veins, track marks, and evidence of clotted or thrombosed veins. Lesions or abscesses at injection entry sites (including *Clostridium botunilum*), or poorly healed lesions due to compromised nutrition and self-care, should be examined. The patient may appear malnourished and be significantly underweight. Lymph glands may be swollen and the liver may be enlarged. The male patient may also report sexual difficulties due to lowered testosterone; this can persist for four weeks after opioid use has ceased. Examination for sexually transmitted disease is also important, given that prostitution is a relatively common means of obtaining money for heroin among those with severe dependence. Typical laboratory findings include evidence of AIDS, hepatitis B, hepatitis C and liver test abnormalities (see chapter 13), decreased globulins, electrolyte abnormalities (often hyperkalaemia), and a relatively high eosinophil count.

Cardiovascular effects due to opioids themselves are typically mild, the most likely effect being orthostatic hypotension. Endocarditis from contaminated needles and emboli, which are capable of producing stroke, are possible. Tuberculosis, which has increased in prevalence over recent years, and lung abscesses are also possible. Bronchospasm and wheezing may be present in those who prefer to smoke heroin.

> In all illicit users thorough physical examination and laboratory investigation of possible exposure to hepatitis B, hepatitis C, and HIV is vital.

Psychosocial history

The psychosocial history of opioid-dependent patients can be very complex. Patients frequently report significant adversity. There is likely to be a history of antisocial or delinquent behaviour. Some users will meet diagnostic criteria for antisocial personality disorder, although many patients will have a history of illegal activity (such as theft or prostitution) that relates only to theft or prostitution to obtain sufficient funds to maintain their opioid supply. Concurrent psychiatric difficulties are more likely to involve dysthymia or depression, and, more rarely, anxiety. Opioids are most unlikely to precipitate psychosis resembling schizophrenia. Depression generally resolves within four weeks or so of abstinence, independent of treatment. Antidepressant treatment should be considered for those with a severe depression or a persistent mood disorder. Good prognostic signs that should be assessed are stable employment history, being married or in a stable relationship, little evidence of dependence on other substances, absent or minor legal history, and being over the age of 40.

The psychosocial history of the prescription opioid abuser may include evidence of abnormal behaviour as part of illness, or somatisation disorder. Most present with chronic pain syndromes and have had numerous investigations. The expectations of these patients regarding their pain management need to be clearly assessed. It is common for such patients to expect their discomfort to be eliminated entirely, and to view the solution to their problems as purely pharmacological or surgical. Particularly challenging are health professionals who have access to opioids, typically doctors or nurses. Such individuals often have a family history of substance dependence.

It is likely that most opioid-dependent individuals will need to make several serious attempts to cease drug use. This is due to both the highly reinforcing nature of the opioids as a group of drugs and the drug-related lifestyle that many dependent users become embroiled in. Many patients will have only drug-using peers, or may be dealing drugs to pay debt, or be in other situations from which it is difficult to extricate themselves. The challenges related to changing lifestyle need to be fully understood.

Past history of treatment is also important. Methadone maintenance has been the mainstay of pharmacotherapy since the 1970s, and many patients will have been on and off methadone. The length of these attempts and the methadone dose used should be noted. More recently, buprenorphine and naltrexone maintenance may also have been attempted. The number of attempts at treatment and their type should be noted, including withdrawal management (detoxification), psychotherapy, support groups, rehabilitation programs, and therapeutic communities.

For the prescription opioid abuser, the high likelihood of psychiatric comorbidity, such as somatisation disorder, means that appropriate psychiatric referral will often need to be sought. Specialist services for health professionals are available, and direct referral to these is advisable as disciplinary proceedings may be needed, limiting rights to prescribe addictive drugs or limiting or revoking registration. Health professionals may also be a challenge to treat given their difficulty in adopting the role of patient.

> Key psychosocial assessment issues include personality, comorbid psycho-pathology (particularly depression), the employment and treatment history, and any history of illegal activities. The extent to which the current lifestyle is drug-related can also be important.

INTERVENTION AND TREATMENT

Intervention for heroin and other opioid use takes many forms. It may include emergency resuscitation of someone who has overdosed, short-term treatment of the withdrawal syndrome (sometimes as a prelude to continuing therapy), long-term maintenance on agonist drugs, abstinence-oriented therapies such as naltrexone (an antagonist), involvement with self-help groups, and psychological therapy. Not all of those who use opioid drugs are in need of treatment, nor will all users respond positively to the offer of assistance. Many heroin users enjoy their drug use and have not experienced significant harm. Furthermore, a high proportion of dependent users recover from opioid use without recourse to formal treatment. However, increasing emphasis is placed on engaging opioid users in treatment in order to reduce their risk of overdose and other harmful consequences of their use.

When assessing a newly presenting opioid-dependent patient, the clinician is faced with an array of issues that need to be assessed in order for treatment to be acceptable, timely, and effective. Important clinical issues include the severity of opioid dependence, pattern of use, coexisting alcohol and other drug problems (such as use of amphetamines, or benzodiazepines), coexisting psychological disorders (such as depression or anxiety), skin and other sepsis, blood-borne viral infections (hepatitis C, hepatitis B, HIV), and a variety of social/legal problems.

Clinicians should adopt a non-judgmental attitude to these often challenging patients, and adopt a treatment philosophy incorporating the principles of harm-minimisation (see chapter 1). It should not be assumed that patients are aware of the various treatment options, and so they may need to be appraised of them.

By contrast, some patients have very clear ideas of their treatment preference (for example not wishing to commence methadone again, but willing to try rapid detoxification with an antagonist). The medical practitioner has a responsibility to discuss the range of approaches with all patients.

The management of opioid overdose

The principal features of opioid overdose include miosis, respiratory depression, reduced level of consciousness, and sometimes hypotension, hypothermia, and hypoglycaemia. Non-cardiogenic pulmonary oedema and pneumonia are not infrequent, particularly with heroin overdose. Opioid overdose is a medical emergency and it should be treated without delay. Treatment should include basic aspects of cardiopulmonary resuscitation, clearance and maintenance of airways, and an urgent call to paramedical services. Treatment is as follows.

- Naloxone intravenously (or intramuscularly if intravenous access is not possible); dose should be titrated to support respiratory function without precipitating withdrawal. Total dose may be in the range 0.4 to 1.2 mg. This should rapidly improve the level of consciousness and respiratory rate, and there should be pupillary dilation. If an acute opioid withdrawal is precipitated the patient may be agitated or angry, and it is not uncommon for the patient to abscond at this stage. This risk has resulted in some services avoiding the use of naloxone and focusing on maintaining life support until the patient is out of danger, or using minimal naloxone doses with frequent observations.
- If naloxone is used as the primary treatment, then repeated doses might be required, as this drug has a relatively short half-life of 1.5 hours.
- Naloxone infusion may be required with long-acting opioids (methadone, slow-release morphine). Usual doses of naloxone are relatively ineffective with buprenorphine overdose, and emphasis should be placed on life support until the level of consciousness improves.
- Treatment may need to attend to the impact of other sedative drugs (benzodiazepines, alcohol) which may complicate opioid overdose.

> Opioid overdose is a medical emergency and it should be treated without delay.

Management of opioid withdrawal

Effective treatment of the opioid withdrawal syndrome has been available for many years and is well researched. Regrettably, such treatment is relatively ineffective in reducing long-term heroin use, and so it needs to be linked with an aftercare program. Relapse is common even with aftercare programs in place, and opioid dependence needs to be understood as a chronic relapsing disorder. Despite these caveats, there are strong demands for withdrawal assistance driven by patients, their family, and the legal system. The reasons for the treatment and the patient's motivation must be appraised, as well as the likelihood of participation in a subsequent longer-term treatment. The management of opioid withdrawal has recently been critically reviewed by Gowing et al. (2000). It is difficult to be prescriptive about the treatment setting and pharmacological approaches, particularly with regard to long-term outcomes, as these practices vary widely across jurisdictions within Australia and New Zealand. Patients undergoing withdrawal require considerable support, reassurance, and information about the nature of withdrawal symptoms. Opioid withdrawal rating scales assist in objective assessment, and these can be of use when titrating treatment to symptoms.

Pharmacotherapies for withdrawal management

Methadone tapering
There appears to be an optimal duration of inpatient stay of about two weeks for methadone treatment of heroin withdrawal, after which many patients opt to leave. The standard treatment approach is to taper methadone at a rate of 5–7.5 mg/day for inpatients from an initial level of 30–40 mg per day. This tapering process is generally longer in outpatient programs, given the standard reduction rate of 1–2 mg/day. Patients typically report the final reductions are the most difficult, and the rate may need to be slowed towards the end of tapering.

Buprenorphine
There is accumulating evidence that buprenorphine, a partial opioid agonist, may offer advantages over methadone tapering because withdrawal distress may be less intense. There may also be fewer side-effects than experienced with adjunct medication such as clonidine. Because buprenorphine is a partial agonist with high affinity for the opioid receptor, there can be problems with precipitated withdrawal with initial doses. First doses should be delayed for at least six hours after heroin and 24 hours after methadone (doses less than 35 mg/day). Buprenorphine withdrawal regimens begin at 4–6 mg/day, may increase up to 10 mg/day after a few days, and are then reduced at approximately 1–2 mg/day for inpatients. More gradual community-based withdrawal is also used, with tapering over four weeks.

Adrenergic agonists and adjunctive medication
An alternative to the use of an opioid is clonidine, an α_2 adrenergic agonist, which has long been established to ameliorate opioid withdrawal symptoms. Effective doses of clonidine are frequently associated with side-effects, including sedation and symptomatic hypotension. Usual dosage is 75 to 150 µg tds; maximal during severe withdrawal and tapered off over one to two weeks. Some clinicians use clonidine skin patches to provide constant blood levels and reduce side-effects. Pulse and blood

pressure should be monitored regularly. Lofexidine is an alternative to clonidine that has less pronounced hypotensive effects.

A large variety of adjunctive medications have been utilised to assist opioid withdrawal in addition to clonidine and methadone tapering, but these have not been subject to evidence-based review. These medications include:

- Benzodiazepines (or zopiclone) as hypnotics, or regularly to reduce anxiety related to withdrawal. In addition, a proportion of those with opioid dependence will have coexisting benzodiazepine dependence. This may entail a tapering benzodiazepine regime, usually with diazepam.
- Loperamide, for controlling diarrhoea.
- Quinine sulfate 300 mg 12 hourly, for muscle cramps.
- Non-steroidal anti-inflammatories, for the management of pain.
- Metoclopramide, for nausea.
- Neuroleptics, for severe agitation and insomnia.

Treatment settings

Withdrawal may be undertaken in outpatient settings (with daily dispensing of medications), such as those offered by certain drug clinics, or home-based programs. Patients with better psychosocial support and less likelihood of contact from the street drug scene may be considered best for this approach. Overall, completion is more likely to occur if withdrawal is managed in an inpatient setting, particularly if there are higher levels of coexistent psychological problems (such as anxiety or depression).

> Opioid withdrawal is uncomfortable. The treatment approaches with the strongest evidence base are methadone tapering with the provision of symptomatic relief using medications such as clonidine. Buprenorphine also shows considerable promise, but has not been as extensively evaluated.

Rapid withdrawal techniques

Rapid withdrawal or detoxification is an approach that has gained considerable publicity. The overall strategy is to administer an opioid antagonist to precipitate and foreshorten the withdrawal syndrome. The antagonist, typically naloxone, but sometimes the orally active naltrexone, displaces opioid drugs from μ receptors, preventing their pharmacological effects. In opioid-dependent individuals this induces a withdrawal syndrome that is likely to be profound and intense. Several other medications are usually administered to ameliorate the more severe antagonist-precipitated withdrawal symptoms. The patient is typically under anaesthetic or heavy sedation for the first few hours. Adjunctive medication includes clonidine, which suppresses many of the withdrawal symptoms, a benzodiazepine for sedation and to control agitation, octreotide (a somatostatin analogue) to reduce gastrointestinal secretions, and an antiemetic such as metoclopramide or ondansteron. Best practice guidelines are yet to be established for these procedures.

Longer-term therapies

Treating opioid dependence in the long term is not easy. It is mainly undertaken by specialist drug services and by private practitioners with a particular interest in the area. There are three broad approaches: substitution therapies, abstinence-orientated pharmacotherapies, and psychological treatments.

Agonist maintenance

If long-term agonist maintenance is to be initiated then managed withdrawal is not appropriate.

Methadone

The most common treatment for opioid dependence is substitution therapy, typically methadone maintenance. Methadone, a synthetic opioid, is active orally and has a longer half-life than heroin or codeine-based homebake. It is thus administered once a day under supervision at a clinic or pharmacy. When stabilised at an appropriate dose (usually between 40 and 120 mg daily), most patients experience few symptoms of withdrawal and have reduced craving. The frequency of injecting opioids and sharing needles also declines substantially. The result is fewer deaths from opioid overdose, as well as lower rates of hepatitis C, hepatitis B, and HIV, and reductions in risky injecting practices. Since users no longer have to support an illicit opioid habit and have more stable lives generally, rates of crime and imprisonment fall. Employment also increases, as does social functioning. The less frequent administration and the minimal cost to the user free up time for family and friends, employment, and further training. Should a lapse occur, high doses of methadone blunt the euphoric effects of illicit opioids so that injecting heroin while on methadone is less likely to be reinforcing. Some users still, however, report a powerful conditioned reaction to the act of injecting that is intensely pleasurable.

Methadone treatment is provided by outpatient methadone clinics, and some GPs, psychiatrists, and other medical specialists. Those on methadone programs need to be registered with the local relevant authority, such as a Health Department. Medication is typically dispensed orally as syrup under observation by a specified local pharmacy or hospital. Methadone is more effective in higher doses (at least 60 mg), as a maintenance therapy, as part of a program that includes treatment of comorbid psychiatric disorders (see chapter 20), and when counselling to deal with personal problems is made available. However, even with these issues attended to, some people will not stay in treatment. Research has identified a variety of factors associated with poor outcomes, including antisocial personality disorder, poor social support, poly-drug dependence, and genetic risk for substance dependence.

Buprenorphine

Buprenorphine is as effective as methadone for people with moderate levels of dependence, and possibly also for those with higher levels of dependence. It is easier to taper buprenorphine than methadone, and, as a partial agonist, it is safer in overdose. Buprenorphine results in less respiratory depression than full agonists such as methadone. The wider safety margin allows for alternate-day dosing for many patients, which is more convenient for those who can, for example, go away for a weekend readily. Buprenorphine is cost-effective and has a low likelihood of being sold on the street, as it can precipitate withdrawal in opioid-dependent people. As a partial agonist it induces a lower level of physical dependence than methadone, so cessation of the drug is easier.

LAAM

Levo-α-acetylmethadol (LAAM), a long-acting analogue of methadone, can be given every 48 to 72 hours. It is an effective maintenance agent after patients have achieved initial stability through a methadone program. Although it is possible to initiate subjects onto LAAM, its very long half-life make this more difficult than induction onto methadone. Concerns about prolongation of the QT interval as a result of LAAM administration are likely to limit its use.

Heroin

Some European countries have tried heroin maintenance for opioid-dependent individuals resistant to other treatments. Reduced illicit drug use and crime, and substantial improvements in psychosocial outcomes, have been found. While supervised administration of heroin to otherwise treatment-resistant patients shows some positive benefits, the cost of treatment is approximately ten times that of methadone maintenance.

> Maintenance therapies using opioid agonists are effective in reducing illicit opioid use, but they are not panaceas. They are associated with improvements in health, social function, and psychological state, and with reductions in criminality.

Long-term antagonist treatment

Naltrexone may be prescribed after conventional withdrawal management as well as after rapid withdrawal (as described above). Drug users maintained on naltrexone will not experience positive reinforcing euphoric effects if they do use an opioid, and craving for opioids is reduced. However, compliance is crucial, as the antagonist effect lasts only about 48 hours after the last dose. Naltrexone may precipitate depression, which fortunately responds rapidly to treatment with selective serotonin reuptake inhibitors (SSRIs). There is a significant risk of opioid overdose after stopping naltrexone because the user may misjudge the level of tolerance to opioids. Tolerance falls after abstinence, a process that may be accelerated by antagonist treatment. If the same amount of heroin is used as when tolerance was high, a fatal overdose may occur. The dropout rate with naltrexone is greater than with substitution therapies such as methadone maintenance. As with methadone, naltrexone is more effective if administered supervised and supported by psychological therapy. Depot preparations of naltrexone may reduce some of the compliance problems associated with antagonist treatment.

Psychological and social therapies

Abstinence-orientated treatments typically entail initial withdrawal followed by a rehabilitation program. This may involve treatment with an opioid antagonist, residence in a therapeutic community, attendance at a self-help group, and individual, family, and group counselling.

Therapeutic communities typically emphasise personal growth and the acquisition of important interpersonal, vocational, and coping skills through collaboration with other community members. The community usually has strict rules regarding rights and responsibilities that vary according to the status of members. Status varies by length of stay, and for new members of the community contact with the outside world is likely to be restricted. Programs can last up to nine months. Lay therapists, many of them recovering addicts or graduates of the program, may be present on-staff, alongside trained mental health professionals. Re-entry to the community for a 'booster' following relapse is also usually possible. Evaluation of therapeutic community programs indicates improved functioning regarding opioid use, improved psychological functioning, and reduced involvement in criminal activity. However, the attrition rate is high, and benefits typically accrue only after extensive involvement in the program. Those who drop out are likely to have had more protracted difficulties, and may have personality features that make it difficult for them to respond to the rules of programs and accept the behavioural consequences of transgressions.

Depression and anxiety disorders are relatively common in those with opioid dependence, especially in women, and may need to be treated either with psychological or pharmacotherapeutic approaches. Treatment outcomes for those with psychological problems are improved by psychotherapy in addition to maintenance pharmacotherapy (for example pharmacotherapy using methadone or naltrexone). Both cognitive behavioural or insight orientated psychotherapy can be effective. However, the dropout rate is again high, and the uptake of those services offered is usually low.

Cognitive behaviour therapy may be useful for both the dependent user on maintenance pharmacotherapy and the non-dependent opioid user who may not require maintenance pharmacotherapy but who is still having difficulty changing chronic patterns of use (see chapter 5). Lifestyle issues may also relate to the subculture associated with procuring or using illicit opioids, or to behaviours such as stealing or sex work that are engaged in to get sufficient money to buy drugs. It is not uncommon for patients to present for help reporting that heroin or other illicit opioid use is still enjoyable, but that they have tired of the lifestyle. Psychotherapeutic strategies that involve redressing imbalances in the user's life are the mainstay with this group of

93

patients. In addition, relapse prevention strategies that encourage vigilance for challenges that may exceed the patient's ability to cope, and that remind patients of the likely negative consequences of a return to use, are important. Given the fragmentation of family relationships that can occur with drug use and associated behavioural problems, family or relationship therapy can also be useful in some circumstances. Many users describe the pleasure obtained from the ritual of preparation and the act of injecting. In an attempt to desensitise individuals to these environmental cues, experimental treatments have involved 'cue exposure' to drug-use instruments without the act of injection. While promising, these treatments do not have sufficient evidence to warrant their use in standard clinical care.

Some of the most challenging patients who require psychological therapy are those with prescription opioid dependence who have chronic pain conditions and who may 'doctor shop' (see chapters 14 and 21). Typically, the collaborative management of a specialist pain service and a consultation–liaison psychiatrist is most beneficial in these cases. Methadone patients with pain problems also pose difficulties regarding pain management, and may have high tolerance to opioid analgesia.

Self-help groups like Narcotics Anonymous (NA) offer support and guidance using 12-step principles, derived from those of Alcoholics Anonymous. The fellowship has meetings that can be either open or closed, involve study, or be for beginners. There is little systematic research examining the impact of NA.

> Psychological therapies can improve the effectiveness of pharmacotherapies such as methadone, and can be used in the treatment of those who do not wish to undertake or who do not warrant such management. Only a minority of people will participate in psychological therapy for extended periods.

EPIDEMIOLOGY AND PREVENTION

Estimates indicate that there are approximately 74 000 dependent heroin users in Australia and 30 000 opioid dependent users in New Zealand.

Considerably greater morbidity and mortality occurs with the use of illicit opioids than with prescription medication. As noted, heroin toxicity is associated with morbidity such as respiratory depression. It is a consequence of high-dose heroin use or the use of heroin concurrent with other CNS depressant drugs. Morbidity and mortality can also result from infections introduced by non-sterile injecting practices. These infections include hepatitis B, hepatitis C, and human immunodeficiency virus (HIV), bacterial endocarditis, and tetanus. Poor injecting equipment or poor injecting technique may cause vascular or nerve damage. Environmental factors such as poor living conditions, exposure to violence, and accidents also pose significant risks.

Morbidity and mortality

Injectors are prone to infection (primarily bacterial) around the site of injection. Bacterial, viral, fungal, and parasitic infections can occur in major organs, including the heart, liver, lung, and brain. Poor injecting technique and local infection can result in vascular damage, with injection into an artery associated with major tissue loss and significant complications. The epidemiology, assessment, management, and prevention of blood-borne diseases, and other morbidities associated with injecting drugs, are dealt with in chapter 13.

The mortality rate for regular intravenous illicit opioid users is approximately 13 times that of the general population. This means that approximately 9% of the total mortality in Australians and New Zealanders aged 15–39 years is due to the use of illicit opioids. As these deaths occur at a young age, the number of person-years lost is extremely high when compared to those lost through the use of other substances. For example, in 1992 the number of Australians who died from tobacco-related pancreatic and oesophageal cancers (570) and causes related to opioid use (562) was similar, but the person-years of life lost to 70 for the tobacco-related carcinomas was 2877 compared to 21 690 for opioids. There is an enormous waste of human life and unfulfilled potential associated with heroin. The major causes of mortality identified through comprehensive research review are accidental overdose (30 to 45%), suicide (15 to 35%), violent death or accident/injury (10 to 25%), and medical complications, often related to drug use (25 to 35%).

Key issues for prevention of harm

Overdose

Accidental overdose is associated with variability in the purity of street heroin and concurrent use of other CNS depressant drugs. The overdosed patient can be administered the opioid antagonist naloxone to reverse the effects of heroin; this is typically undertaken by ambulance officers. Significant mortality is associated with use of opioids alone, either in isolated public places or at home, where there is no one to call for assistance and maintain life until emergency help arrives.

Poly-drug use

Most heroin users have a poor understanding of the risks associated with poly-drug use. Education by medical practitioners must include the risk of mixing CNS depressants such as alcohol and benzodiazepines, which are known to be involved in a large number of fatal heroin overdoses. For this reason benzodiazepines should be prescribed cautiously and in limited amounts to reduce the possibility of concomitant use with heroin. Reasons for poly-drug use are dealt with in greater detail in chapter 14.

> The use of benzodiazepines (or any other CNS depressant) and heroin within eight hours of each other increases the chances of fatal overdose.

Purity and tolerance

Medical practitioners also need to educate drug users about tolerance. Periods of low tolerance are likely to follow abstinence, infrequent use, or following periods of use of low-grade heroin or homebake. Users may be encouraged to test a small dose when they purchase a new batch of heroin in order to reduce the risk of overdose. This advice is more likely to be followed by patients when it is also stated that this is a way to avoid 'wasting' heroin.

> Making heroin users aware of their likely level of tolerance and the likely purity of heroin dose can prevent overdose.

Location

As noted, patients should be discouraged from using heroin in places where help cannot be easily sought or where distress associated with heroin use goes unnoticed. Heroin users should be instructed to use when others are aware that they are using, and when the user can be monitored. Although the provision of safe injecting locations is controversial in Australia, such locations can provide an environment to prevent overdose, and also can contain information about treatment and support.

Providing medical advice as a prevention strategy

It would be naive to suggest that those with established heroin dependence are an easy group of patients to treat. However, the clinical challenges can be magnified by the adoption of negative or punitive attitudes. Such attitudes significantly reduce the likelihood that patients will seek assistance on a subsequent occasion, and an opportunity to prevent possible problems may be lost. As in any consultation, the medical practitioner's language will also need to reflect local or subcultural terminology, and to clarify the language of the patient to ensure that meanings are shared.

A key prevention issue is the provision of information on overdose symptoms, and advice on how to provide resuscitation and what to tell the emergency operator or ambulance officers. Users may sometimes voice a reluctance to call an ambulance for fear of prosecution, and it is important that they are assured that the ambulance officer does not have a policing role. Users also need to be informed that overdoses can occur gradually, and that therefore observation is necessary beyond the period immediately following use. There is a particular risk when other drugs, especially other CNS depressants, have been consumed in addition to heroin. Preventing and responding to accidental overdose in injecting drug users is dealt with in chapter 13.

> It is imperative that medical practitioners reinforce the message that police (or others) will not attend with ambulances.

Heroin use is commonly associated with a broad exposure to health risk through poor living conditions. Chronic unemployment, increased social problems including loss of social and family support, debt, and intermittent incarceration are common features of the heroin user's world. Medical practitioners need to provide advice that aims to reduce exposure to more general risk in order to minimise the harm associated with drug use. Facilitating access to information on health benefits, welfare cards, housing, employment or training opportunities will also help the user move away from the heroin network and reduce harm.

A comprehensive knowledge of treatment options and how to access them is important. These options include managed withdrawal (opioid antagonist-precipitated inpatient or outpatient assisted withdrawal), user support groups such as Narcotics Anonymous, maintenance programs (methadone, buprenorphine and naltrexone), rehabilitation programs, and therapeutic communities. In addition to educating the drug user, it is crucial to assess risks such as depression or suicidality and to provide appropriate treatment or referral. Fear of unwanted involvement of family, police or other authorities can be an impediment to the user seeking treatment, and, again, the separation of the health and criminal justice systems should be emphasised.

> Stabilisation of the dependent heroin user in treatment will significantly reduce morbidity and mortality related to lifestyle and injecting drug use.

Case study

Michelle is 24 years old, and was introduced to heroin by her ex-boyfriend when she was 19. She has used a number of drugs, including marijuana from the age of 12, and ecstasy and LSD from the age of 14. She had her first intra-venous drug experience with amphetamine at 18 after two years of intranasal use. Within six months of her first heroin use, Michelle was injecting daily. When unable to obtain the drug she experiences withdrawal symptoms, including cramps, sweating, irritability, and insomnia. She works as a barmaid part-time, and increasingly in the sex industry. Michelle has had no formal treatment for her heroin use. She is currently using heroin three times a day, but although she says she wants to cease her heroin use she doesn't want to start a methadone program, as a friend has told her that the withdrawal symptoms associated with methadone are worse than those from heroin.

You discuss with Michelle her fears about methadone, explaining that methadone delivered as a maintenance program is designed to suppress withdrawal symptoms, and that the daily methadone dose can, over a period of time, be gradually reduced to a point where she is drug-free without her experiencing significant withdrawal. You also discuss other treatment options, including naltrexone and buprenorphine. Although she is accepting of this advice and information, she insists that she can get off heroin by herself. Michelle is, however, keen to access medication to assist her with heroin withdrawal, and specifically asks for prescriptions for Codeine Forte and diazepam.

You are concerned about Michelle's possible inappropriate use of these prescription drugs, polypharmacy, and her lack of supervision and support to withdraw as an outpatient. Following discussions, Michelle agrees to withdraw at her mother's home, and you arrange for Michelle to drop by the surgery with her mother to pick up her scripts for diazepam, loperamide and metoclopramide, and to provide her mother with instructions to assist Michelle during the withdrawal phase.

Michelle presents to your surgery eight weeks later. Although she has successfully undergone heroin withdrawal at her mother's home, she immediately returned to heroin use, and within a week had reverted to a pattern of dependent use. Her financial situation has become worse and she now owes $4000 to her dealer. She has continued to live with her mother, but her ongoing heroin use, especially in the home, is a source of anxiety and argument between Michelle and her mother.

Michelle now states that her drive to use heroin is too great and she needs some help. Once again, you outline possible treatment approaches. She says that, in all honesty, she would be likely to take any opportunity to use heroin even under treatment. She also retains the same concerns about methadone dependence, and remains unconvinced that buprenorphine would be associated with lesser dependence. As a consequence of her rejection of both methadone and buprenorphine, you discuss with Michelle the opioid blockade and anti-craving actions associated with naltrexone maintenance. You also discuss the high relapse rates that are associated with naltrexone maintenance, and the possible risk of overdose should she relapse after a period of using naltrexone. Nevertheless, she considers this the only option for her other than trying to go cold turkey again at home.

Given Michelle's past motivational relapses and her stated position that she will be likely to take any opportunity to use heroin, you suggest that she involve her mother in supervision of her daily naltrexone use. She agrees to this, and you again discuss withdrawal options. Although precipitated withdrawal under sedation is available, Michelle says that she would rather undertake a slower withdrawal.

You arrange for Michelle's withdrawal to be managed as an outpatient, and ask her and her mother to come to the surgery five days later. At this consultation her withdrawal symptoms are mild, and you decide that she can commence the naltrexone the following day. You provide a script and instruct her mother on supervision of Michelle's naltrexone. Michelle is requested to return the following day, two hours after administration of the naltrexone, to assess whether her withdrawal has been worsened by administration of the antagonist.

Recognising the need for early identification of return to heroin use and for prompt reinstatement of pharmacotherapy treatment following relapse, you suggest that if at any stage Michelle feels an overwhelming desire to use heroin or if she returns to heroin use, she contact you immediately so you can jointly work out the next step forward. An additional appointment is made for two weeks time and you ask both Michelle and her mother to attend.

Case points

Michelle's case illustrates:
- a history of multiple drug use and progression to IV use
- the importance of discussing and offering treatment options
- the need to consider the patient's views
- the complexities of antagonist use
- the need for supervision and for follow-up.

REFERENCES AND FURTHER READING

Gowing, L.J., Ali, R.L. & White, J.M. 2000, 'The management of opioid withdrawal', *Drug and Alcohol Review*, vol. 19, pp. 309–18.

McLellan, A.T., Lewis, D.C., O'Brien, C.P. & Kleber, H.D. 2000, 'Drug dependence, a chronic medical illness', *Journal of the American Medical Association*, vol. 284, pp. 1689–95.

Ward, J., Mattick, R.P. & Hall, W. 1998, *Methadone Maintenance Treatment and Other Opioid Replacement Therapies*, Harwood, Amsterdam.

7

Tobacco

Stuart McLean, Robyn Richmond, Olga Lopatko,
John Saunders & Ross Young

A cigarette is the perfect type of a perfect pleasure. It is exquisite, and it leaves one unsatisfied. What more can one want?

Oscar Wilde 1891, *The Picture of Dorian Gray.*

PHARMACOKINETICS AND PHARMACODYNAMICS

The leaf of the tobacco plant, *Nicotiana tabacum*, contains the alkaloid nicotine. Tobacco leaf is dried, cured, and aged, and these processes affect the concentration of nicotine and other constituents that contribute to the toxicity of tobacco. Cigarettes have substances added during manufacture to improve flavour, control burning, and enhance nicotine delivery, and pyrolysis results in a complex cocktail of hundreds of biologically active substances in tobacco smoke. These include polynuclear aromatic hydrocarbons, aromatic amines, tobacco-specific nitrosamines, and carbon monoxide. The high-boiling-point hydrocarbons constitute the 'tar' in tobacco smoke. These other substances are responsible for much of the carcinogenic and cardiovascular toxicity of tobacco, while it is the effects of nicotine that are sought by tobacco users.

A related drug, arecoline, is found in betel nut, from the Indonesian palm *Areca catechu*. It is chewed, sometimes in combination with tobacco, in South Asia and the Pacific.

Pharmacodynamics

Mode of action

Nicotine is selective for and defines the nicotinic acetylcholine receptor. There are two major subtypes: one at the skeletal neuromuscular junction, and a neuronal acetylcholine receptor (nAChR) in the brain and autonomic ganglia. All nicotinic receptors consist of five protein subunits grouped around a central ion channel, opened when the receptor is activated by binding to acetylcholine, nicotine, or another agonist ligand. Variation in the subunits may give rise to a variety of subtypes of nicotinic receptors that have particular tissue distributions, and that mediate different physiological and pharmacological effects. Although 11 genes have been identified for the α and β subunits of nAChRs, only three nAChRs receptor subtypes can be demonstrated using selective pharmacological antagonists. The various nicotinic receptors are linked to channels for Na^+, K^+ and Ca^{++} ions, serving different functions. Evidence indicates that acetylcholine released into extracellular space diffuses to non-synaptic nAChRs that increase the release of other neurotransmitters (such as noradrenaline, dopamine, serotonin, GABA). However, the physiological roles of nAChRs have yet to be elucidated, in part because of a lack of selective drugs able to stimulate subtypes of nAChRs.

Effects

Studies of the effects of nicotine can be confounded by the effects of other constituents of tobacco smoke, the smoking process, and the subject's tolerance/withdrawal status. In smokers and non-smokers, nicotine increases arousal and attentiveness, and improves reaction time and psychomotor performance. Beneficial effects on memory and learning are less clear, but overall it appears that nicotinic receptors have an important role in modulating higher brain functions. Nicotine can improve mood, for example, by relieving anxiety. The appetite-suppressant effect is often exploited for weight control.

Nicotine stimulates peripheral sensory receptors (for example in the stomach, causing initial nausea and vomiting), and autonomic ganglia. Autonomic effects from sympathetic nerve stimulation and catecholamine release include tachycardia, vasoconstriction, increased blood pressure and cardiac output, and decreased gastrointestinal motility. Secretion of antidiuretic hormone is increased, and urine flow is reduced. Smoking and nicotine suppress the immune system via decreased T-cell activity.

Smoking accelerates atherosclerosis and increases the risk of cardiovascular disease, including angina, myocardial infarction, and stroke. Although other constituents of tobacco smoke are likely contributors, nicotine itself is responsible for some of the increased risk. Short-term use in replacement therapy is still considered justifiable.

Pharmacokinetics

Absorption

Nicotine is a lipophilic amine and is readily absorbed by all routes, as shown by the variety of ways in which tobacco is used: chewing, swallowing, sniffing, smoking, and applying to the skin. The speed and extent of absorption of nicotine is highly dependent on the form and manner in which it is taken.

The fastest route of absorption is by inhalation, with each puff of tobacco smoke delivering a bolus of nicotine to the brain in about 10 seconds. This rapid reinforcement probably contributes to the highly addictive nature of tobacco smoking.

By varying the rate and depth of puffing, a smoker can efficiently produce the desired brain level of nicotine. Absorption is much slower from nicotine chewing-gum, with peak plasma level reached after 30 minutes' chewing compared with 5–10 minutes after smoking. Transdermal patches are even slower, and more variable, giving a peak after 3–12 hours. However, levels thereafter remain constant while the patches are used.

Distribution and elimination

Nicotine has a plasma half-life of one to three hours, so regular smoking through the day results in a plateau after six to eight hours which continues until the last cigarette. Overnight, nicotine levels fall and acute tolerance is lost, so that the first cigarette of the next day (but not later ones) causes tachycardia.

Nicotine is widely distributed into tissues, and crosses the placenta and mammary gland. Usually only about 2% is excreted unchanged, but this can rise to 23% in acidic urine. Nicotine is metabolised to a variety of oxidised and conjugated metabolites (such as cotinine, nicotine-N-oxide, nicotine glucuronide) that are excreted in urine. Metabolic clearance (1.2 L/min) approximates hepatic blood flow. Nicotine is also metabolised in the brain, producing some metabolites with pharmacological activity.

Interactions

Smoking induces many liver enzymes (for example CYPs 1A1, 1A2, 2E1) responsible for the metabolism of nicotine itself and other drugs. This leads to significant drug interactions, with reduced effectiveness of, for example, theophylline, imipramine, and haloperidol in smokers. Nicotine also seems to reduce the sedative effects of alcohol, possibly explaining their common consumption together.

TOLERANCE, DEPENDENCE, AND WITHDRAWAL

Tolerance

Repeated exposure to nicotine results in neuronal adaptations that are reflected in nicotine tolerance, sensitisation, and withdrawal. In smokers, tolerance to the behavioural and cardiovascular effects of nicotine develops within the course of a single day. The first cigarette produces euphoria and tachycardia, but once plasma levels of nicotine have risen significantly, cigarette smoking later in the day produces much less effect on the heart rate and subjective experience. Similarly, acute tolerance develops to the mild muscle-relaxant effect of nicotine. Smokers lose a substantial degree of tolerance overnight while sleeping, and regain it the next day upon recommencement of smoking.

Metabolic tolerance to nicotine develops with repeated exposure to administration of nicotine. Polycyclic aromatic hydrocarbons present in tobacco tar increase the activity of microsomal enzymes and thereby increase the rate of metabolism of nicotine.

The CNS mechanisms of nicotine tolerance are still not very clear. It has been shown that prolonged smoking causes repeated desensitisation of nicotinic cholinergic receptors in CNS that, in turn, produces up-regulation of receptor function and an increase in receptor density. More research is needed to elucidate the mechanisms of nicotine tolerance and dependence.

Dependence and withdrawal

Abrupt cessation of smoking, or a reduction in the amount of nicotine used, causes withdrawal. A number of nicotine withdrawal signs and symptoms have been described. While they are not life-threatening, the withdrawal symptoms can affect behaviour and serve as a very strong motivation for continuing smoking. Withdrawal symptoms start within a few hours of cessation and for most people peak around 24 to 72 hours after the last cigarette.

According to the DSM-IV diagnostic criteria for nicotine withdrawal, the diagnosis of nicotine withdrawal is established if at least four of the eight symptoms and signs (listed in table 7.1) occur within 24 hours of nicotine cessation.

Table 7.1   DSM-IV diagnostic criteria for nicotine withdrawal

1	Dysphoria or depressed mood
2	Insomnia
3	Irritability, frustration or anger
4	Anxiety
5	Difficulty concentrating
6	Breathlessness
7	Decreased heart rate
8	Increased appetite or weight gain

Craving for nicotine is not listed as a diagnostic criterion. However, it is an important element in nicotine withdrawal. There are a number of other signs and symptoms of nicotine withdrawal that have been reported and may be useful in diagnosis of nicotine dependence.

Table 7.2   Other signs and symptoms of withdrawal

Mood changes	Symptoms	Signs
Hostility	Drowsiness/fatigue	Increased peripheral circulation
Impatience	Decreased alertness	Drop in urinary adrenaline,
	Light-headedness	noradrenaline and cortisol
	Headaches	Changes in electroencephalogram
	Tightness in chest	Changes in endocrine function
	Bodily aches and pains	Neurotransmitter changes
	Tingling sensation in limbs	Performance deficits
	Stomach distress	Constipation
	Urge to smoke/craving	Sweating
		Mouth ulcers
		Increased coughing

There is individual variation in the severity of the syndrome and specific promi-nent symptoms. Symptoms usually peak within a few days and then begin to subside over the next several weeks, though the time course may also vary. Heart rate drops and seems to remain low indefinitely, or at least for ten days. Irritability has been shown to extend for five weeks, while hunger and weight gain continue for at least ten weeks.

Smokers commonly maintain blood nicotine levels between 10–40 ng/mL. After overnight abstinence the blood level of nicotine declines to 5–10 ng/mL. Smokers appear to titrate levels of nicotine within certain limits, as the urge to smoke correlates with a low blood nicotine level. The negative symptoms associated with short periods of abstinence can be very rapidly reversed by nicotine use. Some smokers wake up during the night to have a cigarette that ameliorates the effect of low nicotine blood levels. If the nicotine level is maintained artificially by a slow intravenous infusion, there is a decrease in the number of cigarettes smoked and in the number of puffs taken. Thus, smokers smoke to achieve the reward of nicotine effects or to avoid the discomfort of nicotine withdrawal, or most likely a combina-tion of the two.

Withdrawal symptoms are believed to be mainly due to decreased nicotine concentration as the majority of the symptoms can be reversed by re-administration of nicotine. However, other non–pharmacological factors, such as conditioning and expectancy, influence various aspects of behaviour during nicotine withdrawal, and these are therefore important.

Stress and anxiety affect nicotine tolerance and dependence. The stress hormone corticosterone reduces the effect of nicotine. Therefore, elevated levels of corticos-terone mean that more nicotine must be consumed to achieve the same effect. Studies in animals have also shown that stress can directly cause relapse to nicotine self-administration after a period of abstinence.

Reinforcement

Part of the reinforcement of smoking comes from relief of nicotine withdrawal (negative reinforcement). However, nicotine also produces a number of pleasurable effects that are important in positive reinforcement. It has both stimulant and depressant-like actions. The smoker feels alert and active, yet there is some muscle relaxation. Nicotine activates the reward system in the brain that includes the pathways from the ventral tegmental area to the nucleus accumbens (see chapter 2). In several studies in rats, increased extracellular dopamine has been found in the nucleus accumbens after nicotine ingestion. In this species the dopaminergic system is involved in the mechanisms of nicotine-induced locomotor activation and self-administration.

Nicotine is absorbed from the lung extremely rapidly and reaches the brain in a few seconds. Therefore, the smoker gets a dose of nicotine after each inhaled puff, and each puff produces some discrete reinforcement. With ten puffs per cigarette the pack-a-day smoker reinforces the habit about 200 times daily. That will add up to more than 70 000 nicotine shots to the brain in a year.

Nicotine has been shown to increase serum concentrations of β-endorphin. However, it is still not clear whether this effect plays a role in the mechanisms of positive reinforcement.

NICOTINE AND TOBACCO TOXICITY

Acute toxic effects of tobacco smoking

The acute fatal dose for an adult is about 60 mg of the base. The average nicotine intake from a single cigarette is about 1 mg, but sometimes may exceed 3 mg. The typical pack-a-day smoker obtains 20–40 mg of nicotine each day. Acute tobacco or nicotine poisoning results in symptoms such as nausea, vomiting, dizziness, and general weakness. This is quite similar to the experience of many first-time smokers. Severe poisoning can result in convulsions, unconsciousness, and possible death. In fact, unconsciousness, coma, and death may occur before any other symptoms develop.

Acute poisoning usually occurs not as a result of smoking, but as a result of direct skin contact with tobacco infusions or insecticide sprays containing nicotine sulfate, or other preparations with a high concentration of nicotine. Small children might ingest tobacco from cigarettes, cigars or pipes, and this is another source of fatal dosage of nicotine.

Chronic effects of tobacco smoking

Chronic tobacco exposure affects many organ systems. The pharmacological actions of nicotine may contribute to the pathogenesis of smoking-related effects, but direct causation has not yet been determined for all of these effects. In addition to nicotine in the tobacco, smoke tar (particulate matter) and carbon monoxide also play important roles. Table 7.3 describes the chronic effects of tobacco smoking.

Table 7.3 Chronic effects of tobacco smoking

Disorder	Active component and its effects	Possible mechanisms
Cardiovascular system *Atherosclerosis-related disorders*		
Coronary heart disease (CHD)	Nicotine increases risk of CHD (dose-dependent response), contributes to coronary atherosclerosis increases risk of acute ischaemic, thrombotic and arrhythmic coronary events.	Impairs plasma lipid profile, possibly acting via catecholamines (increases low-density lipoproteins and decreases high-density lipoproteins), increasing risk of atherosclerosis. Increases blood clotting by enhancing platelet reactivity and inhibiting prostacyclin. Increases circulating catecholamines. Decreases endothelial nitric oxide content. Adversely alters the myocardial oxygen supply/demand ratio. Produces endothelial injury, leading to the development of atherosclerotic plaque.
	Carbon monoxide impairs oxygen transport and utilisation and causes tissue hypoxia, increases myocardial oxygen needs.	Increases blood carboxyhaemoglobin levels; reduces oxygen transportation by haemoglobin and decreases release of oxygen to tissues; inhibits mitochondrial cytochrome oxidase.
	Tobacco smoking is associated with impaired endothelium-dependent vasodilation and reduced nitric oxide (NO) in the exhaled air of smokers.	Tobacco smoke causes an irreversible inhibition of the activity of nitric oxide synthase. The decreased production of nitric oxide has been shown to contribute to the high risk of pulmonary and cardiovascular disease in cigarette smokers.

Table 7.3 Chronic effects of tobacco smoking

Disorder	Active component and its effects	Possible mechanisms
Cardiovascular system *Atherosclerosis-related* *disorders*		
Ischaemic stroke	Nicotine increases risk of stroke, especially in women using oral contraceptives.	Thromboxane A2 induced by cigarette smoke causes cerebral vasoconstriction. Chronic nicotine treatment enhances focal ischaemic brain injury and depletes free pool of brain microvascular tissue plasminogen activator in rats. Alters platelet aggregation and survival, producing thrombosis.
Cerebral aneurysm and subarachnoid haemorrhage	Tobacco smoking increases risk of subarachnoid haemorrhage in women using oral contraceptives.	Elevates plasma levels of fibrinogen and intravascular fibrin deposition, possibly secondary to increased risk of atherosclerosis (see above); this effect is potentiated by oral contraceptives.
Aortic aneurysm	Tobacco smoking increases mortality in patients with aortic aneurysm.	Possibly secondary to increased risk of atherosclerosis (see above).
Atherosclerosis of the extremities	Tobacco smoking increases risk of atherosclerosis obliterans (very strong correlation).	Similar to the mechanisms for increased risk of atherosclerosis of cardiac and cerebral vasculature.

Table 7.3   Chronic effects of tobacco smoking

Disorder	Active component and its effects	Possible mechanisms
Cardiovascular system *Atherosclerosis-related disorders*		
Thromboangiitis obliterans (Buerger's disease)	Tobacco smoking increases risk of thromboangiitis obliterans (very strong correlation).	It is not known whether tobacco smoking causes this disorder, but tobacco smoking significantly aggravates tissue ischaemia and abstinence from tobacco is the only specific treatment of thromboangiitis obliterans.
Hypertension	Tobacco smoking increases occurrence of malignant hypertension and mortality rate in hypertensive patients.	Possibly secondary to increased risk of atherosclerosis.
Respiratory system *Chronic obstructive pulmonary disease*		
Chronic bronchitis	Tobacco smoking increases risk of this disease dose-dependently.	Impairs ciliary movement, inhibits activity of alveolar macrophages; causes hypertrophy of mucus-secreting glands; stimulates submucosal irritant receptors, and causes smooth muscle constriction leading to airway obstruction. Smoking cessation leads to significant improvement.

Table 7.3   Chronic effects of tobacco smoking

Disorder	Active component and its effects	Possible mechanisms
Respiratory system *Chronic obstructive pulmonary disease*		
Emphysema	Tobacco smoking increases risk of this disease dose-dependently.	Inhibits antiproteases; stimulates release of proteases by neutrophils.
Asthma	Tobacco smoking contributes to the pathogenesis and exacerbation of asthma. Children passively exposed to environmental tobacco smoke have higher risk of developing asthma.	Increases airway obstruction. Increases production of cysteinyl leukotrienes. Children who develop asthma as a result of passive smoking have a higher systemic exposure to nicotine, possibly due to lower clearance rate of nicotine.
Gastrointestinal tract		
Peptic ulcers	Tobacco smoking and nicotine increase risk of development and death from gastric and duodenal ulcers.	Impairs healing processes; inhibits pancreatic bicarbonate secretion; decreases the pressure of oesophageal and pyloric sphincters and promotes reflux; interferes with H_2-receptor antagonist treatment, preventing the inhibition of nocturnal gastric secretion.

Table 7.3   Chronic effects of tobacco smoking

Disorder	Active component and its effects	Possible mechanisms
Gastrointestinal tract		
Cancers	Tobacco smoking is a cause of lung, laryngeal, oral, pharyngeal, oesophageal and bladder cancer; and contributes to pathogenesis of pancreatic and kidney cancer.	A number of constituents of both particulate and gas phases of tobacco smoke are carcinogens or co-carcinogens or tumour accelerators.
Pregnancy and foetal development	Tobacco smoking increases risk of impaired fertility, spontaneous abortions, premature birth, low birth weight, and sudden infant death syndrome.	Possibly impaired uthero-placental circulation.
Myopathy	Nicotine has been shown to produce myopathic effects.	One possible mechanism: nicotinic receptor stimulation produces an increase in NO that results in muscle cell degeneration.
Osteoporosis	Tobacco smoking is a risk factor for osteoporosis.	Impairs calcium metabolism.

ASSESSMENT

Other than caffeine, nicotine is likely to have been the first addictive substance used by many living in the Western world. The routine assessment of cigarette use is therefore an important part of the examination in most medical settings.

On a community-wide basis, smoking is the health status factor most readily changed to decrease morbidity and mortality.

It is particularly important to establish smoking status when respiratory or cardiac health is assessed or where the patient is pregnant, given that smoking has important aetiological and predictive power, and that low birth weight and neonatal complications are associated with smoking in pregnancy. Smoking should not be overlooked in the adolescent health visit, when initial exposure to cigarettes is likely and dependence can occur within a matter of months. The clinical approach with all patients, particularly the adolescent, needs to be empathic. Smokers often feel very defensive about their cigarette use and have probably been lectured regarding the evils of cigarette use by well-intentioned health professionals and family members.

Cumulative risk is related to lifetime exposure to nicotine and the variety of additional toxic compounds that constitute cigarette smoke. Unlike the situation with most other drugs, over 90% of those who smoke cigarettes are nicotine-dependent. Thus, frequency of cigarette use is likely to be daily for most smokers. Nicotine consumption can be estimated by the lifetime quantity, usually measured in pack years, which is the number of year equivalents a smoker has averaged a pack of 25 cigarettes per day. It is important when trying to establish this history that the number of cigarettes per pack is ascertained, as cigarette manufacturers now produce packs of between 10 and 50 cigarettes. It is also useful to assess the current strength of cigarettes smoked in mg of nicotine, as this can assist in selecting appropriate nicotine replacement. However, there is no health benefit in smoking lower-strength cigarettes as smokers of lower-strength cigarettes retain smoke in their lungs for longer to maximise the delivery of nicotine, thereby depositing greater amounts of tar and absorbing more carbon monoxide.

The overall risk for developing significant illness directly related to smoking rises sharply after 20 pack years, but there is considerable individual variation in the time taken to develop smoking-related pathology. Other medical conditions can be important. For example, smokers with pre-existing asthma may rapidly exacerbate their respiratory disease.

Dependence can be assessed by the use of the Fagerström dependence questionnaire, given in table 7.4.

Many patients find answering this questionnaire time-consuming and the information difficult to recall, so it is not always suitable for routine use. A briefer alternative may therefore be used in many situations.

A simple guide for the doctor to assess dependence is a 'yes' answer to one of these questions:
- Does the patient smoke 10–15 or more cigarettes per day?
- Does the patient smoke his or her first cigarette within 30 minutes of rising?

- Did the patient have cravings or withdrawal symptoms in previous attempts to quit?
  If the patient answers yes to any of these questions then there is evidence of nicotine dependence.

While many presentations are influenced by smoking, it is important to examine the key parameters of respiratory and cardiovascular health. Spirometry and blood pressure can be particularly useful as the results can be fed back to patients immediately, and they can also form a baseline against which to measure future change. Additional investigations to validate current consumption may include blood or saliva

Table 7.4   Adapted Fagerström questionnaire and scaling system

Questions	*Answers*	
1 How soon after you wake do you smoke your first cigarette?	6–30 minutes	3
	Within 5 minutes	2
	31–60 minutes	1
2 Do you find it difficult to refrain from smoking in places where it is forbidden (e.g. in buses, trains, the library, church, and cinemas)?	Yes	1
	No	0
3 Which cigarette would you hate most to give up?	The first one in the morning	1
	All others	0
4 How many cigarettes a day do you smoke?	10 or less	0
	11–20	1
	21–30	2
	31 or more	3
5 Do you smoke more frequently during the first hours after waking than during the rest of the day?	No	0
	Yes	1
6 Do you smoke if you are so ill that you are in bed most of the day?	Yes	1
	No	0
Total score = How does the total score rate on the following scale?	Very low dependence	0–2
	Low dependence	3–4
	Medium dependence	5
	High dependence	6–7
	Very high dependence	8+

(From Heatherton et al. 1991)

thiocyanate, urinary or salivary cotinine, or expired carbon monoxide. These measures also make useful measures of outcomes over time.

INTERVENTION AND TREATMENT

Role of the doctor

Doctors are uniquely placed to provide advice about stopping smoking. They have high contact with the general public, and 75% of the community visit a general practitioner each year. Smokers believe that their doctor's advice is an important motivator for attempting to quit. Moreover, 70% of smokers report wanting to quit. Doctors should ask all patients about their smoking at each visit.

Randomised controlled trials present excellent evidence that brief doctor-delivered interventions in general practice significantly increase patients' quit rates. Less intensive interventions such as brief GP advice to quit smoking produce cessation rates of 5 to 10% per year. More intensive interventions, combining behavioural counselling and pharmacological treatment of nicotine addiction, can produce 20 to 25% quit rates at one year.

There are several generally similar smoking cessation interventions, including the program of the National Cancer Institute (US), the American Medical Association, and the Smokescreen program. The program described under 'Behavioural strategies' below is the Smokescreen program, which has been developed in Australia and implemented among general practitioners and other health professionals since 1986. It has been the subject of four randomised–controlled trials and more than 7500 doctors have been trained in these methods.

Behavioural strategies

Identifying stage of readiness to quit

The first step is to ask all patients whether they smoke, and then to identify their stage of readiness to quit. The stages of change model is valuable for assessing a person's readiness to change smoking behaviour. Cessation is a process rather than a single discrete event, and smokers cycle through the stages of being ready, quitting, and relapsing, before achieving long-term success.

The question to ask to ascertain the smoker's stage of readiness is 'How do you feel about your smoking?'

Not ready smokers are not seriously considering quitting in the next six months. They are happy with their smoking. Smokers like these, who are unwilling to try to quit smoking, should be provided with brief advice to increase their motivation to quit, such as raising the issue with them and asking them to consider the pros and cons of smoking.

Figure 7.1   Stages of readiness to stop smoking

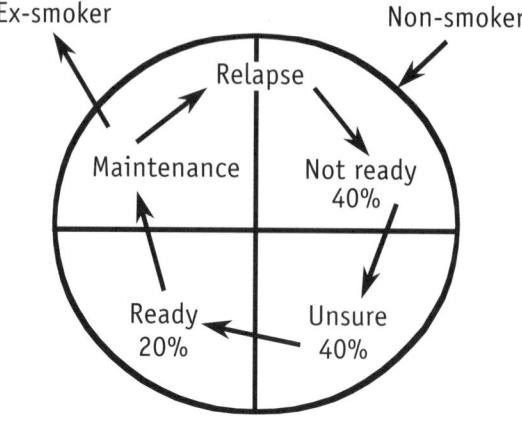

Unsure smokers are uncertain or ambivalent about their smoking, and are aware of both the benefits and disadvantages of smoking. They are seriously considering quitting in the next six months. They should be motivated to weigh up the pros and cons of smoking and to try to make a quit attempt. These smokers should be encouraged to think about the discrepancy between smoking and personal goals, such as health, fitness, improved appearance, and saving money. Discuss their concerns about quitting and relevant health issues.

Ready smokers are planning to quit in the next 30 days. They have made a 24-hour quit attempt in the past year. These smokers are motivated to quit smoking since, for them, the disadvantages outweigh the benefits.

The following steps are relevant for those who are ready to quit.

Cessation strategies

When the smoker has decided to stop smoking, he/she needs to work out how to stick to it.

Strategies are suggested in the mnemonic DEAD:

D The person should try to **delay** the cigarette until the craving passes.

E When faced with a group of smokers, and finding motivation waning, the person should **escape** until the strength to overcome the urge to smoke subsides.

A The person may temporarily **avoid** his/her usual social group particularly if they are smokers.

D He/she may **distract** craving by drinking a glass of water, having a low–calorie snack, or going for a brisk walk.

Other strategies that assist the new ex-smoker are: not drinking coffee; drinking more fruit juice and water and less alcohol; establishing new exercise routines; taking up a new hobby; and substituting healthy, low-fat snacks so that weight gain does not become a problem. Simple advice on healthy eating should be provided to patients to avoid weight gain. The environment should be prepared by removing cigarettes from it.

Giving brief advice to quit and setting a quit date

Smokers who are ready to quit should be offered practical advice and support. This can be personalised to their stage of readiness to quit, level of nicotine dependence, current health status, and social and family background. They should be given advice on the use of nicotine replacement therapy (NRT), encouraged to set a quit date within the next two weeks, and offered a range of cognitive and behavioural strategies (such as 'DEAD' above), and followed up so that their progress can be monitored. The positive aspects of quitting, such as improvement in health and well-being, need to be discussed, rather than using scare tactics.

Pharmacotherapies

Doctors can recommend one of five pharmacotherapies: nicotine patch, gum, nasal spray, inhaler, or non-nicotine bupropion. This provides the patient with a range of options to minimise the withdrawal symptoms associated with cessation. All NRT products have similar success rates. Transdermal patches are the easiest to use and have the greatest compliance, and are therefore a logical first choice unless there are reasons to choose another form of replacement. The aim of NRT is the temporary provision of nicotine from a source other than tobacco while the smoking habit is being broken.

Treatment with pharmacological agents can assist dependent smokers who smoke more than 10 to 15 cigarettes per day. NRT increases quit rates two-fold regardless of setting. It costs less per week than the average cost of smoking.

Nicotine transdermal patch

Patch use avoids the peaks and troughs of plasma nicotine that characterise smoking and, to a lesser extent, other forms of NRT. Once the patch is applied, the patient does not need to do anything active to maintain nicotine levels during the day. The patch has the advantage that it is simple to use. The patch produces blood levels about half those of smoking. At least eight weeks of use are recommended. Both 24- and 16-hour patches are available, and they have about the same efficacy. The 24-hour patches achieve higher blood levels and provide more relief from morning cravings. The 16-hour patch may interfere less with sleep. The nicotine patch can be used safely by patients with a history of cardiovascular disease, as it has been shown not to cause adverse cardiovascular effects.

Nicotine gum

The blood levels achieved by use of the nicotine chewing gum are one-third (2 mg gum) and two-thirds (4 mg gum) those of smoking. Correct chewing technique is important—check the product information. Recommend the use of at least 8–12 pieces daily or a fixed schedule of one piece per hour. Three months of use is recommended, followed by a period of tapering. Dependence on the gum can occur among up to 20% of users.

Nicotine inhaler

The nicotine inhaler consists of a plastic mouthpiece and cartridge containing 10 mg of nicotine. This device delivers a vaporised form of nicotine to the oral mucosa but the vapour does not reach the pulmonary alveoli. The inhaler produces nicotine concentrations that are one-third those achieved with smoking. The inhaler is aimed at those smokers who miss the hand-to-mouth action of smoking, thereby substituting some of the behavioural features of smoking. The recommended use is for 16 weeks.

Nicotine nasal spray

The nasal spray delivers nicotine in a more rapid manner than other NRT. Peak levels occur within 10 minutes, and are about one-half to two-thirds those of cigarettes. The device is similar to those used for nasal decongestant sprays. Each spray delivers 0.5 mg of nicotine, and one dose is a spray in each nostril. Smokers use one or two doses per hour for six to eight weeks, followed by four to six weeks of gradual reduction by halving the dose and decreasing the daily frequency.

Bupropion

Bupropion hydrochloride is an atypical antidepressant that has both dopaminergic and adrenergic action. It is hypothesised that bupropion is effective for smoking cessation because of its dopaminergic activity on the reward pathways in the mesolimbic system (see chapter 2). There is also some evidence that it is a nicotine receptor antagonist. It doubles success rates of placebo with or without NRT as an adjunct. The recommended dose is 150 mg orally once daily for three days, then 150 mg twice daily (at least eight hours apart) for seven to 12 weeks. The drug works equally well in smokers with and without a past history of depression, suggesting that its efficacy is not due to its antidepressant effect.

Combination therapies

Combination therapies can be considered as they produce higher quit rates. The patch can be supplemented by bupropion or gum to relieve intermittent craving. The combination of patch and gum decreases withdrawal symptoms more than either alone.

Table 7.5   Advantages and disadvantages of pharmacological treatments for smoking cessation

Treatment	*Advantages*	*Disadvantages*
Nicotine patch	Easy to use; few compliance problems. Available over the counter.	Half of the users have skin reactions. Some sleep disturbances with the 24-hour patch, but it can be removed at bedtime.
Nicotine gum	2 mg available over the counter; good to use as a safety valve in times of stress.	Provides oral substitute for smoking. Need to spend time explaining correct use. Common adverse effects are mild, and include mouth soreness, hiccups, dyspepsia, and jaw ache. Tends to be under-used so patients don't get the proper effect. Requires special chewing techniques. Dependence on the gum can occur.
Nicotine inhaler	Mimics hand-to-mouth behaviour. Similar to cigarette smoking. Can be used for six months.	Low nicotine levels. Mild symptoms include throat and mouth irritation, and cough.
Nicotine nasal spray	Delivers nicotine in a more rapid manner than the patch and gum. Peak levels of nicotine occur within 10 minutes. Rapid delivery and high plasma concentrations make the spray more suitable for treating withdrawal symptoms in highly dependent smokers.	Contraindicated among those with severe reactive airway disease. About 15–20% of people use it longer than recommended (6–12 months), and 5% use the spray at a higher dose than recommended. Users experience moderate to severe nasal irritation (nasal and throat irritation, rhinitis, sneezing, coughing, and watering eyes) in the first three weeks of use.
Bupropion	Non-nicotine; can be used with patch.	Contraindicated in those with a history of seizure disorder, and a history of eating disorder. Adverse effects are mild insomnia and dry mouth.

117

Newer treatments undergoing testing

A new NRT product, a sublingual tablet that delivers 2 mg of nicotine, is being tested. The method of delivery (transbuccal) is similar to nicotine gum, but the sublingual tablet avoids the problem of improper use associated with the gum.

The antihypertensive mecamylamine (a nicotine antagonist) has been found to assist smoking cessation when used with a patch.

Antidepressant drugs that appear to have promise for smoking cessation include the tricyclic antidepressants nortriptyline and doxepin.

> Tobacco dependence treatments are clinically effective and cost effective relative to other routinely reimbursed medical and disease prevention interventions.

Support and follow-up

For further advice and support, suggest the patient ring the Quit line or the National Heart Foundation to obtain self-help booklets on quitting smoking. There are also other self-help manuals available that can be used between appointments. Enlisting the support of family, friends, or work-mates is also important. It is advisable for the person to inform them of their intention to quit, and to request understanding and support. Ask them to communicate caring and concern, and to be open and patient with any difficulties in maintaining non-smoking.

Quitting is more difficult when other people in the household smoke. The patient should be encouraged to quit together with other smoking members of their household.

Prevention of relapse

Rather than being a discrete event, quitting is a dynamic and continuing process that often involves repeated attempts. Almost half of smokers try to quit each year. Most relapses occur within the first three months after quitting. Successful ex-smokers take an average of four to five serious attempts before finally succeeding in quitting. Ex-smokers who attend for follow-up are more likely to be successful long-term, so follow-up visits should be encouraged.

Tobacco dependence is a chronic condition that often requires repeated intervention. Strategies to use during follow-up visits to prevent relapse:
- Regard slips (occasional smoking) and relapses (return to regular smoking) as learning experiences, not failures.
- Provide praise and encouragement for success.
- Identify high-risk smoking situations. These can be drinking with friends (suggest not drinking alcohol for a limited time), and negative emotional states such as conflict, anger, frustration, and anxiety.

- Identify specific problems, such as weight gain, that may cause relapse. Advice should be given on modifying diet, increasing exercise, and trying stress management techniques. A small increase in weight is less of a risk to health than smoking.
- Plan coping strategies in advance. Discuss problem-solving skills to cope with and anticipate high-risk situations. Discuss how slips were overcome in the past.

The main steps the doctor can take to assist patients to quit smoking are to:

➡ identify the smoker's stage of readiness to quit
➡ discuss behavioural and cognitive strategies
➡ give brief advice to quit and set a quit date
➡ assess nicotine dependence
➡ discuss pharmacotherapies—nicotine replacement and bupropion
➡ discuss social support
➡ suggest follow-up to prevent relapse.

EPIDEMIOLOGY AND PREVENTION

Smoking prevalence

Smoking is the major avoidable cause of morbidity and mortality in our society. It is responsible for more than 18 000 deaths in Australia each year. Recent figures show that 27% of men and 20% of women aged 18 years and over smoke. Highest rates of smoking occur among men (34%) and women (28%) aged 25–34 years. After 34 years of age, the rate of smoking declines with increasing age to be lowest among men and women aged 75 years and over. Adult male smoking rates have declined since the 1960s; among women, smoking rates began to decline in the late 1970s. However, the rate of decline of smoking has slowed in recent years.

Among young people, the smoking rate for those aged 12–15 years in 1996 was 16% for both boys and girls, with the rate rising to 28% among boys aged 16–17 years, and 32% among girls aged 16–17 years.

For more information on Australian data on tobacco use, access the web sites listed following the references.

Smoking-related morbidity and mortality

Almost 3.2 million adult Australians are at risk of developing heart disease and other chronic conditions from smoking tobacco. Of all risk factors for disease, tobacco smoking is responsible for the greatest burden on health. Tobacco smoking increases the risk of a range of diseases, as described above. However, there are significant health benefits of quitting.

After 10 years' cessation, excess risks for smoking-related cancers decrease by about half, and reach non-smokers' levels after 15–20 years. Upon cessation, there is a decrease in lung function decline, and risks are 50% lower after 20 years. In less than a year, risks are similar to non-smokers' risks for cerebrovascular diseases, and the progression of peripheral vascular disease is stopped immediately on cessation. The risk of heart attack falls to the level of a non-smoker after about five years; the risk of ischaemic heart disease drops by half after one year, and reaches the level of a non-smoker after 10–15 years.

> Smoking is the major preventable cause of illness and death in our society and is responsible for more than 18 000 deaths each year in Australia.

120

Prevention

There are many strategies and interventions that are designed to prevent the uptake of smoking.

Supply and demand

Raising the tax on cigarettes and increasing the price of cigarettes reduces demand and use, with large reductions occurring mainly among minors and young people. For every 10% increase in price there is a 14% decline in demand among young people, and a 4% drop in adult consumption. After the effects of inflation are accounted for, excise taxes on cigarettes are well below their past levels. Australia is a relatively low-taxing country compared with many industrialised nations. Increases in taxes, indexed to account for the effects of inflation, would lead to substantial improvements in health.

> Raising tobacco excise taxes and prices are widely regarded as very effective tobacco prevention and control strategies. Taxation and price increases are recommended as components of a comprehensive tobacco-control program.

Advertising and promotion

Evidence shows that advertising and promotion are among the main motivators for recruiting new smokers and maintaining tobacco use. However, attempts to regulate advertising and promotion of tobacco products have had only modest success in restricting smoking. Regulator actions include health warnings on cigarette packages that are designed to be a deterrent to smoking. Warnings are rotated on cigarette packs. Other actions include banning tobacco advertising in magazines, on billboards, and at sporting activities, and substituting sponsorship from other sources for tobacco sponsorship.

Clean indoor air regulation

There is a strong movement to diminish exposure to ambient tobacco smoke and reduce its adverse health effects. Environmental tobacco smoke contains more than 4000 chemicals, and, of these, at least 43 are known carcinogens. Smoking is banned in public places, including airports, and in many workplaces, and restricted in many restaurants. Smoke-free environments have been shown to decrease daily tobacco consumption among smokers, and to increase smoking cessation.

Minors' access to tobacco

Measures that have had some success in reducing minors' access to tobacco include restricting distribution, regulating the mechanisms of sale and enforcing minimum age laws for distribution of tobacco to minors, and providing education and training. Regulation of cigarettes and promotion of tobacco products is used to protect young people from initiating the smoking habit.

Community-based interventions

Educational and health-promotion strategies conducted in conjunction with community and media-based activities can postpone or prevent onset of smoking in 20–40% of adolescents. These strategies require involvement of health authorities, general practitioners, and the media.

Doctors and other health workers have an important role in encouraging tobacco control at all levels of society. The most effective prevention programs are those in which adults reject tobacco, either by stopping its use or not starting its use. Prevention messages and actions must be pertinent and persistent.

The main strategies to prevent initiation and continued smoking include:
- increasing the price of cigarettes through taxation
- placing health messages on cigarette packages to warn of the health consequences of smoking
- restricting advertising and promotion of tobacco products
- substituting sponsorship of sports and cultural events by tobacco companies
- banning and restricting smoking in public places and the workplace
- reducing the access of minors and young people to tobacco by enforcing minimum age laws and regulating points of sale
- implementing multi-component community-based interventions that consist of education, health promotion, media, general practitioner advice, and community-based intervention.

Case study

Tony is a 47-year-old man with chronic bronchitis. You have been treating him for this condition for about five years, and have raised the issue of his smoking on a number of occasions. He commenced smoking at 13 years of age and escalated to a packet (20) per day within two years. From the age of about 25 years to the present he has been smoking about 30 cigarettes per day. He has made several unsuccessful attempts to give up, with the duration of abstinence lasting from two to 10 days.

Tony is married with two children, and is employed as an accountant. His wife used to smoke but stopped three years ago, and his children do not smoke. He is not permitted to smoke in his work environment, but takes frequent breaks in order to be able to smoke outside. He expresses considerable regrets concerning smoking, recognising the link with his bronchitis as well as being concerned about the effect on his children, and the increasing cost of his cigarette consumption.

He expresses a willingness to have another attempt at smoking cessation, but this time with assistance. He mentions the experience of some friends who have been successful in stopping smoking following use of different medications, and asks you for advice. You describe to him the various nicotine replacement therapies, their advantages and disadvantages, and the use of bupropion, comparing this to nicotine replacement therapy. You suggest that in the first instance nicotine replacement therapy using patches is probably the best approach. Tony decides to commence using nicotine patches, and you provide a prescription. You also provide written material that supports the information you have given him about strategies to use in stopping smoking. You emphasise that nicotine replacement therapy only helps alleviate withdrawal symptoms, and that it is necessary for him to minimise his risk of relapse by avoiding high-risk situations, dealing with them when they arise, changing routines that are associated with smoking, and avoiding situations in which other people are smoking. A follow-up appointment is arranged for two weeks ahead.

Tony returns in two weeks with mixed news. He is still using the patches, but has partially relapsed. Over the last week he has smoked an average of five cigarettes per day, considerably less than his usual smoking rate but above his target of abstinence. You discuss the causes of his relapses with him, as well as potential ways in which he may deal with these situations in the future. You also review his medication. An assessment of withdrawal indicates that Tony is experiencing, if any, only very mild symptoms and there does not seem to be any need to increase his dose of nicotine. A follow-up appointment is arranged for the following week.

Tony fails to attend this appointment, cancelling at the last moment. He does not return until six months later, at which point he indicates that he has relapsed completely and had thought that there was no point in coming back. However, he is returning because of further worsening of his bronchitis, and he again expresses a wish to stop smoking. You review the various alternative approaches with him again, and this time it is decided he should try bupropion. The various behavioural strategies that he should use are also reviewed, and you provide him with written information. Follow-up appointments are scheduled and you emphasise the need to return even if he has relapsed. This time, however, Tony is more successful. You see him two weeks, and again three months, after cessation, and he has remained abstinent apart from one or two very minor lapses. At three months you reiterate to Tony the need to be vigilant about his abstinence, and warn him about the risk of relapse, particularly in the following 12 months.

Case points

Tony's case illustrates:
- a history of repeated attempts to quit
- frequency of relapses and the need to re-engage the patient
- the use of different medications if the initial treatment is unsuccessful
- the difficulty of cessation even when smoking is associated with health problems.

REFERENCES AND FURTHER READING

Agency for Health Care Policy and Research 1996, 'Smoking cessation clinical practice guideline', *Journal of the American Medical Association*, vol. 275, pp. 1270–80.

Heatherton, T.F., Kozlowski, L.T., Frecker, R.C. & Fagerström, K.O. 1991, 'The Fagerström test for nicotine dependence: a revision of the Fagerström tolerance questionnaire', *British Journal of Addiction*, vol 86, pp. 1119–27.

Richmond, R. & Harris, K. 1999, *Becoming a Non-smoker*, Hale & Iremonger, Sydney.

The online tobacco encyclopaedia has a great deal of information in all areas of smoking and tobacco and will take you to many useful websites according to the topic of interest: see: http://tobaccopedia.org/

For Australian data on tobacco use: http://www.aihw.gov.au Click on publications, and then click on health, and then open 'The burden of disease and injury in Australia'.

For a global perspective on tobacco, visit the tobacco-free initiative website of the World Health Organisation, which gives the latest updates on tobacco: http://tobacco.who.int

For systematic reviews of interventions and treatments see: Cochrane Tobacco Addiction Group, The Cochrane Library, http://www.cochranelibrary.com

8

Central Nervous System Stimulants

Noeline Latt, Jason White, Stuart McLean, Simon Lenton, Ross Young &
John B. Saunders

Also, he told an astonishing tale about coca, a vegetable product of miraculous powers; asserting that it was so nourishing and so strength-giving that the native of the mountains of Madeira region would tramp up-hill and down all day on a pinch of powdered coca and require no other sustenance.

Mark Twain, *The Turning Point of My Life.*

Stimulant use has emerged in recent years to dominate drug use and misuse in many population groups. Central nervous system (CNS) stimulants comprise a diverse group of natural and synthetic drugs. These include:
- amphetamines and related compounds, including amphetamine (speed) and methamphetamine (speed, crystal, meth, ice), as well as *d*-amphetamine (dexamphetamine), and methylphenidate (Ritalin)
- synthetic amphetamine derivatives, such as 3,4-methylenedioxyamphetamine (MDA, adam), 3,4-methylenedioxymethamphetamine (MDMA, XTC, ecstasy, E, love drug), and paramethoxyamphetamine (PMA, death)
- cocaine
- phentermine and diethylpropion, prescribed appetite suppressants
- ephedrine and pseudoephedrine, contained in various prescribed and proprietary cold and flu preparations
- khat, a plant found mainly in Somalia and Yemen that contains cathinone, an amphetamine-like compound; the leaves are chewed.

Nicotine, the principal psychoactive constituent of tobacco, is also a CNS stimulant. It is covered separately in chapter 7, and will not be discussed further here. Caffeine, theophylline and theobromine, constituents of coffee, tea, cola drinks, guarana and chocolate, are also classed as stimulants, but will not be considered here.

The stimulants include both natural and synthetic drugs. Cocaine is an alkaloid extracted from the leaf of the plant *Erythroxylon coca*; this is chewed by South American Indians for its stimulant effects. Cocaine was widely used in the late nineteenth century, particularly in beverages such as the original Coca-Cola. Adverse effects of cocaine became apparent, and by 1914 its use was strictly regulated in the USA. However, since the 1960s it has become a widely used illicit drug, and it is the most frequent cause of drug-related deaths reported by medical examiners in the USA. Amphetamine and its derivatives are products of the modern pharmaceutical industry, and most street amphetamines are now produced in illicit laboratories.

PHARMACODYNAMICS

Stimulants activate the CNS and have peripheral sympathomimetic actions. CNS stimulation results in euphoria, an increased feeling of well-being, increased energy and confidence, improved cognitive and psychomotor performance, suppression of appetite, and insomnia. Sympathomimetic effects include elevated blood pressure, tachycardia, or reflex bradycardia. Large doses can cause cardiac arrhythmias.

The different stimulants have differences in onset, duration, and relative magnitude of CNS effects and peripheral effects. The effects vary between individuals depending on the amount taken, the manner in which it is taken, the frequency, duration and route of administration, concurrent use with other drugs, past exposure, and the environment in which the drug is used.

The reasons for use relate to the diverse CNS effects of stimulants. Prescribed amphetamines are used as appetite suppressants, and in the treatment of attention deficit hyperactivity disorder and narcolepsy.

The amphetamines increase synaptic concentrations of the neurotransmitters dopamine, noradrenaline, and serotonin. This occurs by two main mechanisms. First, there is increased release of neurotransmitters from storage sites in nerve terminals. Second, these drugs inhibit reuptake by blocking the transporters responsible for removal of neurotransmitter molecules from the synaptic cleft. Increased noradrenaline concentrations contribute to the sympathomimetic effects, while increased dopamine concentrations may be mainly responsible for central stimulant and euphoric properties.

MDMA has a relatively greater effect on serotonin systems than do amphetamine, and this leads to a somewhat different profile of effects, with both central stimulant and hallucinogenic properties. The strength of hallucinogenic effect varies between individuals. Users also report strong feelings of intimacy and 'togetherness' under the influence of MDMA.

Cocaine increases concentrations of noradrenaline and dopamine at the post-synaptic receptor site by blocking the presynaptic reuptake of noradrenaline and dopamine. In addition to its stimulant effects, cocaine possesses potent vasoconstrictor and local anaesthetic effects.

➤ Amphetamines have central stimulant and peripheral sympathomimetic effects.

➤ 3,4-methylenedioxymethamphetamine (MDMA; ecstasy) has central stimulant and hallucinogenic effects.

➤ Cocaine possesses central stimulant, peripheral sympathomimetic (particularly vasoconstriction) and local anaesthetic effects.

➤ Amphetamine-like stimulants release the neurotransmitters dopamine, serotonin and noradrenaline, and block their reuptake.

➤ Cocaine acts mainly by blocking reuptake of dopamine and noradrenaline.

PHARMACOKINETICS

Amphetamine

Oral administration of amphetamine produces peak cardiovascular effects after about one hour, while the CNS effects peak around two hours. These effects last about four to six hours and disappear faster than the blood concentration falls, probably due to acute tolerance. Intranasal administration (snorting) produces effects within a few minutes, while smoking (inhaling the substance as it is vapourised in a heated chamber) and intravenous injection give even faster effects.

Figure 8.1a, b Cocaine and amphetamines can be taken by intranasal administration, smoking, or injection.

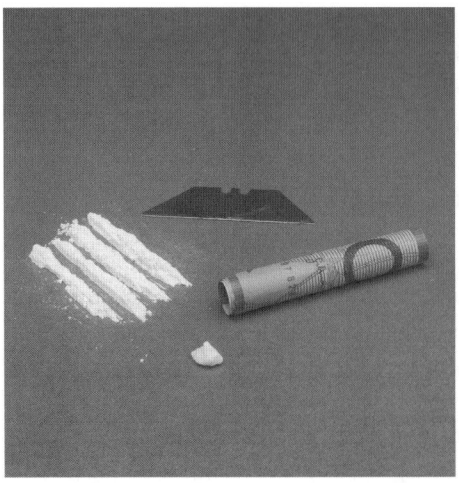 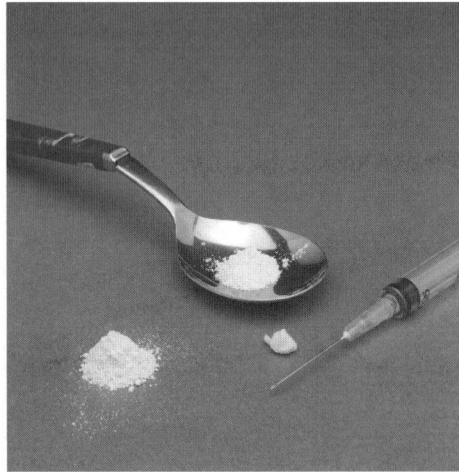

Courtesy Australian Drug Foundation

Amphetamine is eliminated by metabolism in the liver and by renal excretion, including significant excretion of unchanged amphetamine. Being a base, the renal excretion of amphetamine is faster in acidic urine, a feature that can be used to treat overdose. The proportion of amphetamine excreted unchanged can range up to 30%, depending on urinary pH. Active metabolites are formed and may prolong the effects of a dose: methamphetamine is partly converted to amphetamine, and amphetamine partly to the active metabolite 4-hydroxyamphetamine. Several isozymes of cytochrome P450 (CYP) have been implicated in the metabolism of amphetamine and MDMA, including CYP2D6. This enzyme is lacking in some individuals who may, in consequence, be more susceptible to amphetamine toxicity. The half-life of amphetamine is approximately 12 to 36 hours and that of methamphetamine is eight to 17 hours.

MDMA

MDMA is commonly administered orally. Onset of action of MDMA occurs within 30 to 60 minutes with a peak effect at 90 minutes and duration of effect of about eight hours. Its metabolites include the compound MDA, which is itself used as a hallucinogenic stimulant. MDMA also has neurotoxic metabolites that may be responsible for damage to serotonergic neurones (see below). The half-life of the parent compound is around seven to 9 hours.

Cocaine

Cocaine is usually taken intranasally by inhalation (snorting), by smoking the free base (crack) from a heated device, or by intravenous injection of the hydrochloride salt. Cocaine is rapidly absorbed and delivered to the brain, resulting in an intense, but relatively brief, stimulation of the CNS and sympathetic effector sites.

Following intranasal administration of cocaine, onset of effect occurs within minutes, and when inhaled as cocaine free base (crack), or when administered intravenously, onset occurs within seconds. Those who inject or use smokable forms of cocaine experience a powerful and immediate drug effect with a marked rush that is highly pleasurable, followed by a heightened state of cognitive awareness and energy. Duration of euphoria is typically 30 minutes. Because of the intensity of euphoria, speed of effect and short duration of action, cocaine has a rapidly positively reinforcing effect, is highly addictive, and frequently involves a binge pattern of use.

Cocaine is metabolised mainly by liver cholinesterase, and to a lesser extent by plasma cholinesterases, to the inactive water-soluble metabolites benzoylecgonine and ecgonine methyl ester. Only a small fraction (1 to 2%) of the dose is excreted unchanged in the urine. The plasma half-life is 50 minutes (range 45–90 minutes).

When co-administered with alcohol a unique metabolite, cocaethylene, is produced, which itself has stimulant properties.

> → Amphetamine and MDMA have effects lasting four to six hours; the effects of cocaine last around 30 minutes.
> → Active metabolites contribute to the effects of methamphetamine, amphetamine, and MDMA.
> → Inactive cocaine metabolites can be detected in the blood or urine for 24 to 36 hours, and in the hair for weeks to months, after use.

TOLERANCE, DEPENDENCE, AND WITHDRAWAL

Repeated and prolonged use of stimulants leads to the development of marked tolerance, and increasing doses are required to maintain the same effects. Prolonged use results in marked psychological dependence. There is evidence that tolerance develops more to some of the subjective effects than the cardiovascular effects, which suggests that people who take amphetamines at increasing doses for subjective effects are at increased risk of cardiovascular toxicity. Stereotyped behaviour with long-term use of cocaine and amphetamines has been attributed to sensitisation or reverse tolerance.

The acute phase of stimulant induced euphoria is followed by a second phase known as the 'crash'. The crash is thought to indicate the initial phase of the withdrawal state, and is characterised by predominantly psychological symptoms such as extreme lethargy, formication, headache, anxiety, insomnia, irritability, agitation, confusion, and mood lability. Depression is common, and there is the ever-present risk of suicide. Repeated use of cocaine may lead to paranoia and violent behaviour. Depending on the amount and duration of use, the crash starts as the stimulant effects subside, and lasts for hours to several days for cocaine and about three weeks for amphetamines.

There is also a more prolonged phase of withdrawal that may persist for 10 weeks or more. The withdrawal symptoms are predominantly subjective, and include depression (characterised by anhedonia), fatigue and hypersomnia, lack of energy, hunger and excessive appetite, irritability, agitation, and aggression. In the final phase craving becomes episodic and occurs mainly in response to cues previously associated with drug use, a phase known as extinction. Relapse may occur in response to such cues months or years after cessation of use. The last phase may not be observed in an in-patient setting where there are no cues associated with drug use.

> → Stimulant withdrawal symptoms include fatigue, irritability, aggression, depression, and hunger.

TOXIC EFFECTS OF STIMULANTS

Acute toxicity

Acute toxic effects of stimulants are an extension of the pharmacological properties of the drugs, and are determined by the dose, route of administration, and mental state and personality of the user, as well as the environment in which the drug is used. Illicit stimulants are manufactured in non-sterile laboratories by operators who may have insufficient knowledge of chemistry, and who do not practise quality control. The variable potency and presence of potentially lethal adulterants may increase the risk of toxicity.

The toxic effects of amphetamines and cocaine are similar, and arise from increased central nervous system stimulation and sympathomimetic activity. The additional local anaesthetic and vasoconstrictor effects of cocaine may produce more severe toxicity. Multiple organ systems are affected:

- Skin: sweating, hyperpyrexia
- Central nervous system: tremors, excitability, restlessness, apprehension, agitation, muscle twitching, and repetitive stereotyped behaviour. High doses, particularly of cocaine, can result in convulsions, cerebrovascular accidents, such as subarachnoid haemorrhage, cerebral haemorrhage, and cerebral infarction, coma, or even death.

> The possibility of psychostimulant use should be considered in a young adult presenting with seizures or a cerebrovascular accident.

- Neuropsychiatric: manifestations include paranoia, hallucinations, delusions, hyperarousal, and bizarre, violent, and erratic behaviour
- Cardiovascular system: hypertension, tachycardia, dsyarrhythmias, and sudden death. Cocaine use is associated with myocardial ischaemia and infarction (due to marked coronary vasoconstriction, increased myocardial oxygen demand, and enhanced platelet aggregation and thrombus formation), peripheral ischaemia, gangrene of extremities, arteritis, and vasculitis. Bacterial endocarditis may result from intravenous use of psychostimulants.

> The possibility of cocaine use should be considered in young patients with myocardial ischaemia or infarction, arrhythmias, myocarditis, or dilated cardiomyopathy.

- Skeletal muscles: rhabdomyolysis may occur secondary to hyperthermia, seizures, and vasoconstriction, or as a direct effect of the stimulant. This may lead to myoglobinuria and acute renal failure.
- Respiratory tract: inhalation of cocaine may lead to asthma, gas exchange abnormalities, non-specific pulmonary oedema, pulmonary haemorrhage, and

129

haemoptysis due to vasoconstriction. Complications such as pneumothorax, pneumopericardium and pneumomediastinum may occur after free-base smoking with deep, forced, and prolonged inspiratory efforts. Sudden death may result from cardiorespiratory arrest.

- Gastrointestinal system: severe abdominal pain, bloody stools, bowel ischaemia and infarction, and even perforation have been reported with cocaine use.
- Liver: cocaine and MDMA use has been associated with hepatic ischaemia, acute hepatitis, hepatic necrosis and, with MDMA, liver failure.

Acute complications following MDMA use are unpredictable. While most people experience no immediate complications, and MDMA is thought to be a safe drug by recreational users, a number of deaths have been reported following its use. Deaths have been associated with hyperthermia, disseminated intravascular coagulation, hepatic failure, acute renal failure secondary to rhabdomyolysis, and cardiovascular collapse. Hyperthermia is dependent, in part, on ambient temperature: high temperatures increase risk, while low ambient temperatures may result in MDMA-induced hypothermia. Water intoxication and hyponatraemia may result from drinking large amounts of water without salt replacement and increased secretion of antidiuretic hormone.

Chronic toxicity

Chronic stimulant toxicity is manifested mainly by weight loss and such neuropsychiatric complications as poor concentration and attention, memory impairment, sleep disturbances, hallucinations, flashbacks (vivid sense of reliving of a past drug experience), depression, anxiety, and panic attacks.

With repeated use of large doses of stimulants (a run or binge), a psychotic state resembling acute paranoid schizophrenia can develop. This is characterised by severe agitation, anxiety, irritability, restlessness, paranoid delusions, hallucinations (predominantly visual but may be auditory or tactile), repetitive stereotyped behaviour, hostility and violence, and loosening of association and ideas in a setting of clear consciousness. Stimulant-induced psychosis is difficult to differentiate from acute paranoid schizophrenia. Cocaine-induced psychosis may progress to perceptual disturbances, delirium, paranoid delusions, and aggressive or violent behaviour. While the psychotic symptoms generally subside as drug concentration declines, in a few individuals they may persist for weeks to months after cessation of use.

Other medical problems are related to the route of administration. Complications of injecting drug use are discussed in chapter 13. Chronic use of intranasal cocaine may result in rhinorrhoea, nasal ulcers, epistaxis, sinusitis, and perforation of the nasal septal.

Concurrent psychosocial problems—personal, financial, job-related, and legal problems—may progress to social and occupational disintegration. There is evidence that acts of violence are associated with use of cocaine and amphetamines. This can lead to a range of legal and social problems.

Cocaine use during pregnancy is associated with maternal and perinatal complications such as abrupto placentae, miscarriage, prematurity, stillbirth, congenital malformations, impaired brain development, intrauterine growth retardation, and sudden infant death syndrome. In animals, cocaine has several neuroendocrine effects, possibly via actions on 5-HT and dopamine neurones. It activates the hypothalamic-pituitary-adrenal axis, increases vasopressin and luteinising hormone secretion, and reduces secretion of renin and prolactin. The clinical significance in cocaine users has not yet been established.

There is evidence from experimental studies that MDMA is a neurotoxin at serotonergic nerve terminals. Brain-imaging studies in humans have also demonstrated a reduction in the density of serotonin uptake sites in heavy MDMA users, and they have subnormal concentrations of the serotonin metabolite 5-HIAA (5-hydroxyindole acetic acid) in cerebrospinal fluid. These changes are associated with impairment of cognitive functioning, including deficits in memory functioning. There is also evidence of neurotoxicity arising from methamphetamine use: brain-imaging studies in human methamphetamine users show decreased density of dopamine terminals. The pathophysiological implications of this finding are not clear.

> Stimulant induced psychosis needs to be differentiated from acute schizophrenia.

ASSESSMENT

It is important to be aware of CNS stimulant use when assessing patients, as they are commonly used drugs administered by a diverse group of people. Some specific occupational groups such as long-distance truck drivers, shift-workers, students preparing for examinations, and musicians are more likely to abuse psychostimulants. Weight loss may be important for some users, and eating disorders need to be excluded. In others it may be part of a poly-drug use pattern that includes cannabis, alcohol, and other drugs. As stimulant use often starts in adolescence, it should be routinely included in an assessment of drug use among young people. Subcultural membership is important. Some youth may use amphetamines every weekend when attending night-clubs or raves.

> In recent years psychostimulant use has become a common form of substance use among young people.

Different patterns of stimulant use need to be captured in the assessment. The level and frequency of stimulant use are two key aspects of the history. The frequency of use is largely governed by the pharmacology of the stimulant. Intermittent use or recreational use may involve single episodes at weekends, such as MDMA or methamphetamine use at night–clubs or parties. While many users will consume a single tablet only, others use multiple tablets. Use of amphetamine and methamphetamine tends to occur in bursts—a run or binge—that is commonly followed by a crash. The run is usually terminated within one to three days because of the rapid development of tolerance and the emergence of sleep deprivation compounded by exhaustion due to low food intake. At this stage, if there has been repeated or high-dose use, an acute paranoid state may be evident. Methamphetamine may be used in a regular daily pattern (often three times per day) for months at a time.

It is important to assess the quantity, pattern of use, and dependence on the basis of withdrawal symptoms on cessation of use.

Quantification of stimulant used depends on the drug. For stimulants in tablet or capsule form (prescribed or illicit), frequency of use and number of tablets/capsules is sufficient information. Cocaine is usually sold in lines and speed as points or grams/weights. Dollar values can also be used to assess quantities used.

Acute disinhibition due to stimulants, or their effects on decision–making, may lead to unprotected sexual activity. A brief sexual history with appropriate HIV and STD pre-test counselling may be necessary, even in the absence of intravenous drug use.

Clinical examination

The findings on examination of physical and mental state will be determined in large measure by the nature of the clinical presentation. There may be evidence of a hyperactive, psychotic state with signs of sympathomimetic excess, such as tachycardia and hypertension. By contrast, an amphetamine user presenting in a withdrawal state may demonstrate inertia, psychomotor slowing, bradycardia, and a depressed effect. An amphetamine user presenting to a clinic for a scheduled appointment may have no abnormal physical or mental signs.

The overall appearance of a frequent stimulant user may reflect reduced food intake. More specific pointers to intranasal cocaine use (snorting) include a sympathetic rhinitis with erythematous nasal mucosa, and septal necrosis and defects. Stimulant use can cause prominent grinding of the teeth (bruxism), and there may be evidence of this from worn dental enamel. There may be evidence of scratching due to formication.

In an overdose situation, physical complications of stimulant use may be evident. They may include coronary occlusion, cardiac arrhythmias, cerebrovascular occlusion (causing stroke), and seizures. Hyperthermia and muscle tenderness may point to rhabdomyolysis brought on by excessive physical activity and fluid depletion.

The mental state of the patients should be assessed by a brief screening tool (such as the Mini-mental State Examination). Psychostimulant intoxication may be accompanied by agitation, aggression, hypervigilance, and repetitive stereotyped behaviour. Confusion and frank delirium may occur in individuals who have developed dilutional hyponatraemia consequent on over-rapid correction of dehydration. In chronic stimulant users there may be evidence of paranoid ideation, delusional states, and depression. Assessment of depression should include suicidal ideation and intention. Psychomotor slowing may be evident in stimulant withdrawal states. There may be memory deficits, poor impulse control, and poorer performance in higher level cognitive skills.

.Although rare in an amphetamine-related presentation, and probably most typically offered by patients as a rationalisation for their use, undiagnosed attention deficit disorder may be present. Screening for learning difficulties and inattention may require a full specialist assessment. Such patients typically report a paradoxical calming effect of illicit stimulants, similar to that obtained through the medical prescription of these drugs. Referral to a psychologist is necessary for comprehensive assessment.

Laboratory investigations

Urine drug screening may identify recent use of stimulants. The amphetamines and their metabolites can be identified in urine for 48–72 hours after the last use. As cocaine has a short half-life it is not detected in the blood or urine several hours after use. However, the metabolites are detectable in blood or urine for 24–36 hours, and in hair samples for weeks to months after last use. In addition to routine investigations, CPK, cardiac enzymes and serum troponin concentrations should be estimated as appropriate.

INTERVENTION AND TREATMENT

Acute stimulant toxicity

Patients should be nursed in a calm, soothing, and supportive environment. Agitation, anxiety and other central nervous system stimulant effects are controlled with a small dose of diazepam as required. Correction of fluid and electrolyte disturbances and hyperthermia is important. If psychotic symptoms are present, haloperidol may be used. Phenothiazines are best avoided as they lower the seizure threshold. Monitoring of vital signs is essential in cases of stimulant overdose, and ECG monitoring may help detect cardiac disturbances.

Cocaine-induced chest pain and myocardial infarction are best treated with aspirin, benzodiazepines, and nitroglycerine or verapamil. Beta-blockers such as propranolol are contraindicated, but labetalol, an alpha- and beta-blocker, may be used. Thrombolysis is not recommended.

Stimulant dependence

Treatment of stimulant dependence largely relies on psychosocial interventions. Despite considerable research effort, no effective pharmacotherapies have yet been developed. Trials of maintenance with controlled daily doses of oral stimulants (analogous to methadone maintenance with opioids) have produced mixed results.

133

Various medications have been used for symptomatic treatment of stimulant withdrawal. Antidepressants are often prescribed for withdrawal-induced depression, and have been shown to be effective for this purpose. However they have two main problems. One is their delayed onset of action. The second is the potential for drug interaction if the patient relapses, with the possibility of hypertension or the serotonin syndrome, depending on the drugs used. Other medications that have been used include sedatives (short-term use of benzodiazepines and antipsychotics) for control of irritability. This may be particularly useful in the inpatient setting.

Cognitive behavioural therapies for stimulant-dependent patients have been developed. These are extensively employed in the USA for treatment of cocaine dependence, and have been shown to be effective. Programs are typically of several months' duration, with outpatient visits at least weekly. Prevention of relapse through avoidance of high-risk situations (see chapter 5) is particularly important with stimulant users.

It is important to discuss various clinical issues with the amphetamine-dependent patient who has ceased or is about to cease use of the drug. This can help resolve some problems at an early stage, and allay patient fears when symptoms arise. For some issues patients should also be encouraged to return for further intervention if they become problematic. Some of the issues have been mentioned already, but a fuller discussion is given below.

Depression and anhedonia

Patients need to be aware of the likelihood of depression and anhedonia, understand that treatment can help, and be warned that symptoms may last for months. However, in those who have used MDMA excessively, damage to serotonergic terminals may render antidepressants relatively ineffective.

Cognitive impairment

Cognitive impairment is a problem that can arise from use of MDMA and methamphetamine, and probably most other stimulants. The consequences may not become obvious until the person is abstinent, and hence the patient may blame the abstinence for poor cognitive performance. It appears that the brain damage and cognitive impairment is, at best, partially reversible.

Sexuality

Stimulants are used by some people to enhance their sexual performance. In some cases this may result in a pattern of stimulant-induced hypersexuality. Following cessation, loss of the enhancing effect of stimulants can cause concern to patients, who may report reduced libido and diminished sexual performance.

Violence

The irritability and aggression of stimulant withdrawal may be of great concern to some individuals, particularly those with no history of such behaviour. Disruption to families and other social relationships can occur. Strategies for dealing with these symptoms (possibly including medication) may need to be developed.

Conditioned responses

Stimulant users seem to be particularly susceptible to conditioned responses as a result of the association between certain cues or stimuli and use of the drug(s) (see chapter 2). This has important consequences in the person ceasing drug use, as cues may give rise to craving and increase the risk of relapse. Cognitive behavioural therapy may help the patient avoid cues and cope with cravings when they arise (see chapter 5).

Weight gain

Stimulants have anorectic effects. While tolerance develops to these effects, there may be significant body weight loss as a result of stimulant use and consequent weight gain following cessation. For many people, particularly younger women, such weight gain may prove to be a major disincentive to continued abstinence. Strategies to minimise potential weight gain may need to be considered.

> ⇒ Treatment options are limited with stimulants because there are no estab-
>   lished pharmacotherapies.
> ⇒ Antidepressants may be helpful in reducing the severity of depression
>   during withdrawal.
> ⇒ Cognitive behavioural therapy can help patients ceasing use of stimulants.

EPIDEMIOLOGY AND PREVENTION

Epidemiology of stimulant use

It is not easy to describe the epidemiology of stimulants because of the different settings in which they are used by different types of users. Users may, for example, be shift workers, affluent young people who identify with dance culture, or marginalised street injectors. Use includes both illicit stimulants and pharmaceuticals. There have been reports of stimulants prescribed for the treatment of attention deficit disorder being diverted to the black market, especially among those of school age. Truck drivers have been reported to use weight loss medications to help them stay awake and concentrate while driving.

Amphetamines can be used instrumentally, where the stimulant or anorectic effects of the drug are used to achieve specific goals: chronically, usually by a small proportion of users, but often resulting in pronounced health and social problems; and (sub)culturally or recreationally, for example at raves and other dance events where users identify to some extent with a group identity defined by music, fashion, and a shared value system.

Poly-drug use is likely to be the norm for many stimulant users, particularly chronic and recreational users.

Amphetamines

The six national drug household surveys conducted in Australia between 1985 and 1998 have suggested that the proportion of Australians over the age of 14 who have ever used amphetamines has remained fairly stable at rates between 6 and 9%, with 2 to 4% having used the drug in the previous 12 months. Studies of Australian recreational drug users conducted between the late 1980s and the late 1990s consistently identified amphetamine as the most commonly used illicit drug after cannabis. This appeared to change with the rise in heroin use in Australia and other countries in the late 1990s, although as potent forms of methamphetamine crystal became more available in Australia in the early 2000s, amphetamine use re-emerged as a major drug problem. Amphetamine users have tended to be younger than heroin users, and are predominantly males. Amphetamines were identified as the most recently injected drug by 70% of illicit drug injectors surveyed as part of the 1998 national drug household survey, and 51% of injecting drug users said that amphetamines were the first drug they ever injected. Males in the 20–29 age group are most likely to have used amphetamines. According to data from the 1998 national drug household survey, some 25% of this group had ever used, and 16% had used in the last year.

MDMA

Although ecstasy is the stimulant that has attracted the most media attention, its prevalence of use in Australia, New Zealand, USA, and many other Western countries is typically less than that of amphetamines. Despite this, trends indicate that it is becoming more popular, particularly among youth. In 1998, 4.7% of Australians of 14 years and over had ever used ecstasy, and 2.4% had used in the past 12 months. Once again, prevalence is highest among males in the 20 to 29-year-old group, with some 18% having ever used and 12% having used in the last 12 months. Although ecstasy use has been associated with the rave or dance culture and environment, its use is not limited to participants in this scene.

Cocaine

Cocaine use is not common in Australia. In 1998, 4.3% of Australians of 14 years and over had ever used cocaine, and 1.4% had used in the past 12 months. In 1999, cocaine was considered easy to obtain in New South Wales and difficult to obtain elsewhere in Australia. Poly-drug use involving cocaine has been common among drug injectors in Sydney since 1998.

Prevention

Prevention activity to reduce stimulant-related harm can be community-wide (for example primary prevention of stimulant use among the general public), targeted at selected sub-populations (such as prevention programs for long-distance truck drivers), or specific to the setting (for example employing trained outreach workers to provide support for those experiencing problems at raves and dance parties). Ideally, there should be conceptual consistency between macro, community-wide interventions and those employed at more micro levels. However, often strategies and messages employed at one level will not be appropriate at another.

Community-wide public education

The use of the mass media and social marketing, while being effective at raising awareness of an issue, rarely result in changes to individual behaviour or attitudes.

Targeted education

In Australia, education aimed at long-distance truck drivers has been undertaken via distributing postcards at truck stops (including information on the effects of amphetamines on driving, poly-drug use, legal aspects, needle sharing, and coming down), convenience advertising (in toilets and shower cubicles) to provide information confidentially while the drivers were on the road, and advertising and editorials in trucking magazines.

Setting specific strategies

Various strategies have been developed to try to minimise the drug-related harm experienced by some young people attending raves and dance parties. There are three main types of intervention: information campaigns aimed at users; guidelines for night-club owners and rave promoters to help minimise the potential harm attributable to the environment, and employing trained outreach workers to provide support for those experiencing problems at raves and dance parties. Other strategies have included setting up safe houses in some hotels, clubs, and raves in the Netherlands where clubbers can have their ecstasy tablets tested or checked against a register of previously tested pills and capsules.

Integrated strategies

The two national action plans on psychostimulants implemented in Australia in 1991 and 1995 provide examples of coordinated and multifaceted amphetamine prevention campaigns. The 1995 campaign targeted non-users and novice stimulant users in the 15–25 year age group, with a slight bias towards males, those from lower socioeconomic backgrounds, and the unemployed. The program used consistent messages placed within a variety of life contexts. Themes highlighted health risks including overdose, dependence ('Speed catches up with you'), HIV risk ('AIDS hits speed users too'), and the effect of contaminants. The dance party scene was a particular focus.

Elements of the campaign included television and cinema advertisements, billboards, radio, magazines and brochures, sponsorship of dance events, a music CD, school kits, and two monographs circulated to academics and professionals across the country. The national campaign was linked to local initiatives in the second phase. In the third phase, supply control measures and policing were emphasised. So-called 'tribes' intervention which aimed to involve and access specific and hard-to-reach groups of stimulant users were also implemented. These included unemployed young people, injecting drug users, and those in the dance party scene.

➡ A range of public health strategies can be employed to minimise stimulant problems. These include:
➡ prevention programs for the general public
➡ targeted programs for specific sub-populations of stimulant users
➡ interventions in settings where stimulants are used.

Case study

Alan, a 30-year-old male patient, presents at your general practice with insomnia, exhaustion, fatigue, irritability, and depressed mood. His self-reports indicate that he frequently has palpitations and paranoid ideation, although he is not currently experiencing these symptoms. He tells you in confidence that he has been using speed. He has come because of the problems described above, but also because three days ago his wife of six months discovered his drug supply. Up until that time she had been unaware of his stimulant use. He has not used speed since that time.

Alan is self-employed. He first started using speed four years ago as a result of pressures at work; he found he could work longer hours and therefore fill more orders if he used in the second half of the day. For most of these four years his pattern of use has been irregular, using about once per week on average. However, a year ago his use escalated with increasing work pressure, and he is now using most days, usually two or three times per day. He works six days per week and normally tries to abstain from use on his day off, although if he has an important social function he usually finds that he needs to take speed in order to be able to fulfil social obligations.

He now realises that his use of the drug has become counter-productive. He is making mistakes at work, and his performance decreases markedly on occasions when he cannot purchase additional drugs or does not have sufficient time to do so. He had managed to keep his speed use from his fiancée (now wife), but she is very upset at discovering his use. The side-effects are also starting to worry him.

You discuss with Alan both the direct effects of amphetamine-like drugs and also the effects of withdrawal. While he has had some paranoid ideation, there is no evidence of precipitation of major psychiatric problems. You also discuss with him the withdrawal symptoms he is experiencing and is likely to experience over the next days to weeks. While the fatigue, difficulty concentrating, and excessive appetite are likely to resolve soon, you explain that the depressive symptoms and anhedonia of stimulant withdrawal may continue for some time. There is also concern with relapse, particularly if pressures at work continue. Alan has been irritable since stopping his use of speed, but he does not think that aggressive behaviour will be a problem.

You decide to commence him on antidepressant treatment and choose the SSRI sertraline. You discuss with Alan the delayed onset of action of sertraline, and the need for him to avoid using stimulants while taking it because of the possibility of a drug interaction leading to significant hypertension.

Alan returns for follow-up visits in each of the following four weeks and then one month later. He has managed to cease stimulant use, and experienced only mild depression. He would, however, prefer to continue the sertraline for a period of time as he is concerned about his risk of relapse. He is finding difficulty maintaining his level of work without the assistance of stimulants, and is also concerned that work pressures will increase the future risks of relapse. He has, however, with the assistance of his wife, put in a plan to restructure his work time so as to use it more efficiently, and also to obtain additional support in his business. His wife has helped him throughout, and has remained calm despite the initial shock of discovering his drug use. You have discussed the option of referral to a psychologist for cognitive behavioural therapy associated with cessation of stimulant use. At this stage he feels that this is not necessary, but he has the option to use it in the future if continued abstinence becomes difficult.

Case points

Alan's case illustrates:
- stimulant use was to increase work performance and decrease fatigue
- dependence developed only after a long period of stimulant use
- external pressures, such as those from a spouse, are frequently major motivators in breaking a pattern of high-level drug use
- delayed onset of action of antidepressants is a problem; nevertheless they may be helpful in preventing prolonged depression
- follow-up is important, and continued assistance should be given even when the patient has been abstinent for several months. It is particularly important to leave options open for further treatment.

REFERENCES AND FURTHER READING

Crits–Christoph, P., Siqueland, L., Blaine, J. et al. 1999, 'Psychosocial treatments for cocaine dependence: National Institute on Drug Abuse Collaborative Cocaine Treatment Study', *Archives of General Psychiatry*, vol. 56, pp. 493–502.

Gawin, F.H. & Ellinwood, E.F. 1998, 'Cocaine and other stimulants', *New England Journal of Medicine*, vol. 318, 1173–82.

Lange, R.A. & Hills, L.D. 2001, 'Cardiovascular complications of cocaine use', *New England Journal of Medicine*, vol. 345 (5), pp. 351–8.

Warner, E.A., Kosten, T.R. & O'Connor, P.G. 1997, 'Pharmacotherapy for opioid and cocaine abuse' *Medical Clinics of North America*, vol. 81, pp. 909–25.

World Health Organisation 1997, 'Amphetamine-type stimulants', *Program on Substance Abuse*, World Health Organisation, Geneva.

9

Cannabis

Fraser Todd, Stuart McLean, Henry Krum, Jennifer Martin & Jan Copeland

I experimented with marijuana a time or two, I didn't like it, and I didn't inhale.

US President Bill Clinton 1992, reported in *Washington Post*.

Cannabis is the third most popular drug (excluding caffeine) after alcohol and tobacco in developed countries. It is a difficult drug to classify in pharmacological terms, as it has a mixture of mood, cognitive, motor, and perceptual effects and does not clearly belong with any other drug class. Cannabis has also been used for its therapeutic properties: analgesia, bronchodilation, anti-nausea, and the capacity to reduce intra-ocular pressure.

Cannabis has been used for over four millennia. Its position and status within cultures has varied considerably, some cultures embracing it as an important enhancement of the social fabric, while others have regarded it as an evil substance that undermines normal social functioning. Cannabis is currently illegal in most Western countries, while at the same time it is the most popular of the illicit substances. This tension is being resolved in many countries by a steady reduction in the penalties for the possession and use of cannabis, reflecting the widely held belief that it is a 'soft' drug that is less harmful and perhaps less addictive than 'harder' drugs such as stimulants and opioids.

PHARMACOKINETICS AND PHARMACODYNAMICS

The hemp plant, *Cannabis sativa*, produces a resin containing about 60 cannabinoids, of which one, Δ^9-tetrahydrocannabinol (Δ^9-THC or THC), is principally responsible for the psychoactive effects of cannabis. Marijuana refers to the cut-up dried leaves and flowers of the hemp plant. The THC content of marijuana varies greatly (from 0.5 to 12.0%), depending on genetic and environmental factors. The extracted resin, known as hashish, has a higher THC content. When smoked, THC is vapourised and delivered to the lungs together with many other cannabinoids and pyrolysis products.

As with other drugs of abuse, there is a tendency for users to seek forms of the drug with greater potency as their use escalates. Use of indoor hydroponic growing techniques, where the light conditions can be artificially controlled, may assist in maximising THC concentration. Similarly, cannabis may be sought that is reputed to have been grown in tropical areas or areas of high sunshine hours. High THC concentrations are obtained from the heads or flowering buds of the female plant. Over recent years there have also been attempts to breed plants yielding a high concentration of cannabis, such as skunk, much of which is grown hydroponically. The method of smoking may also evolve to deliver a higher dose, for example from a joint (a cigarette containing cannabis alone or cannabis plus tobacco) to a pipe or bong (water pipe), where less side-stream smoke escapes, or in very heavy users occasionally to a bucket bong in which water pressure is used to force smoke into the user's lungs.

Pharmacodynamics

Mode of action

Cannabinoid receptors exist in two forms, CB_1 and CB_2 receptors. CB_1 receptors, found in the brain and peripheral tissues (for example the testes, and endothelial cells), are believed to mediate most of the well-recognised effects of cannabis, described below. CB_2 receptors are associated with the immune system, with their greatest concentration in B-cells and natural killer cells. Cannabinoid receptors are membrane-bound and linked to G-proteins, and use various mechanisms for signal transduction (inhibition of adenylate cyclase, activation of MAP kinase, opening ion channels). Endogenous ligands appear to be esters and amides of eicosanoids, notably N-arachi-donylethanolamide or anandamide ('bliss' in Sanskrit). CB_1 receptors are found in a number of brain regions, including the cerebral cortex, hypocampus, amygdala, and basal ganglia. Concentrations are low in the brainstem and spinal cord. As with other drugs of abuse, cannabinoids facilitate activity in mesolimbic dopamine neurones.

Effects

In common with other psychoactive drugs, the effects of cannabis depend on the dose, the individual user, and the setting. In general, low doses produce a mixture of stimulatory and depressant effects, and high doses are mainly depressant.

The effects of cannabis include euphoria, relaxation, and a feeling of well-being. In addition there are perceptual distortions, such as apparently sharpened senses and altered time sense. Memory, cognition, and skilled task-performance are impaired, although subjects may feel confident and highly creative. Peripheral effects include tachycardia, vasodilatation (especially evident in the conjunctiva), hypotension, reduced intra-ocular pressure, and bronchodilation. Cannabis stimulates the appetite and is anti-emetic—in some countries an oral form of THC is marketed to treat the nausea from cancer chemotherapy. Other potential medical uses for THC and its derivatives are as anticonvulsants, analgesics, and muscle relaxants. There are prospects for the development of more receptor-selective cannabinoids with better effect/toxicity profiles.

> ➟ The major effects of cannabis, including euphoria, relaxation, perceptual distortions, and psychomotor and cognitive impairment, are mediated by the actions of THC at CB_1 receptors.

Pharmacokinetics

Smoking cannabis delivers THC rapidly to the blood and brain. Plasma THC peaks at the end of smoking, and falls to low values within two hours. One metabolite, 11-hydroxy-THC, is active, but remains at low levels and therefore probably contributes little to the effects. The major metabolite, 11-carboxy-THC, persists at high plasma levels for hours after smoking. Carboxy-THC is the metabolite usually measured in blood or urine tests for cannabis, but it is inactive and its presence simply confirms the use of cannabis at some time in the recent past.

Cannabis is traditionally taken orally in some Eastern cultures, in a form often called 'bhang'. Although active when taken orally, its absorption is slower and more variable, and therefore the effects are often less pronounced.

THC is lipophilic, and rapidly taken up by body lipids. This results in a slow elimination of metabolites, which can be detected in urine days after smoking. This long sojourn in the body outlasts the acute effects of THC.

Blood levels and effects

Smoking a standard marijuana cigarette containing 15 mg (1.8%) THC results in a mean peak plasma THC level of 84 ng/mL (range 50–129) at the end of smoking (14 minutes). After two hours, THC levels are below 5 ng/mL. In contrast the effects, delayed somewhat for entry into the brain, are maximal at 20 minutes and last for two to four hours. Thus there is no established relationship between plasma levels of THC and its effects, due to the rapid absorption and disappearance of THC, delay in entry to its central sites of action, and the influence of tolerance.

> Blood concentrations of THC do not correlate well with effects.
> The presence of THC metabolites in urine may not necessarily reflect recent usage.

TOLERANCE, DEPENDENCE, AND WITHDRAWAL

Tolerance

Tolerance to the effects of cannabis has been clearly described in humans. The role of CB_1 receptor down-regulation in the development of tolerance has been demonstrated in animals, and it is likely to be an important mechanism in the development of tolerance in humans.

Dependence and withdrawal

A dependence syndrome associated with cannabis use has been clearly described. While severe dependence clearly exists, the cannabis dependence syndrome is generally thought of as being less pronounced than dependence associated with drugs such as opioids and alcohol, and may take longer to become established. Evidence for this is conflicting, however, and concerns are emerging that dependence on cannabis may develop rapidly in some younger people and be more severe than previously believed.

There has been debate concerning the existence of a specific cannabis withdrawal syndrome. Cannabis withdrawal is not listed as a diagnosis in DSM-IV, but there is now clear evidence that a withdrawal syndrome from cannabis does exist in humans. The great variation between people in frequency, duration, and dose of cannabis use makes it difficult to evaluate the exact nature and frequency of the withdrawal syndrome, and the research literature reports wide variations in the rapidity of development, duration, and severity of withdrawal. It has been estimated that two joints a day for three weeks is sufficient to induce withdrawal symptoms after cessation in some people, while there is also evidence that in others, daily use for several years may not be associated with significant withdrawal symptoms on cessation.

Symptoms of withdrawal include:
- anxiety
- anorexia
- disturbed sleep and an increase in vivid dreams
- nausea
- salivation
- increased body temperature
- tremor
- weight loss
- irritability
- stomach pain.

Use of cannabis will alleviate these symptoms.

> ➡ Tolerance develops to the effects of repeated doses of THC by receptor down-regulation. Dependence and withdrawal do occur in humans.

TOXICITY

Acute toxicity

Acute effects that may cause problems include:

- anxiety, panic attacks, persecutory delusions, visual hallucinations, and overt psychotic reactions in vulnerable people
- impairment of short-term memory and attention
- impairment of motor skills, reaction time, and the ability to perform skilled activities.

A short-lived psychotic state has been reported associated with high-dose use. This generally resolves within a week of abstinence. This cannabis–induced state can be difficult to distinguish from the precipitation of a psychosis in those with a predisposition to mental illness.

Cannabis has relatively weak effects on cardiovascular, respiratory and thermo-regulatory systems. The only notable change in vital signs is an increase of around 20 bpm in heart rate. However, this is not increased further by high cannabis intake. The absence of such effects makes cannabis a comparatively safe drug in overdose.

Chronic toxicity

Chronic use of cannabis has been associated with a range of harmful effects in animal and laboratory studies, but many of these have not been shown to be clinically significant. This lack of evidence does not mean that cannabis is safe but rather that several potential harms have yet to be clarified.

Harms related to chronic use of cannabis include the following:

- Impairment of short term memory, attention, and the organisation and integration of complex information. These effects appear to be relatively mild and of limited clinical significance for the majority of regular cannabis users, but it is likely that those involved in learning and higher education, such as adolescents, might experience significant impairment. There is no evidence to suggest it causes permanent brain damage in adults.
- Effects on major mental illnesses. There is evidence that the use of cannabis increases positive symptoms and rates of relapse and re-hospitalisation in people with schizophrenia. The effects of cannabis on other major mental illnesses have yet to be clarified.
- Chronic respiratory disease. Cannabis has been shown to impair respiratory function in humans, and has been associated with chronic obstructive airways disease and exacerbation of pre-existing disorders such as asthma.
- Effects on pregnancy. Smoking cannabis during pregnancy may reduce birth weight, although this effect has been difficult to disentangle from the confounding effects of concurrent alcohol and tobacco consumption.

In addition, concern has been expressed by clinicians that chronic regular cannabis use may be related to a range of other problems, but the evidence indicating that clinically significant problems arise has yet to emerge.

These potential problems include:

- Psychiatric syndromes. There is debate as to whether cannabis alone is a causative factor in the induction of a chronic psychosis. There is evidence to support the view that heavy cannabis use may precipitate and aggravate a pre-existing condition such as schizophrenia in those people with a vulnerability to psychotic disorder (see above).
  There is great debate as to whether long-term use of cannabis leads to a so-called *amotivational syndrome*. It is probable that this represents the acute intoxication state of frequent users of this drug.
- Fertility. Cannabis use can be associated with changes in the reproductive system. These include a decrease in testosterone levels and sperm production, and inhibition of ovulation. There is no evidence that these changes occur to such a degree that fertility is compromised.
- Respiratory cancer. Concerns have been expressed by clinicians over several cases of respiratory carcinoma in younger regular cannabis users. Cannabis has also been shown to be carcinogenic and mutagenic in vivo and in vitro. However, there is currently no clear epidemiological evidence that cannabis causes increased rates of respiratory cancer in younger people or is related to other forms of cancer.
- Immune function. Immune cells have cannabinoid receptors, and cannabis has been shown to impair the function of immune cells in laboratory conditions. There is no evidence, however, that impairment of immune cell function results in any clinically significant impairment.

Clinically significant harms from chronic cannabis use include:

➡ impaired short-term memory and attention
➡ exacerbation of chronic respiratory airways diseases
➡ increased positive symptoms and acute episodes of schizophrenia
➡ dependence syndrome.

ASSESSMENT

History-taking

There is a wide spectrum of patterns of use in patients concerned about their use of cannabis presenting to services. Some may have experienced a very aversive effect after seemingly low-level use. This is typically seen in naïve users with 'controlled' personalities who find it difficult to cope with the loss of control associated with disinhibited intoxication. Hyperventilation and panic may ensue. Parents can also be alarmed and may seek advice when they learn that their son or daughter has used cannabis, although this use may have been on only a single occasion.

As discussed earlier, as use of cannabis escalates there is a tendency to use preparations that are of greater potency. This includes cannabis plants grown under controlled conditions or in areas with high sunshine hours, hydroponically grown cannabis, high concentration variants of the cannabis plant, and concentrated forms of cannabis such as hash resin or oil.

Heavy users are more likely to smoke the heads (the flowering buds) of the female plant than the leaves, as the heads have a higher concentration of THC than leaf. The method of smoking may also evolve to deliver a higher dose, for example from a joint to a pipe or bong. Ingestion of cannabis as food (for example in hash cookies) is uncommon. It results in a slower onset of intoxication because of slower absorption and passage to the CNS and the effects are more variable than when the cannabis is smoked, as it is more difficult for the user to titrate dose against effect. THC is not water-soluble and is not used intravenously.

In assessing cannabis use the following should be explored:

- whether leaf or heads are smoked
- the source of the cannabis and its growing conditions (garden, plantation, or hydroponically grown; temperate or tropical climate)
- the variant of cannabis smoked
- whether smoked as a joint or with a pipe or bong
- the amount spent on cannabis per week
- the number of hours per day spent intoxicated from cannabis.

Figure 9.1   There are different forms of cannabis and different smoking apparatus.

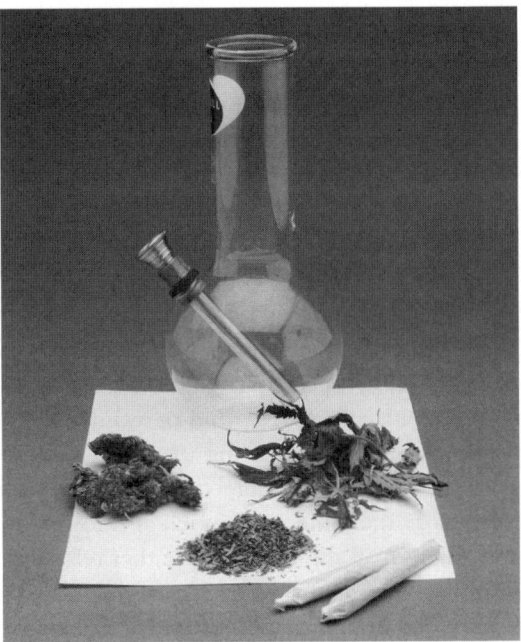

Courtesy Australian Drug Foundation

Cannabis and psychosis

It is particularly important to establish the level and pattern of cannabis use in people who have presented with psychosis. Brief psychosis precipitated by cannabis use is a controversial diagnosis, and it has inconsistent scientific support as a distinct nosological entity. However, a comorbid schizophrenic spectrum disorder may be present, and a psychotic episode in such a vulnerable individual may be precipitated by cannabis. The incidence of schizophrenia peaks in young adult life, when cannabis use is most common. In assessing the possibility of schizophrenia it is crucial to establish current psychotic symptoms through observation, and through interview of the patient and others, such as family members. A family history of major psychiatric illness and evidence of a prodrome also needs to be established. The prodrome is a gradual worsening of symptoms that may start with social difficulties, academic difficulties, or isolation from others, and progress to the development of delusional thought and odd behaviour. It is frequently very difficult to identify whether a psychosis is primarily due to cannabis or a schizophreniform illness. The onset of cannabis use and the possible schizophrenia is often of little use in establishing primacy, given that a prodrome may last for years and it may be difficult to establish the onset with precision. As noted, both the independent onset of schizophrenia and regular cannabis use are likely to occur at the same time during late adolescence and early adulthood.

Investigations

Relatively few investigations are associated with cannabis presentations. Due to the highly lipophilic nature of THC it is readily detectable in urine (mainly via the metabolite carboxy-THC) for periods of several weeks after last use in regular users as it is slowly released from tissues. As discussed, there is a poor correlation between plasma THC levels and clinical effect.

Physical examination

Examination of respiratory function may be useful, and spirometry may be considered to provide feedback to a user regarding the acute consequences of smoking cannabis (alone, or mixed with tobacco). Significant respiratory problems such as emphysema, chronic bronchitis, or exacerbation of asthma may be evident. Sinusitis and pharyngitis may be present. The ongoing exposure to contaminants in smoke and possible decreased host resistance to infection related to cannabis use can result in repeated upper respiratory tract infection, much as is found in tobacco smokers.

Acute cardiovascular signs may also be present, either related to panic (for example hypertension, tachycardia) or as an exacerbation of angina pectoris. Although the long-term consequences of smoking have not been well investigated, an increased likelihood of carcinoma, for example in the nasopharynx and bronchus, is probable. In chronic users weight gain can be present due to appetite stimulation. A reduced sperm count can be associated with chronic use. The effect of any drug use on the developing foetus is of more concern, and it is advisable for women to avoid cannabis if they are pregnant or trying to get pregnant.

The withdrawal state may be due to a combination of psychological factors (including loss of an enjoyable activity, means of coping) and physiological factors (such as decreased density of CB_1 receptors). The primary psychological symptoms are irritability, aggression, boredom, impaired concentration, and anhedonia. In chronic users the cognitive difficulties associated with use may persist for several months until resolving. These symptoms of cognitive inflexibility and impaired higher problem solving are related to frontal lobe impairment. However, the frontal deficits associated with alcohol dependence are considerably more marked than those found in cannabis users.

149

Psychosocial history

Cannabis use is common in Australia and New Zealand, particularly among young people. Statistically and developmentally, experimentation with cannabis is normative behaviour. The use of cannabis, per se, is not associated with psychopathology. This is not to mean that the acute effects of recreational use should not be of concern, and elements of the psychosocial history should aim to clarify these risks. For example, the activities undertaken while intoxicated should be ascertained. The acute impairment of judgment, cognitive flexibility, and reaction time means that driving, operation of machinery, or activities involving physical risk should be avoided. It can be important to enquire about workplace use, as cannabis use during work hours is more common among blue-collar workers, for example on production lines.

Assessment should focus on:

→ the nature and style of cannabis use
→ evidence of psychiatric sequelae
→ withdrawal symptoms
→ medical complications of cannabis use
→ the psychosocial context of use.

INTERVENTION AND TREATMENT

While many people with a substance use disorder do not seek assistance from a health professional, recent data indicate substantial increases in the number of cannabis smokers seeking professional assistance to quit or to manage cannabis-related problems. Unfortunately, on many occasions the problem is ignored, people are told that their heavy use is normal, or they are given poor quality information. It is essential for medical practitioners to arm themselves with up-to-date information, and to be open to the suggestion that their patients are seeking help for a bona fide health problem.

Intervention strategies will vary according to how entrenched use patterns and associated problems have become, and the goals of the individual concerned.

Medical treatment

There is no account of a fatality in a human being with cannabis alone. Pure cannabis abuse rarely requires inpatient or pharmacological treatment. However, care is required during assessment as cannabis dependence rarely occurs in isolation from use of other drugs, and coexisting disorders are common (see chapters 14 and 20).

Even though there are no specific pharmacological treatments, cannabis use may precipitate or exacerbate a number of psychological conditions, which may benefit from treatment with medication:

- Sedative–hypnotic drugs are occasionally needed to treat severe cannabis-induced anxiety or panic. A typical treatment would be diazepam 10 mg orally as a single dose.
- Anti-psychotic drugs such as risperidone or haloperidol are occasionally needed to treat cannabis-induced psychotic states. Anti-psychotic medications ameliorate some of the distressing symptoms associated with this state. These drug-induced states are usually short lived, and completely resolve within a week of cessation of cannabis use.
- Other medication may be considered after careful assessment for coexisting disorders such as depression, anxiety, or phobias.

Pharmacological research on cannabinoid systems is relatively new. With the development of different compounds that are agonists, partial agonists and antagonists at CB_1 receptors, there is the potential to develop pharmacotherapies analogous to those used for treatment of opioid dependence. This could produce a radical change in the way we treat cannabis dependence.

Psychological interventions

Most interventions used for cannabis dependence have been adapted from alcohol interventions. These generally follow the 'brief intervention' format that includes motivational interviewing (see chapters 5 and 10).

There seems little doubt that psychological interventions are of greater benefit than no therapy at all. Even one session of cognitive behavioural therapy is significantly superior to no treatment, and can produce clinically significant reductions in the frequency and amount of cannabis use and related problems among severely dependent users. However, the best treatment is still to be determined. Studies show that there is no difference in outcome between intensive cognitive behavioural therapy compared with brief sessions of social support or motivational enhancement therapy. It should be recognised that specific approaches to cannabis dependency are in their infancy, and further differentiation of the best approach will come with further research.

Here is an example of a six-session intervention that has been developed and trialled with cannabis users.

1 The first session includes motivational enhancement training (see motivational interviewing, chapter 5), goal setting, and an introduction to behavioural self-monitoring.
2 The second session focuses on strategies to manage craving. This session might also cover cannabis withdrawal, social support systems, and an optional section on drug refusal skills if required. A quit date is typically set at this point, if not already agreed.
3 The third session addresses withdrawal management, monitoring urges and cravings, and cognitive restructuring techniques. With respect to the latter, patients might be provided with handouts on awareness and management of negative thinking, common thinking errors, and strategies for handling negative thoughts.
4 The fourth session covers cognitive strategies and skills enhancement. These include discussion of causes of relapse and problem-solving skills. Cognitive behavioural therapy for sleep problems or relaxation training may also be offered.
5 The fifth session should review and consolidate as well as introduce any new skills required. These may include assertiveness, communication skills, or anger management skills.
6 The final session is largely based on the relapse-prevention model. It includes a lifestyle modification component and plans for the future.

Where the clinician believes that the patient may benefit from referral to agencies for other issues, such as depression or childhood traumas, these should be arranged prior to the final session.

Treatment summary

In summary, if medical practitioners provide information on the harms associated with heavy long-term cannabis use, advise on reducing or ceasing use, and adopt brief motivational and cognitive–behavioural techniques to manage withdrawal and craving, they may significantly improve the outcome for patients presenting with cannabis-use disorders. However, some people at the severe end of the dependence spectrum may be helped by more specialised input. A referral to the local alcohol and drug unit or a drug and alcohol specialist counsellor may be required. Here there will be provision for comprehensive assessment of the individual, including the cannabis use and other drug use, as well as coexisting disorders and problems.

Treatment of overdose is rarely required. Pharmacotherapies have not yet been developed for treatment of cannabis dependence. Cognitive behavioural interventions that include motivational interviewing techniques are effective in reducing problematic cannabis use.

EPIDEMIOLOGY AND PREVENTION

Cannabis in its various forms is currently the most widely used illicit drug in developed countries. In most countries, it emerged as a commonly used drug during the 1960s, and the prevalence in its use peaked during the 1970s. While the number of people using cannabis has declined since then, the reduction has been slight, and throughout the 1990s and early 2000s cannabis has remained a popular and widely used drug.

Prevalence

There are a number of ways of examining the rates of cannabis use in the population. Often, the number of people who have ever used cannabis is quoted. More important, however, is the number of people who use cannabis regularly, the amount of cannabis they consume, and especially the number of people who develop problems as a result of their cannabis use.

Patterns of use

Studies over the past decade suggest that between 40 and 50% of Australians and New Zealanders have tried cannabis at least once. Men are slightly more likely to have tried cannabis than are women. Most of those who use cannabis do so only occasionally. Approximately 10 to 20% of New Zealanders use cannabis on a regular basis.

From a health perspective, the most important figures are those relating to problematic cannabis use. Rates of cannabis dependence in the general population range between 1.5 and 5% in most Western countries. Population figures from Australia and New Zealand suggest that our rates for a cannabis-use disorder (abuse or dependence) are in the lower end of that range. Of course, rates are much higher in those who use cannabis regularly, but there is conflicting evidence regarding the frequency of dependence in heavy users. One study of daily users in Australia indicated that 90% had a diagnosis of dependence.

Factors affecting use

Gender

Males have traditionally outnumbered females, both for rates of ever having used cannabis and for problematic use, by a ratio of about 2 : 1 in most countries. This difference has reduced markedly in the USA over recent years, and, while males remain over-represented in Australia and New Zealand, the gap is narrowing steadily.

Adolescence

Cannabis use in adolescence occurs so commonly that trying cannabis is considered normal behaviour. Several recent studies suggest that in some regions 50 to 70% of young people have tried cannabis. Rates of cannabis dependence also appear relatively high, with 5.2% of 18-year-olds in one large cohort reporting symptoms of dependence in the preceding twelve months. High rates of cannabis use in younger people appear to be associated with greater incidence of other problems, such as conduct disorder and depression, parental conflict, lower standards of living, and lower socioeconomic status.

> Cannabis use is very common, particularly among younger people, but cannabis dependence is relatively uncommon.

Ethnicity

Rates of cannabis use and dependence appear higher in some ethnic groups. For example, over 80% of New Zealand Māori people appear to have tried cannabis and rates of dependence in this group are approximately 1.8 times higher than in the non-Māori population. There is less information available on patterns of use by Aboriginal and Torres Straight Islander people, though early evidence suggests increased rates of use in these groups also.

Coexisting mental health disorders

High rates of regular cannabis use are found in people with major mental disorders such as mood disorders and schizophrenia. Cannabis use is likely to worsen the course of these disorders significantly.

Prevention

One of the key issues in prevention of cannabis problems is to identify exactly what it is that is trying to be prevented. Is the goal to prevent all cannabis use, regular use, or problematic use? The main methods of prevention have involved education, early identification and intervention, and legal sanctions.

Education

Traditional drug education packages that attempt to influence the use of cannabis by educating young people about its harms have not been shown to be successful. Approaches that focus on teaching specific and more general life skills, such as drug refusal skills, social and relationship skills, coping skills, and leisure skills, may have more impact, however.

The media are widely used by interested parties to educate and influence potential users towards the view of the educator, but the variable quality of the opinions presented and their inherent biases have undermined the power of such approaches. So, while education should be a powerful tool for prevention, its potential has become seriously limited.

Early intervention

Increasingly, prevention involves intervening as early as possible in the development of problematic drug use. The aim is therefore twofold: first, to identify and ameliorate those factors that predispose to problematic drug use, and, second, to identify and intervene with those at high risk early in the development of their problematic drug use.

Predisposing factors that are related to the development of problematic cannabis and other drug use include family dysfunction and the presence of other mental disorders such as conduct disorder, attention deficit disorder with hyperactivity, and major depressive disorder. Sociopolitical approaches to strengthening families, such as addressing issues of unemployment, inequities associated with lower socioeconomic status, issues associated with child abuse, and providing education that is ethnically inclusive, are likely to have a positive impact in a variety of indirect ways. Identifying and intervening early in the course of the commonly associated mental disorders is also likely to be important.

Early intervention with high-risk groups requires that a wide range of workers, such as teachers and social workers, need to have assessment and screening skills. Access to treatment services needs to be easy and welcoming. Treatment agencies need to focus initially on engaging and retaining their clients, and then to follow them up assertively. Consideration needs to be given to using medication where appropriate, and involving the person's family and peer networks in a supportive role.

Legal sanctions

One of the aims of making a psychoactive substance illegal is to limit its use. In the case of cannabis, there continues to be a gradual weakening of the legal sanctions against its use in many Western countries. That most of the countries that have reduced the legal consequences for cannabis use have not reported significant increases in the prevalence of cannabis use strengthens the argument that legal sanctions do little to limit the amount of cannabis used in a society. Furthermore, the legal consequences of cannabis use in many countries comprise one of the more important harms of cannabis use, and encourage a focus on the moral issues rather than the health consequences of cannabis use.

> → Education about general life skills appears to be more effective at preventing cannibis-related harm than education specifically directed at providing information about the nature of cannabis.
> → Early intervention comprises the early identification of, and intervention with, individuals predisposed to problematic cannabis use.
> → Early intervention may be more effective than education.
> → Legal sanctions are relatively ineffective in preventing cannabis-related harms.

Case study

Matthew, who is 22 years old, attends your general practice with vague concerns about his health and well-being. He is accompanied by his mother, who is also worried about him. He has been studying part-time at university while working in a bakery. He says that he has noticed that he feels run-down and that his energy levels are low; he is falling behind with his assignments, and he is in danger of failing a term. There is no past history of psychiatric illness, and his family is known to you as healthy individuals.

You perform an examination and a series of blood tests, but these reveal no abnormality. You also screen for a depressive illness; this reveals some minor symptoms, but no safety concerns.

A week later Matthew returns, this time by himself. He appears somewhat sleepy, is unshaven, and has hyperaemic conjunctivae but reactive and normal-sized pupils. His movements are clumsy, and sometimes exaggerated and over-deliberate. He is also slow in answering some questions, and tends to wander off the topic of conversation, but he is easily brought back to the item being discussed. Some of his replies are fatuous and irrelevant.

You consider that he is intoxicated and has self-administered a drug prior to his visit to the surgery, so you ask an open question relating his current presentation to the last time he was seen at the surgery, when he came with his mother. Matthew tells you that he has just had a bucket bong of cannabis with his work colleagues at the bakery at the end of the early morning shift. You inform Matthew that his blood tests were normal, but ask him to make an extended appointment within the next few days to discuss his health further.

At the next appointment Matthew talks openly about his cannabis use, saying he is ashamed of the effects that it is having on him and doesn't want his parents to find out. With careful questioning it is apparent that his cannabis smoking started at the age of 15 years, and he remained an occasional recreational user until he started at university and moved out of home. He prefers the intoxication of cannabis to alcohol, mainly because there is little hangover the morning after heavy use. When he smokes through the forced inhalation of a bucket bong he has a tendency to become mildly suspicious of other people and has a feeling of being out of control. He has tried other drugs such as LSD and ecstasy, but these are not currently used. He recognises that he is smoking cannabis too much, but whenever he has stopped he feels very uncomfortable, labile in mood, and cannot sleep soundly; this, in turn, impairs his work and study. Resumption of his cannabis use restores the status quo, but also contributes to his lack of energy and impairs his memory. His consumption has increased markedly after he began working with heavy smokers at the bakery, and he now smokes a minimum of five pipes a day, starting the first thing in the morning.

You consider that Matthew is at an ambivalent stage, but is preparing to make changes, so you begin to discuss with him whether he is motivated to reducing or stopping his cannabis use. You point out in further discussion with Matthew that he is responsible for changing his cannabis use, but that his health deterioration is likely to be related at least in part to his heavy cannabis use. Matthew is pleased that he has been able to talk openly about his drug use, and decides that he is determined to stop smoking cannabis, at least for a period of time.

With Matthew, you review the situations when he is most vulnerable to smoking, and possible action he can take. There is a process of reinforcing the reasons that stopping drug use is beneficial at this time. A simple contract is agreed, and a quit date is set. He finds the first day of not using relatively easy, but on the second day he cannot sleep soundly. He arranges an appointment with you the following day, and, as you agree that lack of sleep is a major problem, you prescribe 15 mg zopiclone for three nights. You acknowledge that Matthew has taken a difficult step, and help him to continue planning for high-risk situations. There are a couple of minor relapses, but with your support and the support of his family, Matthew remains abstinent from cannabis for one month, and subsequently resumes a pattern of intermittent (approximately weekly) use.

Case points

- Matthew was unwilling to mention his drug use with his mother present.
- The presentation was for health reasons and throughout the interviews there is no mention of labelling his drug use, but you are aware that he fulfils the criteria for dependency on cannabis.
- Matthew's health complaints are taken seriously, and you endeavour to exclude serious physical illness.
- Matthew's second presentation has many of the hallmarks of cannabis intoxication. During acute intoxication it is generally unrealistic to embark on a complex therapeutic plan, so another appointment is made to see the patient when he is not acutely intoxicated. If necessary this can be stated directly.
- Matthew's readiness to address his use is assessed (see chapter 7), Matthew would be considered to be contemplating changing his cannabis use, and preparing, with the help from his GP and the practice nurse, to proceed to the action phase.
- FLAGS is a useful acronym to consider when embarking on charging a person's behaviour. Feedback on risks or impairments due to cannibis

use; **L**isten to a patient's concerns regarding their use and possible reduction in use; **A**dvise patients about the consequence of continued cannabis use; **G**oals of intervention should be defined (in Matthew's case to stopping cannabis use for a short period); **S**trategies for treatment are discussed and implemented (in Matthew's case this involves the identification of risk situations and how to cope, as well as a number of items listed below) (see chapters 5 and 10).

- As with cessation of tobacco smoking, setting a quit date can be useful, as can drawing up a simple contract to clarify roles and goals of treatment.
- Symptomatic relief can be a useful adjunct to treatment if withdrawal symptoms are recognised (and problematic). In this case a short supply of a sedative–hypnotic to assist with sleep was prescribed.
- A realistic follow-up period is required, and an expectation that relapses are not uncommon but do not necessarily mean failure.

REFERENCES AND FURTHER READING

Ashton, C.H. 2001, 'Pharmacology and effects of cannabis: a brief review', *British Journal of Psychiatry*, vol. 178, pp. 101–6.

Fant, R.V., Heishman, S.J., Bunker, E.B. & Pickworth, W.B. 1998, 'Acute and residual effects of marijuana in humans', *Pharmacology, Biochemistry and Behavior*, vol. 60, pp. 777–84.

Fergusson, D. & Horwood, L.J. 2000, 'Cannabis use and dependence in a New Zealand birth cohort', *New Zealand Medical Journal*, vol. 113, pp. 156–8.

Hall, W. & Solowij, N. 1998, 'Adverse effects of cannabis', *Lancet*, vol. 352, pp. 1611–16.

Hollister, L.E. 1998, 'Health aspects of cannabis: Revisited', *International Journal of Neuropsychopharmacology*, vol. 1, pp. 71–80.

Johns, A. 2001, 'Psychiatric effects of cannabis', *British Journal of Psychiatry*, vol. 178, pp. 116–22.

10

Alcohol

Olga Lopatko, Stuart McLean, John Saunders, Ross Young,
Geoff Robinson & Katherine Conigrave

No animal ever invented anything so bad as drunkenness—or so good as drink.

G.K. Chesterton 1908, 'Wine when it is red', in *All Things Considered.*

Alcohol is the common name of ethyl alcohol, or ethanol. Alcoholic beverages are made by yeast fermentation of sugars from different plant sources to give a variety of drinks. The alcoholic strength (expressed by volume) varies from about 2 to 5% for beers to 10 to 15% for table wines and, after distillation, 35 to 55% for spirits. Other constituents (congeners) contribute to the flavour. The principal effects of alcoholic beverages are attributable to the amount of alcohol consumed. Usual serving volumes contain approximately 10 g alcohol, termed a 'standard drink'.

Compared to most other drugs, alcohol has a very low potency, and the large doses consequently required to produce its effects are relevant to its toxicity and elimination.

PHARMACODYNAMICS

CNS effects

The effects of alcohol vary with the concentration of alcohol in blood, prior use of alcohol, genetic susceptibility, and the situation. Blood alcohol concentration (BAC) is usually expressed in grams of alcohol per 100 mL of blood (g% or simply %). For example, 50 mg of alcohol per 100 mL of blood is a BAC of 0.05%. Because of the effects of tolerance and other factors, only a general guide can be given on the effects of different BACs (below and table 10.1). At low blood concentrations (around 0.05%) in non-dependent individuals, alcohol causes mild euphoria and stimulates behaviour (from sociability to aggression), possibly via the release of noradrenaline and dopamine, and gives pleasure through the release of dopamine and endogenous opioids. Alcohol also impairs performance, especially of complex tasks that require divided or sustained attention. At higher concentrations (>0.10%) this impairment becomes more noticeable and causes ataxia and slurred speech. Reaction time slows, and the attention wanders. Amnesia can occur at even higher concentrations (>0.15%), and above 0.25% alcohol produces a profound depression leading to, progressively, coma, respiratory failure, and death, at concentrations above 0.3%.

Table 10.1 Effects of different BACs in non-dependent individuals

BAC	Effect
0.02 to 0.03%	Slight increases in talkativeness; relaxation
0.05%	Impairment in some tasks requiring skill
0.06 to 0.10%	Very talkative; speech is louder, acts and feels self-confident. Less cautious and inhibited than usual. Slowed reaction time.
0.20%	Sedated rather than active, may be sleepy. Impairment now includes slurred speech, clumsiness, reduced responsiveness, and marked intellectual impairment. Amnesia.
0.30 to 0.40%	Semiconscious or unconscious. Body functions are beginning to break down. Fatalities occur at and above these concentrations.

Alcohol enhances the effects of the inhibitory neurotransmitter GABA at the GABA-A receptor. GABA opens the chloride channel associated with the GABA-A receptor, allowing chloride ions to enter the neurone, thereby reducing its excitability. By acting via GABA-mediated mechanisms, alcohol produces anxiolytic, muscle relaxant, and sedative effects. Benzodiazepines and barbiturates act at other receptor sites on the GABA-A chloride channel, enhancing the binding of GABA (see chapter 11). In addition to its effects on GABA-ergic systems, alcohol inhibits the excitatory transmitter glutamate through an action on the NMDA receptor subtype. Alcohol blocks the NMDA-linked calcium channel, preventing the influx of calcium ions, which normally activate neurones. This NMDA receptor blockade is thought to contribute to the amnesic and cerebral depressant effects of alcohol.

Stimulation of 5-HT$_3$ receptors has also been implicated in both the pleasure and nausea produced by alcohol. As mentioned above, alcohol stimulates dopamine and opioid systems. The mechanism is not known, but it may be an indirect effect mediated by GABA-ergic or other direct actions.

> Alcohol is a central nervous system depressant.
>
> ➡ The acute effects of alcohol vary with the concentration of alcohol in blood, prior use of alcohol, genetic susceptibility, and the situation (that is, the psychosocial environment).

Other effects

Alcohol dilates blood vessels, producing a feeling of warmth but a loss of body heat. It is an irritant to the gastrointestinal tract, and through various metabolic effects chronic heavy consumption damages the liver and other organs. However, moderate consumption is associated with a reduced risk of coronary heart disease (see below).

PHARMACOKINETICS

Absorption

The ethanol molecule is small and highly water-soluble. It is absorbed from the stomach, small intestine and colon. Absorption may be so rapid that an alcohol effect is felt within a few minutes, or it may be relatively slow, with a gradual rise in BAC over a period of several hours. The overall rate of absorption of ingested alcohol depends on the speed of transit through the stomach (or gastric emptying time). This is because rate of absorption is slow in the stomach, but much higher in the small intestine. If, for example, gastric emptying time is delayed by food, absorption is slowed and the peak BAC will be lower and later than when the same dose of alcohol is taken on an empty stomach (figure 10.1).

The speed of absorption is also affected by the nature of the alcoholic beverage. For example, drinking concentrated beverages (containing up to 30% alcohol) without dilution results in rapid absorption. However, stronger drinks such as spirits (40% alcohol and higher) cause irritation of the gastric mucosa and pyloric spasm, and delay stomach emptying. On the other hand, carbonated beverages neutralise the hydrochloric acid of gastric juice, and speed up stomach emptying.

Although some alcohol is metabolised in the gut and liver during the absorption phase, this accounts for <10% of usual doses.

Distribution

Alcohol distributes rapidly throughout body water, readily crossing the blood–brain and placental barriers. The concentration in blood and other tissues depends on the size of the body's water compartment because alcohol has a low lipid–water partition coefficient. The body water content depends on body weight and composition. In general, females have a smaller proportion of body water than males (about 53%

Figure 10.1 The effect of food on speed of alcohol absorption. Equal volumes (237 mL) of tap water, light cream or glucose (80 g dissolved in water) were given to 14 healthy male volunteers followed 10 minutes later by 45 mL of 95% ethanol mixed with 105 mL of orange juice. Adopted from Sedman et al. (1976).

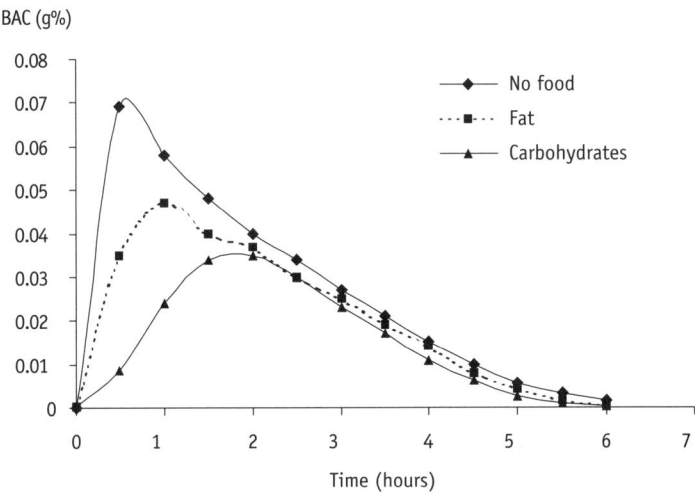

versus 62%), and body water declines with age. Consequently, after drinking the same amount of alcohol, women tend to have higher BACs than men, being both smaller and having a lower proportion of body water.

Metabolism

Approximately 90% of alcohol ingested is metabolised. Alcohol is oxidised sequentially to acetaldehyde and acetic acid, providing energy (29.7 kJ/g ethanol) that can account for half the energy intake in alcohol-dependent patients.

$$CH_3CH_2OH \quad \rightarrow \quad CH_3CHO \quad \rightarrow \quad CH_3COOH$$

ethyl alcohol   acetaldehyde   acetic acid

Two enzymes catalyse the first metabolic step: the cytosolic alcohol dehydrogenase (ADH) and the microsomal enzyme cytochrome P450 2E1 (CYP2E1).

The major pathway of alcohol metabolism is via ADH. Alcohol has a very high affinity for this enzyme, and ADH is saturated even at low alcohol concentrations. This results in a relatively constant rate of metabolism (zero-order kinetics) over a wide range of concentrations. The average rate of alcohol metabolism is approximately 7.5 g/hour.

The microsomal ethanol oxidising system that involves CYP2E1 plays only a minor role in alcohol elimination for most drinkers, but may become important at high BACs. The amount (and activity) of CYP2E1 is increased (induced) by chronic alcohol consumption, and for this reason the enzyme may play a significant role in alcohol elimination in patients with alcohol dependence. This induction can also increase metabolism of other drugs metabolised by CYP2E1.

Both pathways use NAD^+ as a cofactor, and the resulting decrease in the ratio $NAD^+/NADH$ contributes to the adverse metabolic effects of alcohol dependence, such as acidosis. Metabolism via both pathways occurs mostly in the liver, but the enzymes are also present in other body tissues, including the stomach lining and lung parenchyma. The activity of gastric ADH in women is lower than in men. In part, this can explain higher BACs observed in women than in men after consuming similar amounts of ethanol, even after correction for body size. The activity of this enzyme is significantly decreased in alcohol-dependent patients, although it may return to normal levels after a period of abstinence, in patients with *Helicobacter pylori* and/or chronic active gastritis, and in elderly men.

The second step of alcohol metabolism (that is, the oxidation of acetaldehyde to form acetic acid) is catalysed by aldehyde dehydrogenase (ALDH), and is usually so rapid that little acetaldehyde accumulates. The toxicity of acetaldehyde is dramatically evident when ALDH is inhibited by disulfiram, a drug used as an aversive agent in patients recovering from alcohol dependence (relapse prevention). In the presence of disulfiram, even a small amount of alcohol results in a distressing syndrome that includes flushing, tachycardia, hyperventilation, and headache. Even without this disulfiram effect the normally low concentrations of acetaldehyde have been implicated in the toxicity of alcohol, as acetaldehyde binds to proteins and inhibits enzymes, and also initiates immune reactions.

All three enzymes (ADH, CYP2EI, and ALDH) exhibit polymorphisms (inherited differences in structure and function). The frequency of occurrence of genes for the different forms of the enzymes (isozymes) varies between ethnic groups. For example, the ADH2★3 isozyme, which is relatively common amongst African Americans, results in faster metabolism of alcohol than the usual ADH2★1 form. Among Japanese and other Asians, there is a high prevalence of the ALDH2★2 isozyme, resulting in slow metabolism of acetaldehyde which then accumulates after alcohol ingestion, causing flushing, headache, and other effects (see chapter 2).

BAC and rate of elimination

The rate of elimination of alcohol can be followed by measuring the fall in blood alcohol concentration (BAC) with time. Metabolism due to the actions of ADH is saturated at about 3 mM (0.014%), resulting in an approximately constant rate of elimination (V_{max}) at higher BACs. Ingestion of grams of alcohol usually result in a BAC of about 0.02%. The rate of alcohol elimination is about 7.5 g/hour. Therefore, BAC decreases with an average rate (V_{max}) of about 0.015% per hour.

Approximate BACs can be calculated using the following formula:

BAC = (0.02 × number of standard drinks consumed) − (0.015 × number of hours)

For example, someone who drinks two standard drinks every hour will have BAC of 0.075% at the end of a three-hour drinking bout [BAC = (0.02×6) − $(0.015 \times 3) = 0.12 − 0.045 = 0.075$]. Two hours after finishing drinking, the person's BAC will be down to 0.045%. The exact figure will vary according to a range of factors, including body weight, body composition, sex, history of alcohol consumption, and food intake.

There is a two-fold variability in V_{max} (0.01–0.02% per hour) in the population. Women have a faster rate of elimination than men, having a proportionally larger liver volume relative to lean body mass. People with alcohol dependence also have faster elimination rates, as a result of CYP2E1 induction.

Alcohol diffuses very rapidly from blood to alveolar air. The BAC can be conveniently measured by breath analysis, using the equilibrium blood : air distribution ratio of 2100 : 1. Errors can arise from mouth alcohol if measurements are made within 10 minutes of drinking.

MECHANISMS OF ALCOHOL DEPENDENCE AND WITHDRAWAL

Tolerance and physical dependence

Regular intake of alcohol results in the development of tolerance, with larger amounts of alcohol required to produce the same degree of intoxication. Tolerance develops in parallel with physical dependence, and most of the mechanisms are likely to be common to both. The presence of physical dependence is retrospectively established by a number of physiological and psychological disturbances (the withdrawal syndrome) that occur when alcohol intake is stopped.

Pharmacokinetic (metabolic) tolerance

Tolerance to alcohol may be to some extent attributed to metabolic tolerance as the second metabolic pathway (CYP2E1) is induced by heavy or prolonged alcohol intake, resulting in faster oxidation of alcohol in the liver.

Pharmacodynamic (functional) tolerance

The major cause of tolerance is the change in sensitivity of the CNS to alcohol action (functional tolerance). The various mechanisms underlying tolerance to and physical dependence on alcohol are not fully understood, but below are some of the possible neuronal mechanisms.

GABA-A receptor
While acute alcohol administration results in an enhancement of GABA-A receptor activity and increases Cl⁻ flux, chronic alcohol exposure causes a reduction in GABA-A receptor function and a decrease in Cl⁻ flux. GABA-A receptors become gradually less sensitive to the acute effect of alcohol as well as to the effects of other

drugs acting as GABA-A receptors (including benzodiazepines and barbiturates), a condition known as cross-tolerance.

Tolerance to alcohol develops very rapidly. Animal studies have demonstrated that tolerance to alcohol may appear after a single administration of alcohol. The decreased modulation of the GABA-A receptor by alcohol is thought to be the major mechanism of the acute or rapid tolerance to this drug. Changes in GABA-A receptors most likely result in a diminished effect of alcohol on motor coordination and locomotor activity, and a reduction in its sedating and anxiolytic actions.

NMDA receptors

Chronic alcohol ingestion results in adaptation of NMDA receptors to the initial ethanol-induced inhibition of their function. As the effect of alcohol is inhibitory at these receptors the adaptation is an up-regulation and an ultimate increase in their function (that is, an increase in intracellular Ca^{2+}). The number of NMDA receptors increases, but the structure and the properties of the receptors appear to be unchanged. It has been suggested that this increase in the number of NMDA receptors results in tolerance to alcohol-induced motor impairment and hypothermia.

Serotonin receptors

There is some evidence for the involvement of serotonergic systems in alcohol tolerance and dependence. Depletion of serotonergic systems delays the development of tolerance to the motor-impairing and hypothermic effects of alcohol, and slows the development of environment-dependent tolerance.

Vasopressin receptors

Vasopressin receptors affect the rate of loss of tolerance. Endogenous vasopressin is required to maintain tolerance to alcohol. Blockade of these receptors increases the rate of loss of tolerance. Moreover, tolerance does not develop in rats genetically deficient in vasopressin.

Voltage-gated Ca²⁺ channels (VGCC)

Chronic alcohol intake produces an increase in activity of VGCCs. However, the up-regulation of these receptors may not represent an adaptation to the direct inhibitory effect of high concentrations of alcohol, but, rather, a response to alcohol-induced increases in intracellular calcium levels (via other mechanisms) that then block inward calcium flux. The decreased inward calcium flux causes an up-regulation of VGCCs with chronic use.

This receptor up-regulation is thought to contribute to the development of tolerance to the motor incoordinating and other effects of alcohol. It has been shown that VGCC blockers (such as nifedipine, nitrendipine) reduce alcohol tolerance in animal models and block withdrawal seizures.

Alcohol withdrawal syndrome

Just as alcohol intake depresses the nervous system, alcohol withdrawal produces over-excitation of the nervous system. Neuroadaptation to the effects of chronic alcohol use results in decreased activity of inhibitory receptors (GABA-A) and up-regulation of excitatory receptors (NMDA) as well as up-regulation of voltage-gated Ca^{2+} channels. This compensatory hyperactivity leads to a profound hyperexcitability of CNS once alcohol intake is stopped or reduced, and gives rise to the withdrawal symptoms. The severity and duration of withdrawal depend upon the intake level and duration of the preceding period of drinking.

> ➡ When alcohol intake is abruptly stopped or reduced, over-excitability of the CNS becomes pathologically evident (the withdrawal syndrome) as the adaptive neuronal changes are no longer counteracted by alcohol.

Hangover

A mild acute withdrawal (or hangover) can develop following a single intoxicating dose of alcohol or a single short period of drinking (for example during one evening), and is manifested in headache, nausea, tremulousness, and lethargy. Dehydration and sleep disturbances may contribute significantly to the pathophysiology of hangover.

Minor withdrawal syndrome and withdrawal seizures

Many chronic alcohol users begin to experience tremors ('the shakes') within 24 hours after their last drink (usually five to 10 hours after a decrease in alcohol intake or following a night's sleep). Often tremor is accompanied with tachycardia, hypertension, sweating, nausea, diarrhoea, decreased appetite, anxiety, restlessness, headache, difficulty sleeping, and bad dreams. Most patients do not develop all the symptoms. The syndrome peaks on days two to three of abstinence, and the major symptoms subside by day four or five or within a week. Some of the symptoms, however, persist (see the discussion of protracted withdrawal below).

For some individuals the symptoms of withdrawal can become quite severe. After chronic drinking for many weeks or months, a reduction of alcohol intake or abrupt cessation of alcohol use can result in a two-stage withdrawal. One to three days after their last drink, patients can have a generalised seizure. Withdrawal seizures occur in 15% of withdrawing chronic alcohol users, most commonly during the first 48 hours. These are typically of grand mal type, self-limited, with from one to four seizures occurring. They can be an indication of a major withdrawal syndrome.

Major withdrawal syndrome (delirium tremens)

About three to ten days after their last drink, patients can suffer from agitation, disorientation, high fevers and sweating, paranoia, and visual hallucinations. This major withdrawal syndrome is called delirium tremens. It develops in 5% or fewer patients with chronic alcohol problems, and is rarely seen in patients under 30. In most cases the patient has a history of chronic heavy drinking for at least five years, and a recent episode of drinking to intoxication of two or more weeks duration. The symptoms may last from a few hours to two weeks, and be of varying severity. Delirium tremens is a serious medical emergency. Before aggressive modern medical treatment, 15% of patients with this syndrome did not survive. Now, with adequate medication and nutritional support, fatalities from delirium tremens are rare.

> Alcohol withdrawal can be life-threatening. Delirium tremens is a serious medical emergency.

Protracted withdrawal

Research into the protracted withdrawal syndrome, also known as protracted abstinence or late withdrawal, is in the very early stages. There is a lack of agreement on distinctive signs and symptoms and the duration of the syndrome. The usual withdrawal symptoms (see above) are most severe in the first five days following the last drink, but have also been reported to persist for weeks and months (for example six months or longer) following cessation of drinking. Some of the purported symptoms include anxiety, irritability, hostility, depression, insomnia, fatigue, and craving. These persistent mental health disturbances may result in relapse drinking.

> Protracted alcohol withdrawal may be the major trigger for relapse.

A majority of symptoms have been shown to decrease progressively with prolonged abstinence, approximating normal levels for subjects abstinent 10 years or more. It is often difficult to distinguish symptoms caused by alcohol withdrawal from those caused by a patient's underlying mental disorder, if one is present. The signs and symptoms of protracted withdrawal are therefore not as predictable as those of acute withdrawal. Some patients may be predisposed to protracted withdrawal.

Reinforcement

A compulsive desire to use alcohol is in part attributed to its strong reinforcing properties. In those people who are physically dependent, alcohol consumption is reinforced by avoidance and relief of withdrawal symptoms. However, its more general rewarding effects include a mild euphoria and an anxiolytic effect. Specific brain circuits mediate the reinforcing effects of alcohol. A complex, negative feedback system within the mesolimbic dopamine system, also called the brain reward system (ventral tegmental area, nucleus accumbens, central nucleus of the amygdala, and prefrontal cortex), is involved in the regulation of alcohol consumption (see chapter 2). The reinforcing effects of alcohol are mediated by the interaction of multiple neurotransmitters, with dopamine and opioid systems playing major roles in reward. Exactly how these systems are activated by alcohol, and the role of GABA-A and NMDA receptors in this activation, is yet to be determined.

Dopamine

A number of studies in both humans and animals have supported the role of dopamine systems in alcohol reinforcement. Alcohol increases the firing of dopamine neurones in the ventral tegmental area, and the release of dopamine in nucleus accumbens. The alcohol-induced euphoria and stimulant effect in humans is antagonised, and craving for alcohol in chronic users is reduced, by drugs that block the synthesis of catecholamines and deplete brain dopamine. The effects of alcohol on dopamine release may be modulated by brain serotonergic systems.

Opioids

There is some evidence that acute alcohol administration increases the release of β-endorphin and enhances opioid activity, and this may play a role in the reinforcing effects of ethanol. Opioid receptor antagonists (for example naltrexone) decrease alcohol intake in both animals and humans, reduce the high produced by alcohol, and reduce the number of relapses.

Low basal levels of endogenous opioids may play a role in predisposition to the development of alcohol dependence. It has been documented that patients with a family history of chronic alcohol abuse have low basal level of opioids, and that animals with genetic predisposition to high alcohol self-administration have low levels of opioid activity.

> ➭ Low basal levels of endogenous opioids may play a role in predisposition to the development of alcohol dependence.

ACUTE AND CHRONIC ALCOHOL TOXICITY

Toxic effects of acute alcohol administration

Central nervous system

Simple acute intoxication
Simple acute intoxication has been described in the previous section.

Acute alcohol hallucinosis (or alcoholic paranoia)
Auditory and olfactory hallucinations, illusions, and/or paranoid ideation may occur following a prolonged drinking bout, in the absence of any obvious signs of

withdrawal. Patients often experience significant anxiety and depression. They are orientated in time, place, and person, and have a perfect memory for the psychotic episode upon recovery.

Pathological or idiosyncratic alcohol intoxication

In some people, small doses of alcohol (one or two standard drinks) may induce a sudden profound intoxication with visual hallucinations, disorientation, delusions and confusion that lasts from minutes to hours. Severe agitation and hyperactivity, aggressiveness, and violence are common, but depression and suicidal attempts may also occur. This pathological or idiosyncratic alcohol intoxication results in a long deep sleep with amnesia for the episode afterwards. This phenomenon is extremely rare, and is seen almost exclusively in patients with pre-existing severe brain damage.

Blackouts

The term 'blackout' refers to an inability to recall events that occurred while intoxicated. Blackouts are common among alcohol abusers. About two-thirds of alcohol-dependent patients report experiencing blackouts. Blackouts have been considered an early high-risk indicator of alcohol dependence. However, it is now clear that blackouts are also relatively common among non-dependent drinkers, especially among young binge drinkers.

> Frequent binge drinking is usually defined as three or more occasions per two-week period in which six or more drinks are consumed per occasion for males, or four or more drinks are consumed per occasion for females.

Over half (approximately 55%) of those characterised as frequent binge drinkers indicate that they had failed to recall events that occurred while intoxicated. The complete blackout is most likely to occur at blood alcohol concentrations of 0.25% and above.

> Although blackouts may be an important warning sign of problem drinking, they are not sensitive indicators of the risk of developing chronic alcohol dependence.

Sleep disturbances

Alcohol is commonly seen as aiding sleep. While it may induce sleep, alcohol also leads to increased wakefulness and arousal several hours later, and it exacerbates sleep disorders. It is well documented that acute and chronic alcohol consumption cause sleep disturbances. In those with a history of alcohol dependence, sleep patterns may never return to normal, and continuing sleep problems may be a core factor in alcohol relapse. Alcohol's disruptive effects on sleep can cause impaired breathing (sleep apnoea), and are often associated with excessive daytime sleepiness. The latter can result in memory deficits, impaired social and occupational function, and increased risk of car accidents.

While sleep disturbances have been described in patients with alcohol dependence during active drinking and during different stages of recovery, little is known about the underlying biological mechanisms. Serotonin has a prominent role in the regulation of certain aspects of REM sleep and the modulation of onset of non-REM sleep. A number of studies have shown that serotonin dysfunction is involved in alcohol-induced sleep disorders. NMDA antagonists reduce REM sleep frequency in rats in a manner similar to ethanol, implicating glutamate as a selective modulator of sleep.

Alcohol overdose

Profound intoxication with anaesthesia or coma is likely at blood alcohol concentrations of 0.25% and above. Lethal blood levels range from 0.3 to 0.5% in humans, although some highly tolerant drinkers survive these high concentrations. Death occurs as a result of a severe depression of the respiratory centre in the medulla.

Drugs that potentiate or add to the respiratory depressant effect of alcohol and increase the risk of alcohol overdose are:

→ barbiturates and other sedatives
→ benzodiazepines
→ phenothiazines (both antihistamines and antipsychotics)
→ opioids
→ antihistamines.

Cardiovascular system

In healthy individuals alcohol, in a dose equivalent to three to six standard drinks (30 to 60 g), decreases myocardial contractility and causes peripheral vasodilation of central origin (at the level of the thermoregulatory centre in the preoptic area and anterior hypothalamus). This effect results in a mild drop in blood pressure and produces compensatory increases in the activity of the sympathetic nervous system. The latter results in an increase in heart rate and cardiac output. As a result, blood pressure may rise (systolic more than diastolic).

Cardiac oxygen consumption is higher after alcohol intake, especially during exercise, which may lead to acute heart attack in patients with pre-existing coronary heart disease.

Large doses of alcohol consumed over a short period of time (binge drinking) may cause atrial or ventricular arrythmias, especially paroxysmal tachycardia, a syndrome known as the 'holiday heart'.

Gastrointestinal system

Acute alcohol intake can cause acute oesophagitis (secondary). Patients may present with anorexia and abdominal pain. A direct toxic effect of alcohol on the gastric mucosa causing interruption of the gastric mucosal barrier is likely to be due to its lipophilic and lipolytic properties. Direct damage of small mucosal vessels leads to subepithelial haemorrhages with surrounding oedema. This may result in gastrointestinal bleeding in heavy drinkers. Beer and wine stimulate secretion of gastric acid, possibly as a result of the effects of congeners. Ethanol itself is a weak stimulant of acid secretion.

Alcohol can produce haemorrhagic lesions of the duodenal villi, increase small bowel motility, decrease water and electrolyte absorption in the small intestine, and cause diarrhoea.

Haematopoietic system

Days to weeks of heavy drinking cause a reversible increase in red blood cell size (mean corpuscular volume), mild anaemia and leucocytopenia, reticulocytopenia and hyperplastic bone marrow. Alcohol may cause mild thrombocytopenia, decrease platelet aggregation, and inhibit release of thromboxane A_2. All these changes may return to normal within a week of abstinence.

> ➡ Excessive alcohol use, acute or chronic, affects a wide range of body systems.

Effects of chronic alcohol administration

Chronic alcohol use may affect almost every body system. The majority of these effects are detrimental, although some effects of low doses have been shown to be beneficial. The regular consumption of two drinks per day for men and one drink per day for women has been shown to decrease risk of atherosclerosis and associated disorders (for example coronary heart disease, ischaemic stroke, and peripheral vascular disease). The primary mechanisms accounting for these beneficial effects are the increased circulating concentrations of high-density lipoprotein cholesterol and inhibition of blood coagulation. A number of other chronic and acute disorders (intestinal tract infections, duodenal ulcer, gallstones, rheumatoid arthritis, osteoporosis, and type II diabetes mellitus) have been shown to be beneficially modulated by low-level alcohol consumption. Flavonoids present in red wine bring additional benefits by preventing oxidative damage, free radical formation, and elements of the inflammatory response.

It has been suggested further that low-level alcohol users have decreased incidence of anxiety and depression, lower absenteeism from work, improved cognitive functions, and decreased incidence of dementia (including Alzheimer's disease) when compared with abstainers. However, the data available to date regarding these protective effects of low alcohol doses on CNS function are contradictory. More research is needed to confirm or refute these long-term effects of alcohol.

> Regular consumption of two drinks per day for men and one drink per day for women decreases risk of atherosclerosis and associated disorders.

The major toxic and beneficial effects and their mechanisms (where known) are listed in table 10.2.

Concurrent psychiatric problems

Epidemiological and clinical studies have confirmed high comorbidity of chronic alcohol dependence with mental disorders. Many alcohol-dependent patients have coexisting anxiety disorders (about 25%), depression (20 to 40%), and occasionally alcohol-induced hallucinosis. Psychiatric disorders may predispose to alcohol dependence (self-medication hypothesis), but they may also result from chronic abuse of alcohol. Alcohol abuse has been shown to worsen the course of existing psychiatric disorders. However, levels of 'at risk' consumption of alcohol in psychiatric disorders have not been well defined. Light to moderate alcohol consumption has no documented positive effect on the course. Depression usually diminishes with abstinence from alcohol, but may take many months or even years to resolve. Alcohol-dependent patients often have suicidal ideations. One-fifth to one-third of the increased death rate among alcohol-dependent users is explained by suicide. Interpersonal loss within six weeks before suicide is more frequent in alcohol-dependent than in nonalcohol-dependent suicide victims.

ASSESSMENT AND DIAGNOSIS

It is vital for diagnosis and effective management of a wide variety of clinical presentations to consider the possibility that a patient has an underlying alcohol problem. This is especially true given the fact that 15 to 30% of patients seen in general practice have hazardous, harmful, or dependent alcohol use, and 30% or more of patients admitted to hospital are in the same category.

General principles of assessment

A comprehensive alcohol history consists of a series of questions addressing three fundamental issues:
1. the level, frequency and pattern of alcohol consumption
2. symptoms of alcohol dependence, and
3. physical, psychological, and social problems related to drinking.

> It takes approximately 15–20 minutes to elicit an alcohol history in a patient with a drinking problem, but only three to five minutes (and frequently much less) in other patients.

In many consultations it will be appropriate to elicit the drinking history as soon as an alcohol problem is suspected. Alternatively, it is often convenient, and acceptable to patients, if the enquiry about drinking is included with other lifestyle issues such as

171

Table 10.2 Effects of chronic alcohol consumption

Disorder	Symptoms	Mechanisms	Reversibility
Central nervous system *Nutritional problems*			
Wernicke–Korsakoff syndrome		Thiamine deficiency as a result of chronic excessive drinking, possibly together with genetic transketolase deficiency	
Wernicke's disease (acute phase of the syndrome)	Nystagmus or sixth nerve palsy, ataxia, and confusion	Necrotic lesions of mammillary bodies, thalamus, and other areas of brainstem	Reversible, with thiamine therapy
Korsakoff psychosis (chronic phase of the syndrome)	Short-term memory loss (anterograde and retrograde amnesia), confabulation, normal intelligence quotient	Progression of the above	Usually incomplete: only one quarter of patients make full recovery, half make partial recovery, and one quarter of cases are irreversible
Direct toxic effect			
Severe cognitive and memory problems	Long-term impairment of psycho-motor performance and short-term memory (for example blackouts)	May develop in chronic users after an acute alcoholic binge	Improve with abstinence, but long-term memory problems may persist

Table 10.2 Effects of chronic alcohol consumption

Disorder	Symptoms	Mechanisms	Reversibility
Central nervous system *Direct toxic effect*			
Sleep disturbances	Poor sleep efficiency; frequent awakenings; shortened rapid eye movement (REM) periods; reduced non-REM sleep	Possible mechanisms: serotonin and/or NMDA receptor/ neurotransmitter dysfunction; disruption of hormonal and behavioural circadian rhythms in humans	Reversible, but may take years of abstinence to improve; may be irreversible in some cases
Alcoholic dementia	No single syndrome; irreversible cognitive changes with history of chronic alcohol abuse	Possibly a combination of a direct chronic effect of ethanol and nutritional deficiency	Irreversible
Cerebellar atrophy	Ataxia of stance and gait, mild nystagmus	A combination of a direct chronic effect of ethanol and thiamine deficiency; degeneration of all the neurocellular elements of cerebellar cortex, particularly of Purkinje cells in vermis and anterior cerebellar lobes	Improvement in some cases
Cerebral cortical atrophy		Cortical neuronal loss	Reversible in some cases

Table 10.2 Effects of chronic alcohol consumption

Disorder	Symptoms	Mechanisms	Reversibility
Peripheral nervous system			
Peripheral neuropathy	Bilateral limb numbness, paraesthesias, mainly distal	Combination of a direct effect of ethanol and thiamine deficiency	Reversible or partially reversible
Cardiovascular system			
Cardiomyopathy	Symptoms range from unexplained arrythmias to heart failure with dilation of all four heart chambers and low contractility of heart muscle	Direct toxic effect of alcohol: at least 80 g/day over a period of years is necessary to produce cardiomyopathy	Reversible in early disease, high degree of recovery in advanced disease with total abstinence
Hypertension	Increase in blood pressure	30 grams of alcohol a day or more leads to a dose-dependent increase in blood pressure; chronic corticosteroid and catecholamine excess or action through the renin–angiotensin system may be involved	Blood pressure may decrease or return to normal within weeks of abstinence
Strokes	High blood pressure in alcohol-dependent patients increases risk of both haemorrhagic and ischaemic strokes		

Table 10.2   Effects of chronic alcohol consumption

Disorder	Symptoms	Mechanisms	Reversibility
Ischaemic stroke		Alcohol increases plasma high density lipoprotein cholesterol; low levels of alcohol consumption (10–20 g/day) may decrease risk	
Haemorrhagic stroke		Alcohol decreases blood clotting by (a) inhibiting thromboxane production and platelet aggregation, (b) enhancing clot lysis by inducing tissue plasminogen activator thereby increasing risk of stroke. Heavy drinking increases risk of stroke within 24 hours of drinking.	
Coronary artery disease		Alcohol reduces risk at low levels of consumption (10–20 g/day) by increasing plasma high-density lipo protein cholesterol (HDL–C) and decreasing blood clotting (see above). Higher levels are likely to increase blood pressure and predispose to coronary artery disease or a sudden cardiac death. Alcohol-induced increase in HDL–C decreases within weeks if drinking is stopped.	
Peripheral vascular disease		Alcohol reduces risk at low levels of consumption (10–20 g/day) by increasing plasma high-density lipo protein cholesterol (HDL–C) and decreasing blood clotting (see above).	
Gastrointestinal tract			
Fatty liver	Minimal or absent but may cause pain in the right abdomen, dyspepsia, nausea and vomiting; hepatomegaly may be present sometimes with tenderness; abnormal liver function test	Metabolic response to alcohol: impaired fatty acid oxidation, increased production of triglycerides, decreased lipoprotein synthesis and secretion	Reversible over a period of 2 months on cessation of alcohol; 20% develop cirrhosis with continued drinking

Table 10.2 Effects of chronic alcohol consumption

Disorder	Symptoms	Mechanisms	Reversibility
Gastrointestinal tract			
Acute hepatitis	Varies from asymptomatic to fatal liver failure; anorexia, nausea, vomiting, fever, jaundice, weight loss, right abdominal pain may be present; hepato- and splenomegaly, arterial spider angiomas often present; ascites, oedema and encephalopathy present in severe cases	Production of the tumour necrosis factor by activated Kupffer cells; infiltration of liver with leucocytes; liver cell necrosis; hyaline (Mallory bodies) in hepatocytes; central hyaline cirrhosis is suggestive of progression of sclerosis	Protracted recovery even with complete abstinence; >50% mortality with: marked hyperbilirubinaemia, rising serum creatinine, marked prolongation of prothrombine time and encephalopathy; progression to cirrhosis is common
Cirrhosis	May be silent, usually with gradual onset, progressing to jaundice, bleeding from gastro-oesophageal varices, ascites and encephalopathy; liver is firm, nodular, enlarged, normal, or decreased in size	Diffuse fine scarring, uniform loss of liver cells, small regenerative nodules (micronodular cirrhosis); develops in 10–15% of men who drink approximately 150 g/day or more for at least 10 years	Less than 50% have 5-year survival rate if drinking continues; women have about twice the risk of men for any given level of alcohol intake and over a shorter period of time

Table 10.2 Effects of chronic alcohol consumption

Disorder	*Symptoms*	*Mechanisms*	*Reversibility*
Gastrointestinal tract			
• Acute Pancreatitis	Mid-abdominal pain of variable degree, nausea, vomiting, with hypotension and renal failure in severe cases	Most likely a direct toxic effect of alcohol (possibly via initial activation of lysosomal hydrolases) causes activation of proteolytic enzymes, elastase and phospholipase in pancreas, and leads to cell necrosis	In 85–90% subsides spontaneously within 3–7 days of treatment; with continued drinking may progress to chronic form
• Chronic Pancreatitis	Chronic upper abdominal pain, weight loss, exocrine deficiency (steatorrhoea), endocrine deficiency (diabetus mellitus)	As above; usually develops in patients consuming large amounts of alcohol (80 g or more a day), however, may develop with prolonged moderate drinking (50 g/day or less)	Abstinence from alcohol prevents progression; the mortality rate and morbidity are high with continued drinking
Peptic ulcers	*Helicobacter pylori* infection is not more frequent in patients with chronic alcohol abuse than in non-alcohol dependent patients, however, regular use of alcohol increases the risk of peptic ulcer bleeding		
Mallory–Weiss lesion	Can be produced by heavy drinking associated with violent vomiting		

Table 10.2 Effects of chronic alcohol consumption

Disorder	Symptoms	Mechanisms	Reversibility
Endocrine system *Sexual functioning*			
Men	Testicular atrophy, shrinkage of seminiferous tubules, and loss of sperm cells in long-term heavy drinkers; impotence, testicular atrophy, and gynaecomastia	Direct toxic effect, suppression of pituitary and hypothalamic function; increased oestrogen and decreased testosterone in males	Irreversible
Women	Amenorrhoea, a decrease in ovarian size, infertility, spontaneous abortions	Direct toxic effect, suppression of pituitary and hypothalamic function	Irreversible
Endocrine system *General*			
	Increase in cortisol levels via increase in release of adrenocorticotropic hormone; inhibition of vasopressin secretion at rising blood alcohol concentrations, and increased secretion at falling blood alcohol concentrations, resulting in overhydration; decrease in serum thyroxine and triiodothyronine		Reversible

Table 10.2 Effects of chronic alcohol consumption

Disorder	Symptoms	Mechanisms	Reversibility
Foetal alcohol syndrome (FAS)	Changes in craniofacial area, microcephaly with mental retardation	Alcohol and acetaldehyde toxicity; the specific quantity and frequency of alcohol use during pregnancy that causes FAS have not been identified	Irreversible
Immunologic system	Alcohol suppresses neutrophil function, shifts cytokine profiles towards antibody responses, and suppresses cell-mediated immunity. Chronic alcohol exposure predisposes to pneumonia and tuberculosis. Suppression of cell-mediated immunity may be responsible for the higher incidence of several types of cancers		
Cancers	Cancers of the tongue, mouth, pharynx, larynx, oesophagus, cardia of the stomach, pancreas, liver, and breast are strongly associated with alcohol misuse; rate of carcinoma in heavy drinkers is 10 times higher than in the general population		
Gout	Alcohol abuse (particularly by men) is associated with the development of hyperuricaemia and gout		
Osteoporosis	Alterations in calcium metabolism, loss of skeletal collagen		
Alcoholic myopathy			
• Acute	Painful swollen skeletal muscles, increased levels of serum creatine phosphokinase; myoglobinuria and myoglobinaemia (in severe form of acute myopathy); usually a result of a heavy drinking bout		
• Chronic	Gradual loss of skeletal muscle protein resulting in muscle weakness; occurs in up to two-thirds of all ethanol misusers		

smoking, diet, and exercise. One method of broaching the subject is to say: 'We often find that people's eating, smoking, and drinking habits have a significant effect on their health or how they feel about themselves. I'd like to ask you some questions about them.' A more direct approach would be to say: 'Have you ever been concerned about your drinking?'

Careful attention to technique is essential in obtaining the drinking history, otherwise misleading information can be obtained. The usual error is to underestimate consumption. Alcohol histories can, however, be obtained with a reliability and validity that compares favourably with information about other aspects of human behaviour.

Enhancement techniques

The accuracy of the alcohol history can be enhanced in ways that are designed to be non-threatening and non-judgmental, but that encourage the patient to reveal the truth about his (or her) drinking. Useful techniques are included in chapter 4 table 4.1.

Useful techniques when taking an alcohol history:
- introduce drinking as a normal, everyday experience
- give the patient permission to talk about his or her drinking
- acknowledge the possibility of symptoms from alcohol use
- suggest high levels of use.

Building a picture of the patient's alcohol consumption and problems

These techniques can be employed to construct a picture of the typical drinking day. It is usually easiest to ask about drinking after work or in the early evening, and then about drinking later in the evening. Questions about morning and lunchtime drinking, which are potentially more threatening to the individual, can then follow. The number of drinks taken in each session should be established, and the quantity of alcohol (in grams or standard drinks) calculated.

A 'standard drink' is one containing 10 g alcohol. One standard drink is equivalent to one middy, pot or schooner (South Australian usage only) (approximately 300 mL) of regular strength beer, one glass (120 mL) of wine, one small glass (60 mL) of sherry or port, or one measure (30 mL) of spirits (see also table 10.3). Home measures are often two to three times the volume of standard pub measures. Charts and nomograms that indicate the alcohol content of commonly available drinks are available from regional drug and alcohol authorities. Differences in drinking from day to day, and particularly differences between weekdays and the weekend should be established. Questions should also be asked about occasions when six or more drinks are taken in a session, and about drinking to intoxication.

Questions on alcohol dependence are conveniently asked when the picture of the patient's typical drinking day is being pieced together. The elements of the dependence syndrome and examples of appropriate questions are given below.

Table 10.3   Standard drinks contained in common containers of various alcoholic beverages. Alcohol percentages are approximations only.

Light beer (2.7%)

1 can or stubbie	=	0.5 standard drinks

Medium light beer (3.5% alcohol)

1 can or stubbie	=	1 standard drink

Regular beer (4.9% alcohol)

1 can or stubbie	=	1.5 standard drinks
1 jug	=	4 standard drinks
1 slab (cans or stubbies)	=	about 36 standard drinks

Wine (10–15% alcohol)

750 mL bottle	=	about 7 to 8 standard drinks
4 litre cask	=	about 30 to 40 standard drinks

Spirits

1 nip (30 mL)	=	1 standard drink

Pre-mixed spirits (around 5% alcohol)

1 can (375 mL)	=	1.5 standard drinks

Following this, questions are posed about possible social, occupational, and legal problems related to drinking. The extent of the enquiry depends on the information on the level and frequency of consumption obtained at that point.

A convenient screening and brief assessment tool for alcohol use is the alcohol use disorders identification test (AUDIT) described in chapter 4, which covers all these domains.

Issues to consider when eliciting the history

A minority of patients do have well-developed denial mechanisms, and these people can be adept at diverting a challenging line of questioning to a less threatening one. For example, the patient may start to complain about a particular form of treatment or claim that alcohol-related symptoms were, in reality, side-effects of a drug. The clinician must be prepared to redirect attention to the alcohol problems.

Under-diagnosis of alcohol problems may also be related to the clinician's own attitudes. Sometimes this is based on an unjustified pessimism about the outcome of intervention, or pessimism about the nature of alcohol dependence itself, or a more generalised moralistic, judgmental stance. A patient's way of life and behaviour, even when he or she is not drinking, may not conform to the standards the clinician considers acceptable. The clinician should become aware of these attitudes and strive to minimise their impact on the therapeutic process.

It is important to understand the cultural milieu of drinking and the concept of the 'shout' or 'round' where each person in turn will pay for all the drinks ordered by the group of drinkers. The level of consumption in a drinking session will be dictated by the size of the group and the number of shouts. Being involved in a social circle where the shout is the accepted method of ordering drinks will seriously limit the person's chances of reducing his or her alcohol consumption.

It is also helpful to understand the terminology (often in the vernacular), used to describe certain feelings or actions; for example 'the hair of the dog' to describe the first drink in the morning to relieve hangover symptoms.

Medical practitioners who are involved in the treatment of people with alcohol problems must be able to convey a sense of their knowledge and skills to the patient to ensure their credibility. If the medical practitioner fails to achieve this, the assessment is likely to be unsatisfactory and the advice given may well be ignored or only selectively accepted. This may seem so obvious as to need no emphasis were it not for the large number of patients who are able to recount with wry amusement their interactions with inexperienced personnel.

Physical and mental examination

Examination of the patient's physical and mental state may reveal evidence of recent alcohol (or other substance) use such as the smell of alcohol or a withdrawal state, or of the physical and neuropsychiatric complications. In its severe forms alcohol misuse can lead to decline in global functioning, as evidenced by poor general appearance, personal hygiene, overall health, and nutrition. Examination of mental status may reveal patterns of abnormality consistent with the effects of alcohol dependence, such as recent memory difficulties, perseveration, or confabulation.

Physical examination

When undertaking a physical examination the clinician should focus on the following:
1 general appearance—evidence of agitation (due to a withdrawal state), premature ageing, malnutrition, Cushingoid facies
2 signs of intoxication—alcohol on breath, garrulousness, ataxia
3 cutaneous stigmata of harmful alcohol consumption such as conjunctival injection, facial telangiectasia, rhinophyma, thinning of skin, Dupuytren's contractures, bruises (especially of different ages), and non-surgical scars
4 cutaneous stigmata of liver disease, such as spider naevi, palmar erythema
5 signs of withdrawal—tremor and sweating of hands, tremor of face and tongue

6 pulse rate and blood pressure
7 evidence of cardiac enlargement
8 abdominal examination to assess size and consistency of liver, presence of splenic enlargement or of ascites
9 evidence of head injury
10 presence of nystagmus or ophthalmoplegia
11 ataxia, especially of stance and gait
12 signs of peripheral neuropathy.

Mental state examination

In the mental state examination particular attention should be paid to the following:

1 clouding of consciousness
2 abnormalities of perception, especially visual and auditory hallucinations
3 abnormalities of thought, especially paranoid ideation
4 affect, anxiety, dysphoria, depression, blunting, lability
5 suicidal ideation
6 cognition, including awareness of current events, immediate recall, short-term and long-term memory, abstraction, conceptualising, and planning.

Formal cognitive function testing should await the resolution of any clouding of consciousness. The short mental status examination questionnaire is used by some as a simple screening instrument for alcohol-related brain damage. More sensitive screening procedures make use of a short battery of tests, usually under the direction of a clinical neuropsychologist.

> ➡ Physical and mental examination is essential for effective management of alcohol withdrawal and long-term management of alcohol dependence.

Laboratory tests

Laboratory tests may provide evidence of alcohol misuse. This is best detected by the physiological markers of consumption, such as:

- mean corpuscular volume (MCV)
- gamma glutamyltransferase (GGT)
- aspartate aminotransferase (AST)

However, abnormal values are found in only 20–30% of those with hazardous or harmful alcohol consumption, and in about 40% of those with alcohol dependence. Carbohydrate deficient transferrin (CDT) is a more sensitive marker of excessive alcohol consumption than conventional laboratory markers (being abnormal in 40–60% of patients), but the test is expensive. Alcohol consumption is also detectable by blood, urine, and breath analyses, although these will be negative if no recent use has occurred.

Collateral history

The importance of obtaining a collateral history of the patient's alcohol use is detailed in chapter 4.

Making the diagnosis

On the basis of the history, physical and mental status examination, and laboratory tests, the clinician should establish whether the criteria for various alcohol-related disorders are fulfilled.

The guidelines for estimation of low-, moderate-, and high-risk drinking are listed in table 10.4.

While the evidence that alcohol-free days reduce health risk is limited, regular alcohol-free days may help drinkers to remain in control of their drinking and reduce its habit-forming potential. This is especially important for people drinking above the low risk limits.

The major elements to be assessed for a diagnosis of alcohol dependence and the appropriate questions are listed in table 10.5. The most commonly used criteria for diagnosis of alcohol dependence, based on these elements, are the DSM-IV and the ICD-10 Criteria for Substance Dependence. A mild degree of dependence is common in the Australian population. One early sign of this, for example, is finding it difficult to stop drinking after two or three glasses. There is evidence that everyone who drinks, even at low levels, acquires some physiological tolerance to alcohol, but this occurs less in people who drink only intermittently, and they are also less likely to experience withdrawal symptoms.

> The most commonly used criteria for diagnosis of alcohol dependence are the DSM-IV and the ICD-10 Criteria for Substance Dependence.

Following this assessment, the clinician should determine which physical, psychological (neuropsychiatric), and social problems are related to the patient's alcohol consumption. Often it is not possible to determine this at the time of first assessment. Indeed, it may not be possible to determine whether the patient's psychological problems (for example depression) have caused the alcohol problem or are secondary to it. This often has to wait for re-evaluation after a period of abstinence or reduced alcohol consumption. Nevertheless, it is important to record all the possible associated conditions as the basis for an effective plan of management.

INTERVENTION AND TREATMENT

Treatment of alcohol withdrawal

The alcohol withdrawal syndrome is the most common drug withdrawal state. However, coexisting drug abuse is seen with increasing frequency, especially in younger

Table 10.4   Guidelines for low-risk drinking (Australian Alcohol Guidelines: Health Risks and Benefits, NH&MRC 2001)

Alcohol consumption at levels shown below is NOT recommended for people who:
- have a condition made worse by drinking
- are on medication
- are under 18 years of age
- are pregnant[#]
- are about to engage in activities involving risk or a degree of skill (for example driving, flying, water sports, skiing, operating machinery).

Otherwise risks levels for the following patterns are as follows:

Risk of harm in the short-term★

	Low risk (standard drinks)	Risky (standard drinks)	High risk (standard drinks)
Males			
• On any one day	up to 6 on any one day, no more than 3 days per week	7 to 10 on any one day	11 or more on any one day
Females			
• On any one day	up to 4 on any one day, no more than 3 days per week	5 to 6 on any one day	7 or more on any one day

Risk of harm in the long-term★

	Low risk (standard drinks)	Risky (standard drinks)	High risk (standard drinks)
Males			
• On an average day	up to 4 per day	5 to 6 per day	7 or more per day
• Overall weekly level	up to 28 per week	29 to 42 per week	43 or more per week
Females			
• On an average day	up to 2 per day	3 to 4 per day	5 or more per day
• Overall weekly level	up to 14 per week	15 to 28 per week	29 or more per week

★ Note:
1. It is assumed that the drinks are consumed at a moderate rate to minimise intoxication, for example for men no more than 2 drinks in the first hour and 1 per hour thereafter, and for women, no more than 1 drink per hour.
2. These guidelines apply to people of average or larger body size, that is, above about 60 kg for men and 50 kg for women. People of smaller than average body size should drink within lower levels.

[#] see chapter 16 for information regarding alcohol consumption in pregnancy.

age groups. The withdrawal (detoxification) period is only the first step in the rehabilitation process, and offers the opportunity to further motivate and assess the patient.

Blood alcohol levels

It can be useful to obtain a BAC level preceding or at the start of withdrawal. Risks of over-sedation from the interaction of alcohol with prematurely administered sedative medication can thus be minimised. Alcohol metabolism results in a decrease of the blood alcohol level at a rate of about 0.015% per hour, which enables simple calculation of the time required for the blood alcohol to reach zero. In addition, the detection of a BAC greater than 0.15% is helpful in identifying the more dependent drinker. This is particularly so if tolerance to intoxication is evident.

Table 10.5 Elements of the alcohol dependence syndrome

Elements of the syndrome	Examples of relevant questions	Comments
Subjective awareness of compulsion to drink	Do you feel a strong desire or craving for alcohol once you have started drinking?	Craving after a couple of drinks is a characteristic feature of alcohol dependence.
Impaired control	Have you experienced that you were not able to stop drinking once you had started?	'Loss of control' is considered to be a classical early warning indicator of evolving dependence.
Salience of drinking (primacy over other activities)	Do you skip meals because you are drinking? Have you failed to do what was expected of you because of drinking?	Also refers to primacy over activities previously enjoyed and preferred to drinking.
Increased tolerance to alcohol	Have you needed more alcohol than previously to get the desired effect?	One of the more difficult elements to enquire about specifically in a single question. Often best inferred from the speed of drinking and ability to drink large amounts of alcohol without becoming intoxicated.

Table 10.5 Elements of the alcohol dependence syndrome

Elements of the syndrome	Examples of relevant questions	Comments
Repeated withdrawal symptoms or relief or avoidance of withdrawal symptoms by further drinking	Do your hands shake a lot in the morning after drinking? Have you needed a first drink to settle you down the morning after drinking?	Tremor and nausea occasionally after drinking do not necessarily imply dependence. A slightly disguised question such as this is useful before specific questions are asked on relief of morning tremor, sweating, and nausea.
Continued use despite harm	Have you tended to continue drinking even though you knew it had caused you to become unwell or experience problems?	Continuing to drink despite harm is a hallmark of dependence. This criterion is fulfilled when the patient knows (or could reasonably be expected to know) that continued drinking would be harmful.

Predicting severity of withdrawal

The severity of an impending withdrawal syndrome may be difficult to predict. For an individual patient the pattern of clinical features is often similar to previous withdrawals. Thus, a past history of seizures, hallucinations, and delirium may be a guide to a likely severe withdrawal. Factors predictive of more severe withdrawal symptoms include consumption of greater than 150 g of alcohol per day, early morning drinking, hypokalaemia, and recent anaesthesia.

Location of withdrawal treatment

The aim of management is the prevention of a severe alcohol withdrawal syndrome. Those deemed at significant risk should be referred to a medically supervised unit. Other criteria for considering management in a hospital medical setting are significant alcohol-related physical illness, psychiatric disorder, coexisting dependency on other drugs (for example opioids, sedatives), and older age groups. Examination of the patient's physical and mental state is essential to determine whether the patient meets these criteria (see previous section).

The majority of alcohol-dependent patients can be managed without hospitalisation, either at home (outpatient), or in a non-medical unit. Criteria for outpatient home withdrawal include: younger patients, high motivation, good support, suitable supervision from responsible relatives and friends, or domicillary alcohol services. It is necessary to ensure that administration of the prescribed sedative medication is supervised, and that continued drinking is not occurring simultaneously. Sleep disturbance is the most common alcohol withdrawal symptom, and hypnotic medication alone may suffice. Protracted courses of hypnotics are rarely necessary, and medication can usually be discontinued within one week.

Pharmacological treatment

Benzodiazepines

Benzodiazepines have emerged as more effective, less toxic drugs of choice for treating alcohol withdrawal. In Australasia diazepam is the most commonly used treatment. Chlormethiazole (a short acting sedative/hypnotic and anticonvulsant with a mechanism of action different from that of benzodiazepines and barbiturates) is also useful in preventing the development of delirium tremens. However, it appears to have greater potential to produce respiratory depression and physical dependence.

There is considerable variation in the severity of alcohol withdrawal symptoms, and factors such as liver disease may result in marked changes in drug bioavailability when shorter-acting benzodiazepines may be more appropriate. Contraindications to sedatives, such as head injuries, hepatic encephalopathy, and severe obstructive airways disease, should be considered. Thus, strict adherence to 'standard dose' schedules can result in toxicity or ineffective treatment. The severity of withdrawal should be closely monitored and diazepam dosages need to be titrated according to symptoms and rating scales. Rating scales such as the Clinical Institute Withdrawal Assessment for Alcohol (CIWA-Ar) (Sullivan et al. 1989) have been developed as a guide. Prophylactic use of benzodiazepines is recommended in patients with a past history of seizures. In these patients the initial dose of diazepam will be unrelated to the withdrawal rating scale.

There is a considerable range in the dosage required. For moderate withdrawal it is important to give sufficient drug initially to control symptoms, prevent progression to delirium tremens, and retain the patient in treatment. A diazepam oral (or intravenous when necessary) loading technique has been developed to assist in this initial management. Usually, 20 mg diazepam is administered two-hourly to a minimum cumulative dose of 60 mg, or until withdrawal symptoms are controlled. The long elimination of diazepam allows gradual pharmacokinetic self-tapering without the need for additional doses. However, patients who abuse benzodiazepines concomitantly with alcohol should be withdrawn on a more gradual basis, using tapering dosages of diazepam.

In the majority of patients, medication can be decreased after a few days, and discontinued after one week.

> In the treatment of alcohol withdrawal:
>
> Start with seizure prophylaxis if there is a history of seizures.
> → Titrate benzodiazepines according to clinical progress. Do not over-treat (danger of respiratory depression).
> → Do not over-hydrate.
> → Always give thiamine to prevent Wernicke's encephalopathy.
> → Do not discharge on benzodiazepines.
> → Always refer to an alcohol treatment service.

Beta-blockers

Beta-adrenergic blocking drugs can confer additional benefit when combined with sedative–hypnotics, and may be useful in reducing tremor, palpitations, tachycardia and hypertension associated with acute withdrawal. The relative contraindications to beta-blockers of obstructive airways disease and cardiomyopathy are common in alcohol-dependent patients.

Withdrawal seizures

Withdrawal seizures occur in about 15% of patients who do not receive drugs with anti-convulsant properties. Typically these fits occur within the first 48 hours of ceasing alcohol, and are grand mal and single or, at worst, few in number. As discussed above, withdrawal seizures may herald a major withdrawal syndrome and delirium.

In those exhibiting seizures for the first time, blood sugar and neurological investigations should be undertaken before they are attributed to alcohol withdrawal.

A previous history of withdrawal seizures denotes a 70% likelihood of their recurrence. Some medical practitioners recommend that these patients receive a short course (not longer than five to seven days) of an anti-convulsant in addition to oral benzodiazepines. Sodium valproate and carbamazepine are more effective than phenytoin, but they should be used with caution in patients with liver disease because of potential hepatotoxicity.

Withdrawal hallucinations

Haloperidol 2.5 to 10 mg orally or intramuscularly is the preferred drug in the treatment of hallucinations, particularly when they produce agitation and behavioural disorders. A few doses are often sufficient to arrest the hallucinations. Significant hypotension and over-sedation is uncommon.

Major withdrawal (delirium tremens)

The classic full syndrome of profound confusion with agitation and autonomic over-activity preceded by seizures and hallucinations is less commonly encountered nowadays, and is now rarely fatal. Presumably, this reflects improved supportive care and treatment of coexisting medical problems, and the availability of more effective treatment in the earlier stages of withdrawal.

Clinicians are more often confronted with the confused patient without the classic features of the withdrawal syndrome. A thorough investigation for other causes is required before attributing it to alcohol withdrawal. These include hypo-glycaemia, Wernicke's encephalopathy, post-ictal states, head injury (and subdural haemorrhage), hypoxia, and sepsis. Frequent clinical examination, metabolic studies, consideration of the effects of sedative medication (for example in the presence of liver disease), and neurological investigations, including CT scan, may be required.

Optimal management requires a separate room and constant nursing attention. Intravenous fluid replacement may be required if there is severe dehydration and profuse sweating and fever. Specific treatment is required for associated electrolyte disorders (including depleted calcium, phosphate, magnesium, and potassium) and metabolic disorders. There is a paucity of data to suggest that once delirium has commenced any one drug regimen will shorten its duration. Drug treatment is necessary to prevent patient exhaustion, to control agitated behaviour, and to prevent disturbance of other patients. One must be cautious in attempting to suppress all agitation completely, since to accomplish this may require very large doses of drugs with attendant risks of over-sedation.

It may be necessary to use parenteral medication in severe withdrawal states if the usual oral benzodiazepine regimens have been unhelpful. Intravenous diazepam (not well absorbed via the intramuscular route) may prove effective in relieving withdrawal, but disconcertingly high dosages in excess of 60 mg may be required. Anti-psychotic medications such as haloperidol, 5–10 mg, appears to give a more predictable calming effect on behaviour. Infusions of chlormethiazole are effective, but there may be difficulties titrating the dose to symptoms in general wards, and such infusion should be restricted to intensive care situations.

Vitamins and fluids

Multivitamin administration has not been shown to improve the course of the alcohol withdrawal syndrome, but vitamins are given to prevent or treat the Wernicke–Korsakoff syndrome and other nutritional complications. Parenteral thiamine should always precede glucose infusion in alcohol-dependent patients. This is because a glucose load could consume the depleted thiamine stores and precipitate Wernicke's encephalopathy. All hospitalised patients should receive one initial dose of parenteral thiamine followed by a short course (two weeks) of oral thiamine (25 mg twice daily). In nutritional neurological disorders (cerebellar ataxia, peripheral neuropathy, Wernicke's encephalopathy), multivitamin treatment may need to be prolonged. In general, it is important to give a patient adequate nutrition and rest. Patients commonly have normal levels of body water or are slightly over-hydrated. Avoid intravenous fluids unless a patient is hypotensive or has a history of vomiting, diarrhoea, or recent bleeding.

> ➡ Management of alcohol withdrawal can vary from simple reassurance and outpatient management to hospital intensive care.
> ➡ Proper assessment allows the formulation of appropriate individual withdrawal and rehabilitation programs.

Post withdrawal

The management of alcohol withdrawal can vary from simple reassurance and outpatient management to hospital intensive care treatment of the patient with delirium and severe complications. Alcohol withdrawal, however, is only the initial stage of rehabilitation treatment. Proper assessment of alcohol dependence allows appropriate rehabilitation programs to be formulated.

Treatment approaches for alcohol dependence

A broad range of treatment approaches are available (and necessary) for patients with alcohol problems. Patients may present anywhere along the spectrum from early-stage problem drinkers to severe alcohol dependence with major physical complications and cognitive impairment. As this is a complex issue, it is necessary to formulate a basic treatment plan. This needs to address social, medical and psychological issues identified through the assessment process.

General approach

Clearly, it is vital to engage the identified problem-drinker or alcohol-dependent patient into a process of behavioural change. The initiation of the therapeutic relationship requires considerable skill, tact, and opportunistic timing. The assessment itself is usually an ongoing and evolving process, and may, per se, be a powerful treatment tool.

Assessing a patient's motivation and readiness to change generally follows the model of Prochaska and DiClemente, as discussed in chapter 7. Patients in the pre-contemplative stage are unaware of, or denying, alcohol problems, and every effort should be made to remain engaged and provide personalised feedback in the hope of promoting recognition of the problem, and movement to preparation and action.

In working with those in the pre-contemplation and contemplation stages, the clinician should provide objective information on risks and problems, such as the individual's alcohol consumption compared to low-risk drinking guidelines, and psychological, physical, social, or legal issues that have come to the clinician's attention from the history, examination, or blood tests.

Motivational interviewing strategies are very helpful in assisting the patient to recognise attitudes and reasons for their ambivalence regarding problem drinking. This technique is discussed in chapter 5. Key concepts include ambivalence explored through a structured consideration of pros and cons, with an empathetic and reflective approach rather than confrontation. Patients who have urgent and severe problems with complications of alcohol dependence may not be suitable for such approaches, and need concerned confrontation by health professionals, family, or significant others.

A number of key questions need to be addressed at the initial stages of treatment (action stage). These include:

- alcohol consumption goals, for example controlled drinking or abstinence
- management of withdrawal—timing, setting, and knowledge of local facilities
- referral to specialist units
- use of pharmacological treatments
- use of behavioural treatments
- coordination of treatment role, monitoring, and follow-up.

It is important to remember that remission, without treatment, from alcohol dependence is well described. Alcohol abstinence is usually the preferred goal, but there are numerous alcohol-dependent individuals who do not accept this, at least initially, and negotiate with the therapist over controlled drinking programs. An initial option, while retaining the patient in treatment, is for them to attempt to control drinking within set limits. Frequently this cannot be achieved or sustained satisfactorily, and abstinence will come to be accepted. Alcohol dependence is a chronic relapsing disorder, and long-term goals include sustaining social functioning and optimising physical and mental health. Treatment goals include not only abstinence and relapse prevention but, within a harm-reduction model, could also include numbers of abstinence days achieved, reduced use of alcohol on drinking days, and reduction of craving discomfort.

Pharmacological treatments

Prescribing drugs for alcohol dependence requires consideration of the risks and contraindications, including overdose, non-compliance, interactions with alcohol, adverse side effects, medical complications of alcohol dependence such as liver disease, hepatic enzyme induction by alcohol, and the costs of certain newer drugs.

Disulfiram
Disulfiram inhibits ALDH in the liver and, when the patient consumes alcohol, causes an accumulation of acetaldehyde, and hence flushing, nausea and vomiting,

palpitations, and difficulty breathing. The goal is to provide a strong disincentive to drink. It is available as 200 mg dispersible tablets with the usual dose being 200 mg daily. Ideally it is initiated post withdrawal or at least 48 hours after ceasing alcohol (or with evidence of a zero blood alcohol level). The indications are for alcohol dependence in the patient who has a goal of immediate abstinence and who has a clear understanding of the drug and its effects. For successful outcomes it is essential to have some mechanism for supervision of daily doses.

Cautions and contraindications for disulfiram predominantly relate to known cardiac disease (coronary artery disease, history of arrhythmias or heart failure). This is because the aversive reaction may cause tachycardia and hypotension, and precipitate a coronary event or serious arrhythmia. Older patients require a cardiac history and an electrocardiogram prior to commencing disulfiram.

Other cautions include severe liver disease, as disulfiram itself may (rarely) cause a toxic hepatitis. Liver function tests should be done fortnightly for the first two months and thereafter monthly for patients maintained on disulfiram. Patients with major coexisting psychiatric disorders (bipolar, depression, psychotic illnesses) may need close supervision, as disulfiram can potentially worsen these disorders by affecting brain dopamine systems. However, doses of 200 mg per day are generally considered safe with these patients.

Side-effects of disulfiram may include initial drowsiness, fatigue, and a metallic taste. Occasionally rash, peripheral neuropathy, headache, and sexual dysfunction are encountered. The drug is teratogenic and contraindicated in pregnancy. Drug interactions with phenytoin, warfarin, diazepam, and anti-tuberculous medication are recognised.

> Disulfiram is usually prescribed for three to six months following withdrawal and in combination with monitoring, support, and psychosocial interventions.

Acamprosate

Acamprosate (calcium acetyl homotaurinate) is used to prevent alcohol relapse post-withdrawal. The mechanism of action is not yet clearly identified and the drug may have various central nervous system actions, including modification of calcium ion flux, reduction of glutamate (NMDA receptors) activity, and GABA agonist activity. In these respects its actions overlap with those of alcohol, and the major effect of the drug appears to be suppression of protracted withdrawal (see above). The drug is considered not to interact with alcohol if patients drink while taking it. Acamprosate does not have hypnotic, anxiolytic or anti-depressant effects. It is considered generally safe in the absence of severe liver disease or renal insufficiency (renal elimination). Side-effects may include diarrhoea, headache, nausea, and itch. Interactions with other drugs are not described, and it may be given concomitantly with disulfiram. Compliance may be an issue as the dose is generally two tablets (300 mg each) three times a day.

Studies with acamprosate show beneficial outcomes, including increases in non-drinking days and a near doubling of abstinence rates, although a majority of study subjects return to drinking. It may be concluded that acamprosate has a modest overall benefit in the treatment of alcohol dependence. It is not yet possible to predict subgroups of patients who may particularly benefit from this drug.

Opioid antagonists

Opioid antagonists were studied using the hypothesis that alcohol increases the functional activity of brain opioid systems and that antagonists should reduce alcohol consumption, its reward effects, and possibly craving. Naltrexone, 50 mg daily, shows positive outcomes with regard to relapse rates, craving, and number of non-drinking days, together with evidence of diminished reward effects after drinking. The principal contraindication for the use of naltrexone in alcohol dependence is coexisting use or dependence on opioid drugs. Naltrexone is generally well tolerated and does not have an abuse potential. Side-effects are reported as nausea and headache. This drug may be hepatotoxic, and caution is required if transaminases are above three times the normal range. Monitoring of the liver profile is recommended during the course of naltrexone treatment, which is usually three to six months.

Context of pharmacological treatment

It is desirable that pharmacological treatments be delivered in structured clinical formats and integrated with psychosocial treatments, rather than as ad hoc quick-fix treatments. It is hoped that in the future it will be possible to identify sub-populations of patients who have better response rates to a particular medication or combination of medications. Drug treatment for alcohol dependence should be routinely considered within the treatment plan.

Non-pharmacological treatment options and services

Brief interventions

Over the last decade there has been considerable emphasis on brief interventions in accordance with the broad aims of early identification of those with alcohol problems, and the need for simple and cost-effective treatment approaches delivered from primary care settings.

These treatments are tailored specifically to non-dependent problem drinkers. Brief interventions have a framework of two to three sessions on assessment, advice, and counselling, and goals are usually for moderation or harm-free drinking with an educational emphasis rather than diagnostic labelling (see chapter 5).

Very brief interventions may be confined to five-minute sessions, and can incorporate an update of the current alcohol use, motivational interviewing techniques, advice on cutting down, safe-drinking guidelines, and self-help manuals. For patients in the action stage, brief advice on relapse-prevention can be given (see chapter 5).

Brief interventions have been subject to considerable positive evaluation and should be integrated into primary care and other health and specialist practice in order to reach the huge population of hazardous and problem drinkers. The components of brief and more significant interventions have been summarised using the acronym FLAGS (table 10.6).

Table 10.6   The FLAGS approach

Review AUDIT score		
Low-risk range	*Risky or harmful range*	*Alcohol-dependent range*
Feedback results of AUDIT	**Feedback** results of AUDIT	**Feedback** results of AUDIT
Reinforce safe drinking behaviour	**Listen** to patient's concern	**Listen** to patient's concern
	Advise patient about consequences of continued alcohol use	**Advise** patient about consequences of continued alcohol use
	Goals of treatment should be defined:	**Goals** of treatment should be defined:
	• reduce alcohol consumption to within safe limits	• advise on the importance of a period of abstinence
	• have 2 alcohol-free days per week	
	Strategies for treatment should be discussed and implemented:	**Strategies** for treatment should be discussed and implemented:
	• gain a greater understanding of situations that trigger drinking	• consider the need for detoxification
	• offer a self-help booklet for reducing drinking	• consider pharmacotherapy in conjunction with supportive therapy
	• offer a follow-up appointment	• advise on the importance of compliance with treatment
		• encourage attendance at a self-help group
		• offer a follow-up appointment
		• refer to a specialist if necessary

Outpatient alcohol treatment units

It is a reasonable objective to motivate moderately to severely alcohol-dependent patients to accept referral to an outpatient alcohol service. Some of these services are well staffed with a variety of health professionals, including psychologists and psychiatrists who are well placed to assess and treat coexisting disorders. In general, the treatment unit will provide a comprehensive assessment and outpatient treatment.

Much of the outpatient alcohol treatment unit's work involves one-to-one counselling that may be described as generally supportive, but that is increasingly tailored to more specific behavioural treatments. These are an extension of the motivational interviewing and behaviour change strategies discussed in chapter 5.

Family involvement

Although family therapies (systems theory, problem-solving, marital therapy) have been used in treatment of alcohol dependence, the important factor is that involvement of significant others in recovery can enhance treatment outcomes.

Alcohol dependence remains a disorder that affects members of the dependent person's family, and these family members may themselves develop social or psychological problems needing treatment. These issues include self-blame, guilt, covering up, facilitating drinking behaviour (co-dependence), inability to focus on individual family members' needs, and preoccupation with being responsible for the alcohol-affected family member.

A joint interview with partners and family should be sought as soon as possible in the treatment process. There may be particular cultural reasons that put greater emphasis on family involvement from the start of treatment interventions (for example for indigenous populations; see chapters 17 and 18).

Residential (inpatient) treatment

The appropriateness of residential treatment programs (excluding withdrawal management) have been subject to increasing scrutiny over the last decade. Issues have included cost effectiveness, the duration of treatment, and selection criteria for residential treatment. However, there are some alcohol-dependent patients who require residential treatment.

Commonly cited criteria for residential treatment include:
- failure to respond to outpatient treatment, or non-compliance
- lack of social supporting structure
- important psychiatric or medical complications
- rural domicile with no outpatient services
- severe life crises
- coexisting drug dependencies.

Exclusion criteria for intensive inpatient programs include impaired cognitive function and a record of disruptive behaviour, for example through severe personality disorder.

Alcoholics Anonymous (AA)

Alcoholics Anonymous is an organisation that has operated internationally for more than 60 years. It is an important component of alcohol dependence treatment. AA is based on the principle that alcohol dependence is a physical, mental, and spiritual disorder that requires lifelong abstinence and participation in a recovery program. The program includes regular meetings, a 'buddy' system, fellowship, and a potential new social structure involving non–drinkers.

All patients attending health professionals should be offered encouragement to attend AA. Ideally, therapists should have contact with appropriate local AA members who could take patients to meetings, and an insight into which local meetings may best fit a client, for example women, or young people.

The AA approach does not suit all, and it may have a lower acceptance among women. Clearly, involvement of a patient in AA does not preclude the need for comprehensive assessment or the need to address coexisting disorders or provide other concomitant treatments.

Al-Anon and Alateen are associated organisations, developed to variable degrees in regions of Australia and New Zealand, which provide education and support for partners and families of patients with alcohol dependence.

EPIDEMIOLOGY AND PREVENTION

Epidemiology

Impact of alcohol use

The majority of Australians and New Zealanders drink alcohol at least occasionally, and 70 to 80% of the population report drinking in a way that causes few problems. For those people who do drink to excess, alcohol can cause a broad range of physical, psychological, and social problems. The effects of alcohol dependence can be devastating, and in severe cases can lead to disintegration of social, physical, and/or psychological function. Because of the impact of intoxication and dependence on behaviour, alcohol-dependent people may lose both self-respect and the respect of the community, and this makes the condition particularly disabling.

While the impact of alcohol dependence on health is widely recognised, the effects of non-dependent excessive drinking are often underestimated by the community and the health-care system. The number of non-dependent heavy drinkers far outweighs the number of dependent people, so has a greater influence on the community burden of alcohol problems. Episodic heavy drinking is associated with trauma and violence, crime, drownings, burns, suicides, unwanted pregnancy, unsafe sex, and many other complications.

> Episodic heavy drinking is associated with trauma and violence, crime, drownings, burns, suicides, unwanted pregnancy, and unsafe sex.

Excessive alcohol use is estimated to cost Australia \$4.5 billion, and New Zealand between \$1.4 and 4.6 billion, per year. This involves both direct costs, such as provision of detoxification services and treatment of alcohol-related liver disease, and indirect costs, such as lost productivity of individuals affected by alcohol, and enforcement of drink-driving regulations. Excessive alcohol use is estimated to be a causative factor in over 6000 deaths per year in Australia.

Prevalence of alcohol use and alcohol-use disorders

Australia and New Zealand have two of the highest rates of alcohol consumption of the English-speaking world, with only the United Kingdom higher. In 1999 they ranked 21st and 22nd , respectively, against all countries of the world for recorded per capita consumption data. Nevertheless, consumption in both countries has fallen since 1970. The majority of the population drink alcohol at some time in each year. Over 80% of men in both countries report some drinking in the past year. In New Zealand, 85% of women report some drinking in the past year, while 64% of Australian women reported drinking 12 or more times in the past year. Four per cent of survey respondents report symptoms of dependence on alcohol (5% men, 2% women). While these rates are similar to those of other countries, they are likely to be underestimates, as alcohol-dependent people are less likely than non-dependent people to respond to surveys.

It is difficult to estimate accurately the proportion of the population drinking to excess but not dependent on alcohol. Just under one in five (18%) men report drinking seven or more drinks on one occasion at some time in the past year, with 11% of men drinking that amount twice a week or more often. This number would include both dependent and non-dependent heavy drinkers. Among women, under one in ten (7%) report drinking seven or more drinks on one occasion at some time in the past year, and a further 6% drink five or more drinks on one occasion at least twice a week. Almost half of New Zealand men aged 20 to 24 report drinking at least six drinks per occasion on a weekly basis, and one in three women report drinking at least four drinks per sitting at least weekly.

> Just under one in five men and one in ten women report drinking seven or more drinks on one occasion at some time in the past year.

Moderate- and high-risk drinking and dependence are more common in men than in women, and are more common in those aged 45 or younger than in older people. The rates of drinking reported by people in the Northern Territory are higher than in other areas of Australia. Certain populations are at higher risk of alcohol problems than others. In both Aboriginal and Māori populations, drinking tends to be polarised: there are higher proportions of abstainers than in the general community, but heavy drinking is more common among those who do drink. Alcohol problems are more common among unemployed than employed people, and in people who have never married than in married people. It is difficult to discern from cross-sectional surveys whether factors such as unemployment or marital status are the result of heavy drinking or are risk factors contributing to its development. People with psychiatric illness are at increased risk of alcohol-use disorders.

Aetiological factors

A variety of genetic and environmental factors can predispose people to the development of alcohol dependence. The role of genetic factors in the development of alcohol dependence is well accepted, and appears to be stronger in men. In most studies the children of alcohol-dependent fathers who have been adopted out at an early age display a significantly increased risk of alcohol dependence. Greater similarities have also been shown between the drinking patterns of identical (monozygotic) twins than between non-identical (dizygotic) twins.

> Both genetic and environmental factors may contribute to the development of an alcohol use disorder.

A variety of biochemical, physiological, and genetic studies since the 1980s have continued to shed light on the possible mechanisms of genetic transmission of risk. Potential factors include a reduced physiological response to alcohol, so that more alcohol is consumed before intoxication is evident. Various aspects of neurotransmission have been studied, and differences may affect risk of alcohol dependence. In up to 40% of Japanese people and 10% of Chinese people there may be a clear, genetically determined difference in the way alcohol is metabolised. Those affected may display flushing, palpitations and headaches 20 minutes after only one or two drinks of alcohol. This response is due to decreased activity of ALDH, causing a build-up of alcohol's metabolite, acetaldehyde. Those who have this reaction are protected against the development of alcohol dependence because of their aversive reaction to alcohol. Paradoxically, people who are heterozygous for this defect may be able to continue drinking and even become heavy drinkers. If this happens they are at greatly increased risk of the physical complications of drinking, in particular alcoholic cirrhosis and cancers of the upper gastrointestinal tract, pointing to a link between acetaldehyde and physical complications of drinking. This enzymatic variant is rare in Caucasians.

While men are at higher risk of alcohol-use disorders, women are at greater risk of the physical complications of drinking for the same quantity and duration of drinking. This increased rate of complications largely relates to women's lower lean body mass, which means that women have a lower volume to absorb the alcohol, and hence have a higher effective blood alcohol concentration.

A variety of personality factors may impact on use of alcohol. For example, a thrill-seeking personality may be inclined to increased experimentation and risk-taking with alcohol, particularly in youth. There has been considerable interest in other personality types that may predispose to alcohol dependence, but there is not yet broad agreement on findings.

Environmental factors

A variety of environmental factors may predispose to the development of alcohol use disorders. These include childhood separation, major psychological trauma such as childhood abuse, and chronic stress. In a person with a history of alcohol-use disorders, a variety of social or psychological stresses can trigger a relapse. Peer pressure and the availability of alcohol are important factors that influence drinking levels. This is particularly the case among teenagers and young adults, where a pattern of episodic heavy drinking, and group drinking with the aim of intoxication, is common. In adults of all ages there may be significant pressures to drink with friends, particularly at pubs or parties, and also with colleagues at business lunches. These influences may encourage the development of an alcohol problem or hinder its treatment.

Comorbidity

Heavy drinking is commonly associated with smoking, and, particularly in younger persons, may be associated with use of other substances. Combined use of a number of sedative substances, such as alcohol, benzodiazepines, and heroin, is an important factor in opioid overdoses. Psychiatric disorders (particularly schizophrenia and depression) are commonly associated with alcohol dependence or harmful alcohol use, creating considerable challenges in management. In the case of depression it may be difficult to discern whether the depression is the result or cause of the alcohol-use disorder. However, in a significant proportion of cases, depression resolves with sustained abstinence.

> Combined use of a number of sedative substances, such as alcohol, benzodiazepines and heroin, is an important factor in opioid overdoses.

Impact of alcohol consumption on health

Alcohol's effects on health can be divided into those effects resulting from acute intoxication and those arising from chronic excessive drinking. Because acute intoxication leads to disinhibition, impaired judgment, and impaired coordination, it is associated with trauma of every kind (including work-related, domestic, motor vehicle, and violence), drownings, burns, and suicide. In addition, the social effects of acute intoxication are all too apparent. An intoxicated person may become involved in arguments, domestic violence or neglect, crime, or drink driving. Unplanned and unguarded sexual liaisons may lead to unwanted pregnancy or sexually transmitted disease.

Chronic, regular, heavy alcohol consumption is associated with a range of medical disorders. The most widely known of these is alcohol-related liver disease, and in particular alcoholic cirrhosis. The cirrhosis rate of a country is directly related to its alcohol consumption, but despite this clear link, and the severity and notoriety of the condition, alcoholic cirrhosis occurs in only 10 to 15% of dependent drinkers. Risk of cirrhosis steadily increases with consumption level in men drinking six or more drinks per day, and women drinking four or more drinks per day. It is generally found after 10 or more years of heavy alcohol consumption. Once complications of cirrhosis have occurred, the prognosis is poor if drinking continues, with only 50% surviving at five years. Abstinence significantly improves survival. Patients with cirrhosis are at increased risk of hepatic carcinoma.

The other liver changes that are seen in heavy drinkers are fatty change and hepatitis. Fatty liver is common in heavy drinkers and is generally asymptomatic, detected only as hepatomegaly on physical examination, or raised liver enzymes, and it is fully reversible. Episodes of alcoholic hepatitis, which may be triggered by episodes of heavy drinking, may vary from being clinically mild to acutely life-threatening. Repeated episodes of hepatitis may result in cirrhosis.

A less well-recognised but more common consequence of excessive alcohol use is hypertension. It is estimated that up to 30% of what is otherwise classed as essential hypertension is in fact related to alcohol consumption. Blood pressure generally improves with reduction in consumption or abstinence. Alcohol is also a factor in a number of cancers, particularly of the liver, mouth and oropharynx, and colorectal region. It appears likely that alcohol is also a factor in breast cancer. In addition to these complications, chronic excessive alcohol consumption affects virtually every system in the body: neurological, immunological, gastrointestinal, musculoskeletal, renal, and cardiovascular. (See the discussion of acute and chronic toxicity above.)

> Up to 30% of cases of essential hypertension are associated with excessive alcohol use.

Because of its broad effects on health, excessive alcohol use or related problems are found more often in sick people than in the general community. While community surveys show 10 to 20% of people drink to excess and one in six general practice patients admits to drinking heavily, up to 30% of hospital inpatients and 40% of emergency department patients have been found to show some evidence of excessive drinking or related problems. Heavy drinking significantly increases the workload of hospitals: it is associated with an increased rate of return visits to the emergency department or trauma ward, and is an often unrecognised factor in a wide range of complications of elective surgery.

> One in six general practice patients, and up to one in three hospital inpatients, have evidence of a drinking problem.

Heavy alcohol use in pregnancy may result in foetal alcohol syndrome, with typical facies and impaired cognitive function. Risk increases with the amount of maternal consumption. As there is no clear lower threshold for increase in risk, advice to women who are pregnant or intending become pregnant tends to be cautious, precluding heavy drinking, and suggesting either light or no alcohol consumption (see chapter 16).

Benefits of alcohol in moderation

Despite the risks associated with heavy drinking, alcohol has an accepted role in most societies. Alcohol has been used as a social lubricant for millennia, and has ceremonial and religious roles in many cultures. In moderation, alcohol has also been shown to be associated with health benefits: in particular a reduced risk of ischaemic vascular disease (ischaemic heart disease, ischaemic stroke, and peripheral vascular disease), and probably a reduced risk of type II diabetes. Indeed, the mortality rate for moderate drinkers is generally lower than for abstainers, and this effect seems to be independent of any prior health problems in abstainers. The lowest risk for overall mortality is estimated to lie at relatively low levels of consumption: one to two drinks per day for a man, and up to one drink per day for a woman. It should be emphasised that many of the studies showing health benefits of alcohol have been conducted in middle-aged men in whom the risk of ischaemic vascular disease is high. In a 20-year follow-up of young Swedish army recruits, alcohol consumption was linearly associated with risk of death. Death in these cases was most commonly due to violent causes (including motor vehicle accidents and suicide).

> In middle-aged men, moderate consumption appears to be beneficial, while in young men alcohol consumption is directly related to mortality rate.

Natural history of alcohol dependence and excessive use

The risk of alcohol dependence increases with the amount of alcohol consumed, but not all heavy drinkers go on to become dependent. There is a degree of natural flux from heavy drinking back to lower levels. In particular, episodic heavy drinking and related problems are relatively common in young adults, but only a small proportion go on to develop long-term alcohol dependence.

Once a person becomes dependent, the majority follow a pattern of remission and relapse, similar to that of a chronic condition such as rheumatoid arthritis. Without pharmacotherapy, one-year abstinence rates average approximately 20%. The rate of alcohol dependence peaks in the age group 30–49, and declines thereafter through a combination of increased mortality, adoption of abstinence, or, in a small proportion, return to controlled drinking. Spontaneous remission may occur for a variety of reasons, including religious conversion, the development of a strong new relationship, or health problems related to alcohol.

Many of the complications of alcohol-related disease can be arrested or reversed by abstinence. Alcohol-related cardiomyopathy and cirrhosis, and, to some extent, cognitive damage, can all improve with abstinence. Although cirrhosis often involves irreversible elements, some improvement may occur through liver regeneration.

There may be interaction between alcohol and other agents in causation of disease. Alcohol markedly exacerbates the hepatic damage arising from hepatitis C and various toxins; it also increases the chance of oropharyngeal cancers in smokers.

➡ Alcohol exacerbates the hepatic damage arising from hepatitis C and from liver toxins.

Prevention

Methods for prevention and treatment of alcohol misuse can be divided into primary, secondary and tertiary interventions. Primary interventions include measures to prevent the initiation of excessive drinking, such as education campaigns and limits on supply of alcohol (table 10.6). Secondary interventions minimise the impact of heavy drinking on health, prevent progress of heavy drinking to alcohol dependence, and, where possible, return the person to a safe level of drinking. A typical example is early intervention for risky alcohol consumption. Tertiary interventions are treatment measures directed at those with established alcohol dependence or complications of their drinking, and aim to minimise harm, promote remission, and prevent or delay relapse.

It is difficult to assess fully the effectiveness of education campaigns, as many other factors can impact concurrently on a community's drinking. For example, the rate of alcohol consumption in Australia has tended to fall in recent years, but it is difficult to be certain what has caused this reduction. Education campaigns are likely to impact differentially according to the socioeconomic class of the recipient: better educated people of higher socioeconomic status are more likely to respond to health promotion messages than their less educated peers.

Sometimes education programs are limited in their impact because they affect knowledge without affecting behaviour. Nevertheless, this can itself be important. Anecdotal evidence suggests a reasonably high level of ignorance of safe levels of

daily alcohol consumption in the Australian community, and heavy drinkers typically judge their own drinking against that of their peers rather than against any
national recommended limits.

Table 10.7 Examples of primary, secondary, and tertiary interventions

Primary	*Secondary*	*Tertiary*
Public education on sensible drinking limits, labelling on alcohol containers (for example number of standard drinks, strength)	Public education campaigns on drinking and driving	
Policy/Legal controls		
Blood alcohol limits for young drivers	Random breath testing★	Punishment and prevention of further drink-driving, for
Supply limitations	Blood alcohol limits	example fines, imprisonment,
Age limits on buying alcohol	for drivers	licence suspension, ignition interlocks
Licensing controls		Controls on serving alcohol
Controls on cost and availability, for example tax, pricing, licensing		to intoxicated people
Controls on advertising and promotion		
Local or community initiatives		
Geographical limits on drinking (no-drink zones at sporting venues or parks)		Server responsibility: refusing further alcohol to intoxicated persons and
Community-imposed alcohol bans in selected Aboriginal communities		facilitating their safe transport home
Supervision of teenage parties		
Workplace initiatives		
Industry guidelines on avoiding drinking before working with machinery	Employee assistance programs	Employee assistance programs

Continued

Table 10.7   Examples of primary, secondary, and tertiary interventions

Primary	Secondary	Tertiary
Medical practitioner actions		
	Early detection and brief intervention for hazardous and harmful alcohol use	Treatment services (general medical or drug and alcohol services) for treatment of alcohol dependence
Advice on alcohol consumption in patients with newly diagnosed hepatitis C and in pregnancy	Counselling to reduce alcohol consumption before elective surgery	Management of complications of alcohol dependence

★   Note: Some interventions may act as both primary (preventing problems ever occurring) and secondary (limiting extent or severity of problems in those who already might drink to excess)

Secondary interventions

Early intervention for excessive alcohol consumption by doctors and other primary health care workers has been shown repeatedly to be both effective and highly cost-effective as a method of treating non-dependent hazardous or harmful drinking. Early intervention involves active case detection by taking an alcohol consumption history or using a screening questionnaire, followed by provision of brief advice or counselling. As little as five minutes of advice has been shown to have a significant impact on drinking six to nine months later. Intervention typically involves feedback of any evidence of alcohol-related harm or risk, education about safe drinking, and enhancing skills in reducing alcohol consumption. Brief intervention can be integrated with routine clinical practice, and checking of other health risk factors such as blood pressure.

> As little as five minutes of advice from a health practitioner can significantly reduce drinking six months later in a non-dependent person.

In the field of public policy and policing, random breath testing has been a striking example of how a prevention/intervention measure can impact on alcohol-related harm. Following the introduction of random breath testing in 1982 there was a striking fall in the rate of fatal road crashes, and this was accompanied by a change in the reported drinking habits of those intending to drive. The great success of random breath testing as a deterrent to drink-driving has been attributed to the high visibility of testing leading to a perceived high risk of apprehension and punishment. This was combined with consistent efforts to change public attitudes regarding the acceptability of drink-driving.

A wide variety of other interventions have been implemented to reduce drink-driving. These include server-responsibility programs in hotels, where bar staff are instructed to refuse alcohol to intoxicated persons and to consider the safety of patrons leaving the hotel. These have been publicised, and appear to have been implemented in at least some centres.

Tertiary treatments

Tertiary treatment involves intervention at the stage when alcohol-related harm is already evident. In the case of drink-driving, this would include efforts to reduce recidivism in offenders. Rehabilitation programs, though widely implemented, have met with mixed success. Skills-based programs for drink-drivers have sometimes been more successful than knowledge-based education. Licence revocation has been shown to reduce risk-taking on the road even if driving continues, and innovative measures such as ignition interlocks have shown some promise.

A wide variety of treatment facilities are available for those with established alcohol dependence or alcohol-related complications. These are dealt with in more detail in the section on treatment. In general, tertiary treatment services are considerably more expensive than prevention and early intervention programs, and lifelong abstinence is difficult to achieve in people with established dependence who may be experiencing physical, psychological, and/or social complications of drinking. It is also difficult to ensure access of all the needy population to appropriate treatment services.

Case study

Xavier, a 46-year-old university professor, is married and lives with his wife and two daughters. He presents to your general practice complaining of frequent headaches, early morning waking, sweating, tremor, and anxiety in the last three days. He has also noticed a decrease in his energy and ability to concentrate and a decrease in appetite.

Xavier has a history of mild hypertension. His blood pressure has increased in the last few years despite the initiation of therapy with ramipril. This is his second visit over the last month.

His physical examination reveals fine tremor, at least 10 spider naevi, early gynaecomastia, tachychardia (90/min), elevated blood pressure (170/100 mm Hg), and a liver that was slightly enlarged but of normal consistency, and not tender.

Although on all previous visits Xavier denied excessive alcohol use, you suspect that it could be the cause of some of medical problems, and three weeks ago you ordered detailed laboratory tests. The results indicated slightly elevated levels of aspartate transaminase (90 U/L; [N: 10–45 U/L]), gamma-glutamyl transpeptidase (100 U/L; [N: 0–60 U/L]), and carbohydrate-deficient transferrin (35 U/L; [N: 0–20 U/L]). His blood test results revealed mild anaemia (erythrocyte count 3.8×10^{12} cells/L; [N: 4.5–6.5×10^{12} cells/L]) and increased mean corpuscular volume (110 fL; [N: 80–100 fL]). You have not discussed the results of the laboratory tests with him as he missed his previous appointment.

During the current visit you explain the meaning of the laboratory test results in an empathic way, and suggest that his current symptoms are likely to be a consequence of physical dependence on alcohol. His high blood pressure is also likely to be related to excessive alcohol use.

Xavier admits that he has been under gradually increasing pressure at work and at home for the past five years, and that his alcohol intake has increased. You therefore elicit a more detailed history of his alcohol use.

Pattern and context of drinking

Xavier started drinking when he was 15 and used to binge drink when he was in his twenties. However, these binges ceased after he married at age 27. He smoked tobacco and cannabis recreationally in his twenties, but has never used any other illicit drugs. None of his parents or close relatives has a drinking problem. He has no history of seizures.

In his thirties Xavier's alcohol consumption was about one small bottle (375 mL) of light beer and two glasses of white or red wine on weekdays (three standard drinks a day) and two to three bottles of table wine on weekends with friends and family. His share was about 500 mL of wine a day on weekends (five standard drinks a day). He, therefore, used to drink 25 standard drinks a week or less than four standard drinks per day on average.

He started to increase his alcohol intake about five years ago when he was promoted at work. He felt that he needed to relax after a busy and stressful day, but the amounts previously used did not suffice. His drinking escalated, especially during the last 12 months. A year ago he was drinking two to three small bottles of medium-strength beer on his arrival home, shared a bottle of wine with his wife at dinner (his share was about two-thirds of a 750 mL bottle), and had one or two nips of Scotch whisky on an average day (nine to 10 standard drinks a day). Now he is drinking two bottles of red or white wine (14 standard drinks) on weekdays. On weekends he drinks mostly Scotch whisky (about two-thirds of a bottle, that is 15 to 16 standard drinks). Therefore his weekly alcohol consumption is about 100 standard drinks. He often skips his breakfast and takes a sip of wine or Scotch before leaving for work.

Problems related to alcohol use

His wife and daughters object strongly to his drinking. His wife became especially concerned with his health and well-being a while ago, after she noticed him having a nip of Scotch early in the morning. They often argue when he is intoxicated, but otherwise they have a good relationship. However, five days ago she threatened him with divorce if he continued drinking. Earlier that day he had an argument with a university colleague who complained about his poor supervision. He got very annoyed, left home, and drank all night in the pub, consuming about double the amount he usually had. On his way home he was arrested for impaired driving with a BAC of 0.19%.

He has not drunk alcoholic beverages from that time. He has felt miserable and anxious with headaches and sleep difficulties, and has been shaky and sweaty.

Xavier has tried to stop or cut down many times before, with little success. His periods of abstinence did not last longer than three weeks. He would start drinking heavily again because he felt a strong craving for alcohol, and he felt so much better after a drink. He also reported recent morning drinking, which caused problems at work and at home.

He realises that he probably drinks excessively and this could be a cause of problems and a loss of prestige at work. He has often taken unpaid sick leave this year, and his number of work hours and productivity have decreased lately. He often feels depressed and has difficulties concentrating.

He is likely to be fined for drink-driving and to have his licence suspended.

Despite a long history of family problems related to his excessive alcohol use, Xavier believes that his wife and daughters would support him if he decides to quit drinking. They are on much better terms now, as he has not drunk for several days and is determined to stop. He still meets socially with the same group of friends he has been with for a number of years, although they have met much less often during this year. They are all moderate drinkers.

You summarise the information obtained and reflect it back to your patient. Xavier agrees that his serious health, social, professional, and legal problems are associated with his alcohol use.

Diagnosis of dependence

You question Xavier further in order to make a diagnosis of dependence (using DSM–IV criteria) and learn that (before his recent decision to stop drinking):

1 compared to last year Xavier had to drink larger amounts of alcohol to achieve the relaxation he was seeking
2 in the morning he woke up early feeling shaky and sweaty, and had to have a drink before he went to work; he also had difficulty with falling asleep when he stopped drinking, and took benzodiazepines (though with little effect)
3 he found it difficult to stop drinking once he started, even if he made a decision to drink less
4 he had made several unsuccessful efforts to abstain during this year, and had a persistent desire to control his drinking

5 he did not spend much time obtaining alcohol and appeared to recover from alcohol intoxication (or withdrawal) relatively quickly, although he had taken sick leave

6 he did not give up his usual activities because of his drinking, as he still maintains his everyday routine and he has never been very much involved in recreational activities

7 he continued drinking excessively after he realised that his morning drinking had been noticed at work and caused some problems.

As Xavier satisfies five out of seven DSM-IV criteria, you conclude that he meets the criteria for diagnosis of alcohol dependence.

Motivational interviewing and goal-setting

You discuss the diagnosis with Xavier and ask him how he feels about his physical dependence on alcohol. He is very much concerned about the effects of his drinking on his health, on his family relationships, and on his professional status, and he is willing to do something about his drinking. He is, therefore, at a stage of preparation for change. Using motivational interviewing techniques, you encourage him to talk about the possible benefits of changing his drinking pattern. You advise him that he needs to have a period of abstinence of at least three months' duration, mainly because of his impaired liver function. You also explain that you will prescribe a higher dose of ramipril but it is unlikely that the drug would lower his blood pressure effectively unless he abstains from alcohol.

Xavier agrees with you that moderate drinking is not appropriate at this stage, and that abstinence is the most appropriate treatment goal.

Treatment strategies

Given that Xavier still experiences withdrawal symptoms and feels a strong craving for alcohol, you consider a prescription of acamprosate or naltrexone. You explain to Xavier that naltrexone would significantly reduce his enjoyment of alcohol and possibly his craving for it, and acamprosate would reduce protracted withdrawal. However, the use of acamprosate requires strong motivation to take it three times a day. As Xavier is concerned that he could forget to take the drug regularly, you recommend naltrexone. You also prescribe a short course of diazepam (four days) to help relieve his current withdrawal symptoms. You explain that benzodiazepines are commonly used to treat alcohol withdrawal, both inpatient and outpatient, as they have a mechanism of action similar to that of alcohol. You also inform him about the danger of benzodiazepine dependence.

Xavier agrees that in addition to naltrexone he will need to develop skills that will help him to abstain from alcohol. You present these skills in an empathic and positive way, and discuss with Xavier his high-risk situations and how he might deal with them.

You also discuss with Xavier the importance of his social support in maintaining long-term abstinence. Xavier states that his wife and his daughters would probably be his most reliable support. He also suggests that his family friends would support him as they had been concerned with his behaviour lately, and many times had expressed their willingness to help. Previously, he would only get angry and annoyed with their supportive attitude.

At the end of the visit you summarise Xavier's goals and also reinforce and help him to clarify his reasons for deciding to change.

Xavier agrees to come to see you again in two weeks' time for you to assess his progress, monitor his blood pressure, and repeat his liver-function tests.

Case points
Xavier's case illustrates the following:
- tolerance to alcohol
- cross-tolerance with benzodiazepines
- withdrawal and physical dependence
- behavioural (psychological) dependence
- chronic alcohol toxicity (organ damage)
- laboratory tests suggestive of alcohol abuse
- social, professional, and legal problems related to excessive alcohol use
- increase in alcohol consumption in response to specific life events
- abstinence in response to specific life events
- relapse
- state of change
- diagnosis of dependence
- treatment plan (treatment of withdrawal, relapse prevention)
- social support.

REFERENCES AND FURTHER READING

Fauci, A.S. et al. (eds) 1998, *Harrison's Principles of Internal Medicine* (14th edn), McGraw-Hill, New York, pp. 2503–8.

Garbutt, J.C., West, S.L., Carey, T.S., Lohr, K.N. & Crews, F.T. 1999, 'Pharmacological treatment of alcohol dependence. A review of the evidence', *Journal of the American Medical Association*, vol. 281, pp. 1318–25.

Mayo-Smith, M.F. 1997, 'Pharmacological management of alcohol withdrawal: a meta-analysis and evidence-based practice guideline. American Society of Addiction Medicine Working Group on Pharmacological Management of Alcohol Withdrawal', *Journal of the American Medical Association*, vol. 278, pp. 144–51.

National Health & Medical Research Council 2001, *Australian Alcohol Guidelines: Health risks and benefits*, Commonwealth of Australia, Canberra. Also via http://www.health.gov.au/hfs/nhmrc/publications/synopses/ds9syn.htm

Nutt, D. 1999, 'Alcohol and the brain. Pharmacological insights for psychiatrists', *British Journal of Psychiatry*, vol. 175, pp. 114–19.

Sedman et al. 1976, 'Food effects on absorption and metabolism of alcohol', *Journal of Studies on Alcohol*, vol. 37 (9), pp. 1197–214.

Sullivan, J., Sykora, K., Schneiderman, J., Naranjo, C. & Sellers, E. 1989, 'Assessment of alcohol withdrawal: The Revised Clinical Institute Withdrawal Assessment for Alcohol Scale (CIWA-Ar)', *British Journal of Addiction*, vol. 84, pp. 1353–7.

11

Sedative–Hypnotics

Gavin Cape, Gary Hulse, Geoff Robinson, Stuart McLean, John Saunders, Ross Young & Jennifer Martin

Benzodiazepines—The opium of the masses

Malcolm Lader 1978, title of a commentary in the journal *Neuroscience*.

The sedative–hypnotics are a group of drugs whose effects include anxiolysis at low doses and sedation and sleep (hypnosis) at higher doses. The benzodiazepine family of drugs is the main focus of this chapter.

While safer than the barbiturates that they have largely replaced, benzodiazepines may induce a dependence syndrome and have physical and psychological side-effects. These drugs are also implicated in more serious harms, including overdose deaths, when used in conjunction with other drugs. Barbiturates have a strong association with misuse and abuse, but have not been readily available in Australia and New Zealand for several years.

The drug gamma-hydroxybutyric acid (GHB or grevious bodily harm/GBH) is a manufactured street drug that has similar action to the benzodiazepines and has become fashionable. In high doses profound sedation and seizures can occur.

Some newer therapeutic agents, for example zopiclone and zolpidem, are chemically different from benzodiazepines, but have similar sedative–hypnotic effects. It is suggested that they will have less association with problems of dependence, but this is yet to be determined.

The first benzodiazepine, chlordiazepoxide (Librium), was marketed as a safe tranquilliser in 1959 and started a new era in the 'control of personal and emotional problems'. Along with lavish promotional campaigns many other benzodiazepines were developed, with diazepam (Valium), the best known, being released in 1963. During the 1970s and early 1980s benzodiazepines became the most commonly prescribed class of drug in the world. The prescribing of benzodiazepines declined subsequently, due to increasingly negative attitudes to these substances associated with concerns over side-effects and the recognition of a specific dependence syndrome. Another concern has been the diminishing clinical effect that comes with the development of tolerance to these drugs.

While benzodiazepine dependency can result from illicit or street use, it is more commonly a result of over-prescription by doctors, and in this sense it is an iatrogenic entity.

PHARMACOKINETICS AND PHARMACODYNAMICS

The name 'benzodiazepine' refers to a characteristic 7-membered nitrogenous ring, but some newer sedative–hypnotic agents (for example zopiclone, zolpidem) that lack this structure are pharmacologically similar. Most are poorly water-soluble, requiring an organic solvent (such as propylene glycol) to make a soluble formulation in capsules or for injection. Unless well diluted, mixing these solutions with water or blood can result in precipitation. A notable exception to this is the ultra-short-acting benzodiazepine midazolam, which is readily dissolved in water. This characteristic makes it ideal for brief anaesthesia induction, and in a more sinister application (as it is tasteless and odourless) it has been used to spike drinks, giving it a reputation as one of the date-rape drugs.

Mode of action

Benzodiazepines enhance the effects of gamma-aminobutyric acid (GABA), the main inhibitory neurotransmitter in the central nervous system (CNS). GABA binding to postsynaptic GABA-A receptors opens the chloride channel resulting in hyperpolarisation and inhibition of the neurone. Benzodiazepines and GABA bind to different sites on the GABA-A receptor macromolecule, allosterically enhancing each other's binding, but only GABA can open the chloride channel. The protein subunits of GABA-A receptors vary in different parts of the brain, suggesting that there may be a range of receptor subtypes. This raises the prospect of the development of more selective drugs in the future. In addition, two other types of ligand bind to the benzodiazepine receptor site. Inverse agonists (for example β-carbolines) decrease GABA binding and cause anxiety and convulsions. Antagonists (for example flumazenil) block both agonists and inverse agonists, and can be used to reverse the effects of benzodiazepines after overdose. The existence and role of endogenous benzodiazepine ligands remains uncertain.

Pharmacokinetics

Absorption

The benzodiazepines are all relatively lipophilic drugs that are well absorbed orally. However, the more lipophilic agents (for example diazepam) are absorbed faster than the relatively more hydrophilic drugs (for example oxazepam). This difference may be important for sleep induction, but not for relief of anxiety, where continuous effect is more important than rapid onset. For acute seizures, the intravenous or rectal route is preferred. Intramuscular injection of diazepam results in slow and erratic absorption.

Midazolam can be formulated into an aqueous solution for intravenous administration, after which it cyclises at the neutral pH in vivo to a lipophilic form that rapidly enters the brain and produces anaesthesia.

Distribution

Benzodiazepines readily enter the CNS, giving rapid anaesthesia after intravenous administration. Under these circumstances, recovery is due to redistribution to less vascular tissue rather than to elimination from the body. This explains the paradoxically brief action of IV diazepam, whose effective elimination half-life is over 100 hours.

All benzodiazepines can cross the placenta and result in neonatal depression if used in high doses during labour. Prolonged use during pregnancy can result in withdrawal symptoms in the newborn infant.

Elimination

Benzodiazepines must be converted into water-soluble metabolites before they can be excreted renally. The more lipophilic drugs require oxidative metabolism (which can result in active metabolites) before conjugation to inactive and excretable glucuronides. For example, diazepam can undergo N-demethylation, ring-hydroxylation, or both reactions, to form nordiazepam and oxazepam, both active drugs. The active metabolites, which can have longer half-lives than the parent drug, can accumulate and result in prolonged effects, especially with chronic dosing.

Plasma levels and effects

There is no simple relationship between plasma levels and effects, as there are influences of the route of administration, speed of absorption, rate of distribution, formation of active metabolites, and degree of tolerance. Furthermore, the potency of benzodiazepines varies greatly, as seen by the 100-fold variation in doses typically used.

> ➡ Benzodiazepines bind to receptors on the GABA-A receptor complex, enhancing the inhibitory affects of GABA.
> ➡ Benzodiazepines differ mainly in their pharmacokinetics, although newer sedative–hypnotic agents (for example zolpidem, zopiclone) may have different retention.

TOXICITY

There is a range of acute and chronic side-effects, including performance deficits and emotional blunting. A range of other effects has been reported.

Chronic use predisposes to physical dependence (see below). Many of the acute toxic effects of benzodiazepines persist, although tolerance to some effects occurs. There is no known organ toxicity.

Performance deficits

Most benzodiazepines have a marked effect on memory, particularly anterograde amnesia (the consolidation of memory). This effect may be useful prior to endoscopy/surgery as the patient has little memory of the procedure taking place, but it may be a great hindrance in continued use.

Specific brain functions are also affected, leading to motor incoordination, decreased reaction time, and ataxia. This can lead to performance on complex tasks being impaired, for example an increase in motor vehicle accidents with people taking benzodiazepines.

The elderly are particularly prone to the performance deficits from a cognitive perspective (for example confusional states) and neuromuscular perspective (for example frequent falls).

Emotional blunting

With arousal being inhibited by benzodiazepines, many long-term benzodiazepine users complain of being unable to feel the normal highs in life. Benzodiazepines may also inhibit the normal grieving process.

Paradoxical effects

An uncommon side-effect may be extreme disinhibited behaviour leading to actions uncharacteristic to the user, sometimes called the paradoxical rage reaction. This side-effect has been linked with child battering, assaults, and shoplifting. A common saying in those people who take large doses of street benzodiazepines is that the user feels '10 foot tall, bullet-proof, and invisible'.

Other effects

Other effects of benzodiazepines that have been reported include:
* muscle weakness or hypotonia
* headaches
* sensitivity reactions
* potentiation of other intoxicating drugs, for example alcohol, opioids
* menstrual irregularities, breast engorgement
* euphoria, restlessness, and hypomanic behaviour.

When used as an hypnotic, benzodiazepines may increase the incidence of night-mares, especially during the first week of use.

Overdose

Benzodiazepines are relatively safe in overdose (compared with barbiturates), but they can cause respiratory depression if taken in very large amounts or when administered intravenously. When benzodiazepines are taken with other CNS depressants (for example alcohol or opioids), their respiratory depressant effects are greatly magnified.

TOLERANCE AND PHYSICAL DEPENDENCE

Tolerance

The development of tolerance to the sedative and psychomotor effects of benzodi-azepines is well documented, but there are conflicting reports about the development of tolerance to the anxiolytic and memory effects.

Tolerance is thought to be related to the action of benzodiazepines at their receptor sites, and not to pharmacokinetic changes—benzodiazepines do not stimu-late microsomal hepatic enzymes (whereas barbiturates are potent enzyme inducers). Receptor-mediated mechanisms that may lead to the development of tolerance include changes to the intrinsic sensitivity to GABA, altered functional properties of the GABA-A receptor complex, and up-regulation of neuronal calcium channels (increasing cellular excitability).

Dependence and withdrawal

Benzodiazepines used for three to six weeks at therapeutic doses can be associated with the development of dependence and clinically significant withdrawal symptoms upon cessation or dose reduction. The withdrawal syndrome for benzodiazepines usually lasts for several days or weeks, but a small proportion of patients complain of withdrawal symptoms for months.

Dependence is a major problem with continued use, resulting in a withdrawal syndrome after sudden discontinuance (or even between doses of short-acting agents such as triazolam). Benzodiazepines also have a street value, which is usually a good indication of a propensity to dependence—they are commonly sought-after drugs. It is important to recognise that withdrawal syndromes do occur following cessation of benzodiazepine administration, and it is not merely the return of the condition being treated in the first place. New symptoms arise, for example perceptual changes, there is a characteristic peaking of withdrawal symptoms/signs, and the syndrome occurs when patients have stopped taking benzodiazepines for epilepsy. There is debate about incidence, and there is wide variation in the severity and type of symptoms experienced in withdrawal. In general, reports indicate that approximately 40% of people on benzodiazepines for more than six months will have a moderate to severe withdrawal, and the remaining 60% will have a relatively mild withdrawal syndrome, if the drug is stopped suddenly.

The cause of withdrawal is largely unknown, although there is some evidence for down-regulation of benzodiazepine binding sites in the GABA complex, and for increased calcium and 5-HT flux during withdrawal. Supporting evidence for non-GABA involvement includes the finding that the calcium channel antagonist verapamil, the GABA-B agonist baclofen, and the 5-HT$_3$ receptor antagonist zacopride, have all prevented withdrawal responses in rats.

Symptoms and signs of withdrawal

The absence or presence of withdrawal symptoms should be assessed. Withdrawal symptoms can largely be divided into three main groups: anxiety and anxiety-related symptoms, perceptual distortions, and major events.

Anxiety and anxiety-related symptoms

These include:
- anxiety, panic attacks, hyperventilation, tremor
- sleep disturbance, muscle spasms, anorexia, weight loss
- visual disturbance, sweating
- dysphoria.

Perceptual distortions

These include:
- hypersensitivity to stimuli, for example hyperacusis
- abnormal bodily sensations
- depersonalisation/derealisation.

Major events

These include:
- seizures—grand mal type
- precipitation of psychosis, for example hallucinations, delusions, and delirium.

> ➡ The molecular mechanisms responsible for the development of benzodi-
> azepine tolerance, physical dependence, and the withdrawal syndrome are
> not well known. In addition to changes at the GABA-A receptor complex,
> there is evidence for non-GABA-ergic involvement in withdrawal, that is
> 5-HT and calcium channel activation.
> ➡ Dependence on benzodiazepines can occur after several weeks of
> continuous use.
> ➡ Tolerance does occur, but is often symptom-selective.
> ➡ Withdrawal symptoms are not simply the re-emergence of the original
> condition treated.

THERAPEUTIC USE

Benzodiazepines do have a limited place in the pharmaceutical armoury of the
medical practitioner and can be useful for short-term prescribing (two to four
weeks, generally much shorter). They have the following therapeutic benefits:
- relief of severe anxiety
- sleep promotion, for example to ward off jet-lag
- muscle relaxation after injury
- anti-seizure activity, for example to abort status epilepticus
- surgical or medical procedures as a pre-med or induction of temporary anaesthesia, for example for dental or endoscopic procedures (amnesic properties can
  be useful)
- withdrawal regimes from alcohol dependence and other drugs
- rapid tranquillisation in psychiatric emergencies.

Caution must be exercised before prescribing benzodiazepines, as once a
prescription is started it can be difficult to stop. Special care is indicated in the
following groups of patients, and constitutes a relative contraindication to their use:
- grief reactions—possibility of prolonging the grief reaction
- brain-damaged patients—risk of exacerbating cognitive impairment
- drug-seeking patients—assisting in maintenance of a dependence
- the elderly—risk of falls and other complications (see chapter 19)
- alcohol- and drug-dependent patients—risk of overdose, inappropriate use
- patients with personality disorders—risk of increased behavioural problems.

In clinical practice there are three main groups where benzodiazepine dependence is likely to occur:

- long-term prescribed patients who take therapeutic doses
- the elderly (usually when prescribed as a hypnotic; see chapter 19)
- younger street users who are likely to be abusing other drugs such as alcohol or opioids (see chapter 14).

There are few, if any, indications for long-term treatment with benzodiazepines. In this respect all dependent patients need to be assessed for a withdrawal regime.

ASSESSMENT

A comprehensive assessment should be undertaken prior to the investigation of benzodiazepine dependence and to determine the need for withdrawal management. This initial assessment should include the original reasons for prescription of benzodiazepines and a determination as to whether this situation still exists. The next step in the assessment process involves determining if the patient is dependent, and, if so, if the patient is currently showing signs of withdrawal or if he or she is likely to in the near future.

Dependence can be ascertained by reviewing:

- the duration of regular use
- the dosage
- the type of benzodiazepine used
- the presence of signs of withdrawal following short periods of abstinence.

Common withdrawal symptoms will include sleep disturbances, and early morning wakening, often accompanied by anxiety, tremor, and sweating. Panic attacks and hyperventilation may also be reported. Relief of these symptoms following use is also a marker for physical dependence.

Having identified that the patient is currently dependent and requires managed withdrawal, the practitioner needs to determine the most suitable withdrawal treatment plan. This will include identification of those patients who are likely to have a severe withdrawal, and who therefore may require inpatient treatment. Withdrawal from benzodiazepines is usually done on an outpatient basis through a general practitioner or specialist. However, if severe withdrawal is anticipated then advice from or referral to a specialist may be required, and an inpatient withdrawal setting considered.

The commitment and ability of the patient to adhere to a withdrawal treatment plan should also be assessed. Those who have poor social support or unstable social conditions, or who have low levels of motivation to adhere to treatment, may also be candidates for inpatient withdrawal.

The practitioner will also need to identify those patients where change to a longer-acting benzodiazepine is indicated. By substituting a long-acting benzodiazepine, usually diazepam for the short-acting benzodiazepines, the clinician avoids

Table 11.1 Common benzodiazepine equivalent doses to 10mg diazepam

Benzodiazepine	*Common tradenames*	*Half-life in hours (approx)*	*Equivalent dose to 10mgs diazepam*
alprazolam	Xanax	6–12	0.5mgs
chlordiazepoxide	Librium	5–200	25mgs
clonazepam	Rivotril, Klonopin	18–50	0.5mgs
diazepam	Valium, Pro-Pam	20–200	10mgs
flunitrazepam	Rohypnol	18–200	1mg
lorazepam	Ativan	10–20	1mg
midazolam	Hypnovel	2–5	1 – 2mgs
nitrazepam	Mogadon	15–38	5 – 10mgs
oxazepam	Serax, Ox-Pam	4–15	20mgs
temazepam	Normison, Euhypnos	8–22	20mgs
triazolam	Halcion	2	0.5mgs
zopiclone	Imovane	5–6	15mgs

the frequent dosing schedules required with a shorter-acting benzodiazepine, and the longer action promotes stable benzodiazepine blood levels. This leads to a more controlled and graduated reduction in benzodiazepine dose, which in turn translates into a withdrawal that is easier to manage and is more acceptable to the patient. The practitioner will need to establish an equivalent dose level of diazepam for the benzodiazepine it is to replace (see table 11.1). This movement to a longer-acting benzodiazepine is less necessary with medium half-life benzodiazepines or for those patients who only take benzodiazepines at night.

Predictors of severe withdrawal

There are several predictors of those who will suffer significant withdrawal:
- those who have been taking benzodiazepines for extended periods of time
- those who use doses above the recommended therapeutic level
- the type of benzodiazepine taken—there are more likely to be problems with those with a short half-life, such as lorazepam and triazolam, and those benzodiazepines with high receptor efficacy, such as flunitrazepam
- patients with a past history of complicated withdrawal, for example seizures, delirium, or psychosis
- patients with a past history of uncompleted or failed withdrawal
- patients with coexisting severe psychiatric or physical disorders.

INTERVENTION AND TREATMENT

Engagement

As part of the assessment the practitioner will have reviewed the patient's motivation to address the overuse of benzodiazepines and dependence. Where motivation is marginal or low, the first step is enhancement of motivation for change. The patient may perceive great benefit in continuing benzodiazepine use, so various strategies may be required to encourage the uptake of treatment.

The patient (and the prescribing practitioner) needs to be assured that withdrawal from benzodiazepines is the best treatment. As indicated above, there are many reasons that long-term use of benzodiazepines is contraindicated and discussion with the patient is usually useful. A rationale can contain the following information:

- If benzodiazepines have been taken for a prolonged period then it is likely that, due to the development of tolerance, they will no longer be effective for the original condition.
- Side-effects (for example memory impairment) are also likely to be present (see above, under toxicity), and will almost certainly be impairing the patient's functioning.
- Dependency symptoms, such as taking the drug merely to avoid withdrawal effects, may be present.
- Medical authorities have also determined that maintenance prescribing of benzodiazepines for dependency requires authority from a specialist (benzodiazepines have a controlled drug status in those patients judged as dependent).

Introducing the withdrawal regime

Patients need information about the manner and nature of withdrawal, and it is usually best provided in oral and written form. Reassurance should be given that the great majority of patients in a withdrawal program can manage it successfully and with little impact on their day-to-day lives. Involvement of significant others can also be a great source of support.

Rate and timing of withdrawal

Benzodiazepines must not be stopped abruptly in patients at risk of withdrawal, as there is a danger of precipitating major events such as psychosis and seizures.

The timing of withdrawal is an important part of therapeutic engagement. Ideally withdrawal should be planned for a time when the patient is ready, has gathered sufficient supports and information, and when other stressors are minimised. A written contract may be helpful.

For patients on long-term stabilised high or therapeutic doses of benzodiazepines, gradual withdrawal over weeks or months is recommended. Some authorities have

221

suggested a month of withdrawal for every year the patient has been dependent on benzodiazepines. Such approaches may be reasonable for socially unstable persons with coexisting psychiatric disorders and ongoing crises, but gradual withdrawal, although ameliorating symptoms, does not prevent them. Many patients prefer a shorter withdrawal (over two to three months) rather than the long-term protracted process. In general, decrements of 5% of a stabilisation dose per week are tolerated.

With 24-hour supervision and medical support, inpatient withdrawal may be rapid, decreasing from 40 mg of diazepam equivalents to zero in a week to 10 days. It is important to note that withdrawal symptoms may peak up to five days after cessation of diazepam, so further close monitoring is essential.

Prescribing considerations

As noted in the discussion of assessment, a long-acting benzodiazepine is often substituted for a shorter-acting benzodiazepine to promote more stable blood levels during withdrawal management. This leads to a situation that is generally easier to manage, and a more graduated reduction. The transition to a longer-acting drug can, however, be a difficult period in management, not only from pharmacological considerations but also in dealing with the patient's psychological dependence on the previous benzodiazepine tablet and more frequent dosing.

Other medications may be useful, and some authorities have recommended the use of antidepressants (particularly sedative tricyclics and the selective serotonin reupstake inhibitors) or propranolol (20–160 mg/day), which may lessen the severity of withdrawal symptoms. Carbamazepine has also been used, particularly in those patients who have a history of seizures, and clonidine may be useful for restlessness and agitation.

Prescriptions may need to be endorsed under close control, with restrictions as to the amount dispensed by the pharmacist at any one time. Some patients require dispensing two or three times per week, and some users of street drugs who are unstable or unreliable on higher doses may merit daily dispensing similar to the provisions of a methadone program.

Monitoring withdrawal

Regular monitoring is essential to detect any emerging underlying condition, to adjust the rate of withdrawal, and to offer advice, information, support, and, if necessary, the use of other medications as above.

Psychological and community support may be helpful. Consider a referral to a counsellor or psychological therapist for stress/anxiety management, and encourage attendance at self-help groups such as Tranx.

It is important to attempt to follow up benzodiazepine-withdrawn patients and to identify psychosocial stressors that could bring about relapse. Many patients can be successfully withdrawn from benzodiazepines, but, as with other addictions, relapse is not infrequent, particularly for street drug users who may still be able to purchase benzodiazepines or who may engage in doctor shopping. Further action is advised if doctor shopping is suspected, as discussed in chapter 21.

Special scenarios

The benzodiazepine-dependent patient on methadone maintenance

Benzodiazepine-dependent patients on methadone maintenance can be withdrawn in the usual manner. Participation in a methadone program carries an advantage of supervised frequent dispensing. It is important not to ignore the methadone patient who is dependent on benzodiazepines, because the benzodiazepines may cause more social and behavioural problems than opioids. Being on methadone is not an indication for prescribing maintenance benzodiazepine.

The benzodiazepine-dependent patient who injects benzodiazepines

A small but troubled subgroup of street drug users injects benzodiazepines. They appear to inject temazepam most commonly, but they are frequently IV opioid users as well. It is important to try to attempt to engage them and to encourage oral use of benzodiazepines, preferably with observed consumption. Continuing temazepam prescriptions are contraindicated (also see chapters 13 and 14).

The pregnant benzodiazepine-dependent user

Benzodiazepine dependency in pregnancy is a concerning scenario, as there is evidence (not unequivocal, however) that benzodiazepines may cause foetal malformations (for example dysmorphogenesis) that may be dose-related. It is preferable to indicate such concerns to the patient and to persuade the pregnant woman to withdraw at a gradual and steady rate.

The elderly on long-term hypnotic benzodiazepines

The decision to withdraw hypnotics gradually in the elderly patient may be difficult due to patient resistance, but continuing efforts to do so are advised. Various important factors to weigh up include the disposition to falls and frailty, cognitive impairment, alcohol use, and issues of control of chronic pain (see chapter 19).

➡ The original reasons for the prescription of benzodiazepines may have been superseded by dependency.
➡ Patients must be informed about benzodiazepine dependency concerns, and be strongly encouraged to accept a withdrawal program.
➡ Identify which benzodiazepine-dependent people will need referral to specialist services or require inpatient management of withdrawal.

> ⇒ Develop a treatment plan and contract for gradual withdrawal. Do not stop the benzodiazepines abruptly.
>
> ⇒ Substitute diazepam if multiple dosages of shorter acting benzodiazepines are being taken.
>
> ⇒ Consider referral for psychosocial supports and skills-training for anxiety and insomnia.
>
> ⇒ Monitor, reassure, and provide information to the patient.
>
> ⇒ Accept that some patients will require adjunctive drug treatment for emerging anxiety and depression.

EPIDEMIOLOGY AND PREVENTION

Prescriptions

In Australia and New Zealand benzodiazepines remain one of the most prescribed of all medication groups, and there are significant concerns with over-prescription of this class of drug. It is estimated that approximately 4% of all prescriptions from general practice are for benzodiazepines, which are prescribed to approximately 7% of patients. Pharmaceutical records indicate that enough benzodiazepines are prescribed to maintain approximately 3% of the adult population on daily continuous medication.

Predictors of benzodiazepine prescription include being female, being elderly, being an established patient, having chronic illness or disability, attending a busy doctor, or attending a doctor working in an inner urban area. The elderly appear to be particularly likely to receive a prescription of benzodiazepine, with over 40% of prescriptions being for those over 70 years of age.

Illicit use

With high levels of prescription, it is not surprising that benzodiazepines find their way into illicit use. It is estimated that 6% of the population have used benzodiazepines for non-medical purposes, with 3% having used in the last 12 months. This recent use is primarily among younger age groups with a mean age in the mid twenties.

While most illicit use is via oral administration, IV administration is reported among approximately 5% of males. Most users see benzodiazepines as a second-choice drug, which may explain why its illicit use is often associated with the use of other drugs such as alcohol and heroin. Benzodiazepines are also used to mitigate the withdrawal effects of alcohol, stimulants, and opioids.

Rationalising benzodiazepine use

Reductions in benzodiazepine dependence could follow if prescribing for insomnia, anxiety and depressive disorders was more judicious.

Sleep disturbances

Insomnia is commonly a symptom of an underlying problem. Benzodiazepine treatment is often ineffective in these cases and may aggravate the problem. Such problems include sleep apnoea, narcolepsy, disturbances of circadian rhythms, and sleep disturbances associated with shift work, poor sleep habits, psychiatric illness, or psychosocial stress such as recession, unemployment, personal problems, and financial problems. Also included here are presentations resulting from inappropriate expectations about sleep. For example, in the elderly early bed times, due to loneliness or lack of activity, result in early morning wakening, and this may be interpreted as insomnia (see chapter 19).

225

The first line of treatment for any sleep disturbance should be non–pharmaceutical, including counselling with structured advice on sleep management (Mant & Walsh 1997), and, where available, access to relaxation tapes and videos on sleep.

Anxiety and depression

Most anxiety disorders, including agoraphobia, panic, post-traumatic stress, and generalised anxiety disorder, are best treated with cognitive-behaviour therapy. This non-pharmaceutical intervention incorporates a number of behavioural techniques such as graded exposure to feared situations, relaxation techniques, and coping strategies, and verbal interventions aimed at correcting the patient's interpretation of inert situations as dangerous or undesirable.

Only in severe cases should co–drug treatment be initiated. Benzodiazepines are, however, not the only option, with selective serotonin reuptake inhibitors and tricyclic antidepressants of proven efficacy. Short courses of benzodiazepines may be required to mitigate anxiety initially heightened by antidepressants.

Benzodiazepines have no place in the management of social or specific phobias and obsessive compulsive disorders for which cognitive-behaviour therapy has proven efficacy. SSRIs or moclobemide, or beta-blockers, may be prescribed as co-therapy. For some anxiety disorders (except panic disorder) buspirone, a drug with anxiolytic but no sedative/muscle relaxant properties, may be efficacious. Onset of action is slower than with benzodiazepines, with significant improvement noted after four to six weeks. Buspirone has less potential for producing sedation, psychomotor impairment, abuse, or dependence. While it has few drug interactions, its use may lead to the serotonergic syndrome or worsening of anxiety when used with SSRIs, and it should not be used with monoamine oxidase inhibitors.

Reducing non-prescription and illicit use

Benzodiazepines are frequently used contrary to medical advice. In some instances they are used as recreational drugs, and they are commonly implicated in accidental and intentional overdose, usually as part of poly-drug use. Major groups at risk include young women, the elderly, people with psychiatric morbidity, and problem users of alcohol, heroin, and other drugs. These groups often have a poor understanding of poly-drug pharmacy, and should be educated on the risk of mixing benzodiazepines with other CNS depressants.

Benzodiazepines should be prescribed in limited amounts to reduce the likelihood of future non-prescription or illicit use, alone or in association with alcohol, heroin, or other drug use.

Avoiding dependence

Where indicated, benzodiazepine treatment should be initiated at the lowest possible dose and in general not exceed two to four weeks. Tapered use is recommended over this period. In rare instances where longer use is indicated, regular reviews of the underlying condition, use patterns, and tapering, are essential. Interrupted courses of treatment of two to four weeks should be considered.

Initiating review and reduction

Given the high level of benzodiazepine prescriptions over many years, in any community there will be a reservoir of patients who have been using benzodiazepines for prolonged periods and have both pharmacological and psychological dependence. In such cases frequent reassessment is needed, and, if indicated, benzodiazepine withdrawal should be initiated.

A large proportion of long-term benzodiazepine users will, with encouragement and support, reduce or cease consumption, irrespective of age, sex, duration of use, or despite initially indicating they did not wish to cease.

- ➡ Benzodiazepines are frequently inappropriately prescribed to manage insomnia, anxiety, or depressive disorders.
- ➡ Identify and treat the underlying causes of the sleep disturbance with the first line management non-pharmaceutical intervention.
- ➡ Most anxiety disorders are best treated with cognitive-behaviour therapy.
- ➡ For most anxiety disorders, buspirone has equivalent efficacy to benzodiazepines.
- ➡ Poly-drug use involving benzodiazepines is commonly practised and is frequently implicated in accidental and intentional overdose.
- ➡ Restrict benzodiazepine use to short courses (two to four weeks) at the lowest possible dose.

➡ Where longer use is indicated, ensure frequent reassessment of need, consider interrupted courses of treatment of two to four weeks, and whenever possible initiate tapered withdrawal in a supportive environment.

Case study

Mary, a 43-year-old nurse, presents at your general practice with a six-year history of taking lorazepam 1 mg three times a day and 1–2 mg at night. She started benzodiazepines nearly 20 years ago to assist with previous shift work, and has taken them intermittently ever since. Her longest abstinence was for one year, during which time she took amitriptyline primarily for insomnia. She drinks one or two glasses of wine per evening and does not smoke. She claims never to have used hospital supplies of benzodiazepines. One year ago her husband, who had a major psychiatric illness, died. Three weeks ago her prescribing doctor retired from practice, so she has come to you instead.

Mary has had no significant past medical history and no contact with psychiatric services. She agrees she is dependent on lorazepam and that she is now free from the previous social stressors. She consents to a six-month withdrawal regime after gathering information and ensuring good social and medical support. You initially convert her lorazepam to an equivalent dose of diazepam—10 mg in the morning, 15 mg at night. These doses are then gradually reduced in a step-wise fashion. Mary continues to work throughout the withdrawal period, during which her main adverse symptom was insomnia. Over the last three months you assist her in the management of this problem by prescribing low-dose doxepin and regular medical reviews.

Case points

Mary's case illustrates:
- occupational risk (nursing and shift work)
- a long history of social stress (husband's illness)
- the new prescriber recognises the need to encourage withdrawal
- supportive withdrawal can often be successful, and there was no development of major psychiatric symptoms.

REFERENCES AND FURTHER READING

Mant, A. & Walsh, R.A. 1997, 'Reducing benzodiazepine use', *Drug and Alcohol Review*, vol. 16, pp. 77–84.

227

Marriot, S. & Tyrer, P. 1993, 'Benzodiazepine dependence: Avoidance and withdrawal', *Drug Safety*, vol. 9, pp. 93–103.

Norman, T.R., Ellen, S.R. & Burrows, G.D. 1997, 'Benzodiazepines in anxiety disorders: Managing therapeutics and dependence', *Medical Journal of Australia*, vol. 167, pp. 490–5.

Salzman, C. 1997, 'The benzodiazepine controversy: Therapeutic effects versus dependence, withdrawal and toxicity', *Harvard Review of Psychiatry*, vol. 4, pp. 279–82.

12

Hallucinogens

*Jason White, Jennifer Martin, Henry Krum, Stuart McLean, Ross Young &
John Saunders*

*After a while she remembered that she still held the pieces of mushroom in her hands,
and she set to work very carefully, nibbling first at one and then at the other, and
growing sometimes taller, and sometimes shorter, until she had succeeded in bringing
herself down to her usual height.*

Lewis Carroll 1865, *Alice's Adventures in Wonderland.*

Hallucinogens are also called psychedelics or psychotomimetics. They produce distortions of thought, perception and mood. Hallucinogens comprise several chemical and pharmacological classes of drug, with multiple actions on various neurotransmitter systems. Other drugs, such as cannabis and amphetamines, can produce hallucinogenic effects at high doses, but these effects are not the reason for use of these drugs, and may arise as adverse side-effects.

Hallucinogens differ from many of the drug classes described in this book. In particular, they are not usually associated with problems of dependence arising from long-term high-level use. Most of those who use these drugs will have a pattern of only a few lifetime occasions of use. Thus, there is no necessity for treatment of withdrawal or of the dependence syndrome as there is for alcohol, opioids, and other drugs.

Hallucinogen use tends to be a hidden problem. There is very little information on the extent of use of these drugs, and any information is likely to be very unreliable. Nor has the incidence of problems arising from hallucinogen use been well documented. Use of these drugs is known to be predominantly among people in their mid-teens to late twenties. Use of hallucinogens in people over the age of 30 years is minimal.

The drugs that comprise this class differ in origin (plant or synthetic), pharmacology, and effects. For these reasons, and because of the differences from other drug classes described above, this chapter will focus on description of the respective types of hallucinogens followed by a general approach to management of acute toxicity.

INDOLEAMINE DERIVATIVES

LSD

Lysergic acid diethylamide (LSD) is a complex indoleamine derived from ergot, a fungus that affects rye. LSD is a partial agonist at 5-HT_{2A} and 5-HT_{2C} receptors in the locus coeruleus and cerebral cortex. LSD is also a partial agonist at D_1 and D_2 receptors, and can activate inhibitory autoreceptors, so its overall effects may be due to multiple receptor actions.

LSD is one of the most potent of the hallucinating drugs, producing hallucinatory effects after doses of 100–200 μg. As for other psychoactive agents, the effects of LSD vary with the user's personality and expectations and the setting in which it is taken, and may be modified by any coexisting psychiatric condition. Typical effects include euphoria and other emotional changes, time distortion, visual and auditory hallucinations, synaesthesia (for example seeing sounds), and detachment from reality. Dysphoria and panic attacks can also occur. The effects develop rapidly and last for from three to 12 hours.

LSD is absorbed orally and is metabolised by hydroxylation and demethylation. Both the drug and its metabolites are present at very low levels in the blood and are therefore difficult to detect.

Tolerance and physical dependence

A high degree of tolerance to the behavioural effects of LSD develops after three or four daily doses, but this dissipates with periods of abstinence. As most users are occasional users only, the magnitude of tolerance development is not usually sufficient to result in marked dose escalation. There appears to be less tolerance to the cardiovascular side-effects.

There is cross-tolerance between LSD, mescaline, and psilocybin, but none between LSD and amphetamine derivatives, anticholinergics, or ketamine/phencyclidine (PCP). These two latter drugs are discussed later in the chapter. Physical dependence and withdrawal on cessation of use are not known to occur.

Acute toxicity

Acute toxicity includes somatic effects that are largely sympathomimetic:
- pupillary dilatation
- increase in blood pressure
- tachycardia
- hyper–reflexia
- tremor
- nausea
- piloerection
- muscular weakness

- increased body temperature.
  Non-sympathomimetic effects are:
- dizziness
- weakness
- drowsiness
- nausea
- paraesthesia
- emotional lability.

The subjective effects typically peak several hours after ingestion. While they are usually pleasant, they may be followed by dysphoric experiences. Table 12.1 gives a typical time course of these effects, if they occur.

Table 12.1 Typical time course of LSD dysphoria

2–3 hours after ingestion	*After 4–5 hours*	*After 12 hours*
visual illusions	sense of panic	syndrome settles
perceptual changes	feelings of loss of control	afterimages
synaesthesia (confusion		
in sensory modalities)		
hallucinations		

Chronic toxicity

Flashbacks (recurrence of drug effects some time after use of the drug) occur in more than 15% of users. The incidence of flashbacks is related to the number and magnitude of doses that the person has taken over the previous months or years. These events are precipitated by a number of factors, including marijuana use, anxiety, and fatigue. They may persist intermittently for several years after last use.

As LSD is not commonly used on a regular basis, its real chronic toxicity is not known. There is little evidence for long-term personality changes, but there have been some reports of a reduction in the capacity for abstract thinking with repeated use.

> For LSD:
> - Symptoms of intoxication last for 12 hours, and may include perceptual disorders of different sensory organs.
> - Acute psychotic-like symptoms are due to activation of serotonin receptors.
> - Tolerance occurs to the subjective and behavioural but not the sympathomimetic effects, but there is little evidence of marked dose escalation.
> - Withdrawal and dependence do not commonly occur.
> - The incidence of flashbacks is 15% and is dose-related.
> - Use is mainly sporadic, so it is difficult to know the real chronic toxicity for many hallucinogenic compounds.

Psilocybin

Psilocybin is another indoleamine, specifically N,N–dimethyl–4–hydroxytryptamine. This compound is pharmacologically active, but, in addition, an active metabolite, psilocin, is formed. Psilocybin is found in *Psilocybe* and other species of mushroom. The drug content of the mushroom varies with age and light conditions, and other drugs that can cause sympathomimetic effects can be present, such as the phenylethylamines.

Psilocybin is a mixed $5-HT_{2A}$ and $5-HT_{1A}$ receptor agonist. Its effects depend on the number of mushrooms ingested and their potency. Typically, two to four mushrooms produce relaxation and feelings of well-being, while 20 to 30 mushrooms will elicit a full LSD-like response. Psilocybin can produce symptoms that resemble psychosis.

The effects of an oral dose (for example 0.2 mg/kg) develop 30 minutes after eating the mushrooms, or five minutes after drinking an extract, and last for from four to eight hours, followed by drowsiness and sleep. The oral bioavailability (as psilocin) is 50%, with a maximum blood level of 8 ng/mL after 100 minutes.

Acute toxicity

The most common toxic effects are agitation, panic attacks, psychosis, and ataxia.

PET scans during acute intoxication show overactivity in the prefrontal and inferior temporal regions of the right hemisphere, but underactivity in the subcortical regions.

The active ingredients in mushrooms can cause CNS and cardiac toxicity. The mechanism is unknown, but histochemistry analysis shows shifts in the activity of enzymes involved in the cytoplasmic and mitochondrial redox processes, and in enzymes involved in nerve tissue metabolism.

Chronic toxicity

As mushrooms are not usually taken on a regular basis, chronic toxic effects have not been well documented in humans.

Other indoleamines

N,N–dimethyltryptamine (DMT) is found together with cyclic tryptamines (harmine alkaloids) in the traditional Amazonian beverage hoasca, which is used for religious purposes. DMT is a short-acting hallucinogen, which perhaps uniquely displays no tolerance. After an IV dose, the effects are maximal in approximately two minutes and dissipate by about by 30 minutes, paralleling the blood levels. DMT is an endogenous substance, of unknown significance, in humans. Bufotenine (N,N–dimethyl 5-HT) is found in the skin of *Bufo* toads, but its hallucinogenic effects are controversial, especially as other toxins are present.

PHENETHYLAMINES

Mescaline

Mescaline (3,4,5-trimethoxyphenylethylamine) is found in the buttons on the Mexican cactus *Peyote*. Although from the phenethylamine class, its mode of action and effects are similar to those of LSD. Mescaline is deaminated to inactive metabolites, principally the corresponding trimethoxyphenylacetic acid. Mescaline is commonly taken orally.

Acute toxicity

The acute toxicity is similar to other hallucinogens, but mescaline requires a larger dose to have effects and it is longer-acting than LSD.

The simultaneous physiological and psychological effects of oral mescaline appear in about half an hour. These can include nausea, vomiting, dizziness, headache, palpitations, chills, flushes, polyuria, hunger, stomach cramps, restlessness, and physiological signs of sympathomimetic arousal. Perceptual alterations occur with small doses, and are manifest by spatial and time distortions, alterations in body image, and visual hallucinations. Larger doses produce more florid visual hallucinations, depersonalistion, auditory hallucinations, and emotional alterations.

Tolerance

Tolerance does develop, and there is cross-tolerance between mescaline and LSD. This is likely to be related to a similar pharmacodynamic interaction with serotonin receptors.

Mescaline withdrawal symptoms have been described to occur within three to four days after discontinuation of the drug. However, few users are likely to ingest the drug sufficiently often to develop physical dependence.

Chronic toxicity

There has been little study of chronic toxicity. Mescaline may be teratogenic.

AMPHETAMINE DERIVATIVES

MDMA (ecstasy), MDA (Adam) and MDE (Eve) are chemically related to mescaline and the amphetamines, and have hallucinatory and stimulant properties. However, the hallucinogenic effects are not as prominent as those of mescaline and LSD. Some have suggested they be put in an intermediate class called entactogens. They produce pleasant emotional effects, euphoria, and increased energy, as well as autonomic effects (hypertension, tachycardia, hyperthermia), and toxicity to sero-tonergic neurones. MDMA is discussed in chapter 8.

CYCLOHEXYLAMINES

Phencyclidine (PCP) and ketamine

The two major drugs in this class are phencyclidine (PCP) and ketamine (super k, special k). Although more is known about PCP and its effects, ketamine is more widely used in Australia and New Zealand. Both drugs produce a feeling of detachment from the body, disorientation, loss of proprioception, and disordered thoughts. PCP was briefly used as a dissociative anaesthetic, but delirium and hallucinations during recovery were troublesome, and it was replaced by ketamine. Ketamine has fewer of these side-effects and a briefer action and is still used in human anaesthesia and, particularly, veterinary anaesthesia.

PCP and ketamine are potent non-competitive antagonists at NMDA receptors, and this is believed to mediate most of their effects. However, both drugs have additional actions, including agonist activity at δ receptors (which may mediate some of the psychotomimetic effects), opioid actions (which may mediate the respiratory depressant effects of high doses), and enhanced dopamine activity. Withdrawal symptoms may involve depletion of 5-HT, noradrenaline, and dopamine.

PCP and ketamine produce a range of schizophrenic-like symptoms, including flattened affect, thought disorders, depersonalisation, and catatonia. They can also exacerbate pre-existing schizophrenic states. Both drugs have been used to induce an experimental schizophrenic state. This effect is associated with NMDA receptor blockade, and supports the hypoglutaminergic theory of schizophrenia.

PCP and ketamine can be swallowed, smoked, snorted, or injected. Onset of action varies with route of administration. For ketamine this ranges from 30 seconds (IV) to 10 to 20 minutes (oral). Typical duration of action is one to three hours for ketamine and four to six hours for PCP. These values may be much greater following an overdose. PCP is eliminated by a mixture of metabolism and excretion, with a half-life of seven to 16 hours. Several enzymes are involved in its metabolism, including CYP3A. Ketamine has a half-life of three hours, with CYP2B6 the major enzyme in its metabolism.

Acute toxicity

For both ketamine and PCP the clinical spectrum in the patient with acute toxicity depends on the dose ingested. Lower doses produce a state resembling alcohol intoxication, with the prominent symptoms being ataxia, slurred speech, nystagmus, numbness of extremities, and euphoria.

At higher doses the prominent symptoms are:
- distorted sensory processing
- disorganised thought
- drowsiness
- apathy
- hostile and bizarre behaviour
- marked anaesthesia and catatonic-like muscular rigidity
- increased heart rate and blood pressure
- hypersalivation
- sweating
- fever
- myoclonus
- convulsions
- respiratory depression
- coma.

Altered pupils, nystagmus, diplopia, decreased pupillary light reflexes, absent corneal reflexes, and bilateral ptosis may occur at any level, and are usually accompanied by cholinergic symptoms such as dilated pupils, hypersalivation, sweating, and flushing.

Other reported effects are sinus tachycardia, arrhythmias, hypotension, and bradycardia.

The recovery period from ingestion of a high dose may be prolonged (several days) and is marked by alternating sleep and waking illusions and with features of the lower dose state.

Chronic toxicity

Effects of long-term use of these drugs have not been well researched. Nevertheless, there is some evidence of adverse changes, particularly for PCP. Chronic psychotic sequelae in the form of organic brain dysfunction and behavioural effects may follow prolonged exposure. These may manifest as personality changes, and persistent difficulties with recent memory, speech, and thinking. Flashbacks have been reported, but are probably not as common as with LSD.

Tolerance and physical dependence

Tolerance develops to some of the behavioural and toxic effects of PCP and ketamine, and this may lead to dose escalation in chronic users.

Abrupt withdrawal after long-term use is followed by fear, tremors, facial twitches, and craving. Animal studies have shown seizures, irritability, and weight loss during ketamine withdrawal.

For ketamine and PCP:
- Low doses produce a state resembling alcohol intoxication.
- Chronic psychotic sequelae in the form of organic brain dysfunction and behavioural effects may follow prolonged exposure.
- PCP and ketamine can block the cation channel of the NMDA receptor, but also affect opioid and dopaminergic systems.
- Tolerance does occur to some of the behavioural and toxic effects of ketamine and PCP, and physical dependence can develop.

ANTICHOLINERGICS

Hyoscine (scopolamine) from *Datura stramonium* is a competitive inhibitor of muscarinic receptors of acetylcholine in the CNS and peripherally. It produces a state of delirium in which awareness fluctuates, cognition and memory are impaired, and delusions can occur. While most people find this unpleasant, some seek to repeat the experience.

Other plants that contain the antimuscarinic substances hyoscine and atropine and which have been used for hallucinogenic effects are Jimson weed, Angel's trumpet (*Datura sauveolens*), and the nightshade plants (*Solonaceae*). The Australian corkwood, *Duboisia*, has a traditional Aboriginal use to produce altered consciousness and heightened suggestibility to facilitate tribal education. Therapeutic drugs with antimuscarinic side effects, such as antiparkinsonian agents, antihistamines, and tricyclic antidepressants, have been taken to produce hallucinations.

Peripheral antimuscarinic effects include dry mouth, blurred vision, mydriasis, urinary retention, and tachycardia. The hallucinogenic effects occur in the higher end of the dose range. Such doses are not uncommon with plant preparations. Drowsiness or agitation can occur, and there is a danger of hyperthermia, coma, and death. Physostigmine is the appropriate reversing agent, but most cases respond to conservative treatment.

ASSESSMENT

Clinical features and assessment

The majority of presentations related to hallucinogen use are acute complications of intoxication. Physical signs may include dilation of the pupils, tachycardia, quickened deep tendon reflexes, elevated body temperature, hypertension, and tremor consistent with mild sympathonimetric stimulation. Toxic effects have been associated with mushroom ingestion and include arrhythmias, myocardial infarction, nausea, and vomiting. However, these may be due to a mixture of compounds and even different types of mushrooms being ingested, some of which are poisonous. Anticholinergic toxicity may also be associated with temporary loss of vision.

More commonly, the presentation is predominantly psychological and associated with the acute panic of a bad trip. This may be elicited by a high drug dose or because the setting in which the drug was taken was not conducive to a relaxing intoxication (for example, being questioned by a parent or police officer). The early effects of the hallucinogen may be associated with perceptual illusions, pseudohallucinations (where the user is aware that the visual objects perceived are not real) or synaesthesia (where an object in one sensory modality is perceived in another, such as seeing sound). Emotional response may include exaggerated laughing or tearfulness.

In the second phase of intoxication, loosening of associations is likely and establishing a coherent history may be difficult. A thorough mental status examination, and, if there is another person available, a collateral history may be most appropriate at this stage. The interview with the intoxicated patient should be calm, with a relaxed tone employed and a slow pace taken to avoid exacerbation of anxiety. The patient may be illogical and obsessed with fantasy.

The third phase of intoxication involves derealisation or depersonalisation, often with the patient exhibiting little movement and appearing to be sedated. Catatonia has been described. The derealisation can also be related to a sense of oneness with the environment and profound experience of meaning, which can be elevated to paranoid grandiosity at times. Acute panic can occur at this stage, but its occurrence is difficult to predict. Panic usually only lasts for several hours.

Chronic problems may relate to ongoing schizophreniform signs and symptoms; however this may be due to an underlying psychotic vulnerability that has been triggered by drug use. Auditory hallucinations are rarely triggered by hallucinogenic drugs, and those with schizophrenia very rarely have visual hallucinations. Ongoing auditory hallucinations should therefore be investigated as a highly likely sign of an underlying psychosis which may need treatment with an antipsychotic.

Treatment

Treatment of the bad trip usually involves talking down and placing the patient in a quiet peaceful environment that is adequately lit. Having someone sit with the patient for support is preferable, and the patient should be gently reminded that the drug ingested has produced these changes in thinking and feeling, and that the changes will soon disappear. It is sometimes also useful to let the patient know that the symptoms may seem to be slow to abate, and that this is because of altered time perception. The patient should not lie down with eyes closed, as this exacerbates the hallucinosis. Rather, they should sit up with eyes open, if possible talking to provide some distraction from obsessing on cognitive or perceptual changes. A busy accident and emergency centre on a Saturday night may pose too many challenges for a patient who is acutely panicky, and being in a familiar environment like home, with support, may be preferred. Reassuring the patient of doctor–patient confidentiality can also assist in reducing general stress, as patients can be paranoid regarding police involvement.

The pharmacotherapy of a bad trip is inadequately researched; however benzodiazepines (for example 20 mg diazepam) and clonidine have been used effectively. Haloperidol may be administered if the benzodiazepine is ineffective. There is a low risk of adverse effects with each drug class: benzodiazepines may disinhibit the patient and cause acute distress, while antipsychotics may paradoxically increase panic.

Use of medication depends partly on risk to the patient and to others. Occasionally the hallucinations may be associated with considerable risk (for example, the thought that the patient can fly). Increased physical strength has been reported with PCP intoxication, and sedation of the patient and observation is warranted.

Anticholinergics comprise the only hallucinogen class for which there is an effective antidote. However, while physostigmine is able to reduce anticholinergic toxicity, the dangers associated with its use mean that more conservative procedures (for example benzodiazepines, calming) are usually employed.

Continuing psychological symptoms are relatively uncommon following cessation of hallucinogen use. Anxiety (not associated with any psychosis) should be treated symptomatically with relaxation techniques. Post-hallucinogen persisting perceptual disorder has been treated with benzodiazepines and antidepressants (for example sertraline). Again, exacerbations by antipsychotic therapy have been noted. Relaxation techniques may be helpful in facilitating acute coping with the flashbacks, which may not be completely eradicated by pharmacotherapy. It is prudent to recommend abstinence from other psychotropic drugs during treatment as these may precipitate flashbacks.

REFERENCES AND FURTHER READING

Pechnick, R.N. & Ungerleider, J.T. 1997, 'Hallucinogens', in Lowinson, J.H., Ruiz, P., Millman, R.B. & Langrod, J.G. (eds), *Substance Abuse: A comprehensive textbook* (3rd edn), Williams & Wilkins, Philadelphia, pp. 230–8.

White, J.M. & Ryan, C.F. 1996, 'Pharmacological properties of ketamine', *Drug and Alcohol Review*, vol. 15, pp. 145–55.

PART 3

Specific Populations

Part 3 is devoted mainly to specific populations of drug users. These chapters address the particular problems faced by groups such as adolescents, women, indigenous Australians, Māori people, and the elderly. More complex problems of injecting drug users, multiple drug users, and those with coexisting mental health disorders are also covered. In each case it is assumed that the reader is familiar with the general material presented in parts 1 and 2.

The final chapter addresses several important professional issues for medical practitioners. These include some of the problems associated with working with patients who have drug and alcohol problems, and the specific difficulties associated with problematic use of alcohol and other drugs by medical practitioners themselves. While the focus is naturally on patients, it is also important to consider colleagues at risk for problems of this nature.

13

The Injecting Drug User

Gary Hulse, Maria Basso & Alex Wodak

INJECTING DRUG USE

Injecting as a mode of drug administration

Injecting drug use refers to the administration of drugs, normally by the user, with a needle and syringe. This practice was first noted soon after the invention of the hypodermic syringe in the nineteenth century. Today, the drugs most commonly injected are heroin, amphetamine, cocaine, and anabolic steroids, although prescription medications such as benzodiazepines are sometimes injected.

As noted in earlier chapters, most drugs can be administered by non-injectable routes. For example, heroin and cocaine can both be administered very efficiently in base form by inhalation of vapour, while amphetamine is well absorbed when taken orally. However, despite alternative modes of administration, injection is the favoured mode for heroin and is increasingly popular for amphetamine use. Many users' favoured mode of administration is via injection because they believe it gives maximum effects for the minimal amount of drug.

Routes of administration

Individual drugs are commonly associated with a specific route of administration. Heroin, cocaine hydrochloride, and amphetamine are usually injected intravenously, while anabolic steroids are usually injected intramuscularly. Occasionally other drugs intended for oral administration are injected intravenously, such as benzodiazepines, methadone and other opioids, and antihistamines.

The route of administration has a major impact on the rate of increase in concentration of the drug in the brain, and therefore on the impact of the drug on mood and cognition. Of the injecting modes of administration, the quickest onset of action is associated with intravenous, followed by intramuscular, and then subcutaneous administration. It should also be noted that the more rapidly the concentration of the drug increases in the brain the greater the risk of harmful effects, such as accidental overdose.

Prevalence of injecting drug use

It is estimated that approximately 100 000 Australians inject drugs regularly, and an additional 175 000 inject drugs occasionally; in New Zealand there are approximately 30 000 drug injectors. The number of drug injectors in Australia is estimated to have doubled every 10 years since the 1960s. In the 1990s, the rate of increase of injecting drug use in Australia and New Zealand appears to have been even more rapid than in the previous quarter century. The age of initiation of injecting drug use in Australia and New Zealand has been declining for several decades. Most males begin to inject drugs between the ages of 17 to 24, with females commencing injecting at a slightly later age.

The majority of injecting drug users in Australia are heroin or amphetamine users. Intravenous opioid users make up the majority of all drug injectors in New Zealand. Although heroin is the most commonly injected opioid in Australia, it has been relatively unavailable in New Zealand since the 1980s, with morphine and homebake the most commonly injected opioids (see chapter 6).

The process of injecting drugs

It is important for doctors who wish to work effectively with injecting drug users to have some knowledge of the drugs injected and the injecting apparatus used, and to be aware of potential risks associated with each step of the injecting process.

Heroin, cocaine, and amphetamine are bought from the black market in powder form, which is then combined with water and mixed into a solution in a spoon or foil prior to injection. The solution is then drawn up through a filter into a syringe, and is commonly injected through the skin directly into a vein or muscle, or subcutaneously.

There is a risk of moving bacteria and other microorganisms from the epidermal layer to deeper tissue or into the vascular system. Drug injecting can therefore be the portal of entry of microorganisms that later cause morbidity, such as bacterial or fungal endocarditis, septicaemia, or skin abscess. Injecting drug users often continue to inject into favoured sites even when an abscess has developed. This carries an increased risk of transmission of bacteria into the blood, and of serious infection such as endocarditis.

A skin abscess can result from the injection of compounds such as talc used to cut drugs, frequent injection into the same site without allowing time for the vein or skin to heal since the last injection, or injection into soft tissue such as when an injection accidentally misses the vein or when the substance is intentionally injected into subcutaneous tissue. The development of a skin abscess following an unhygienic injection may also result in microorganisms entering the blood system.

The most common veins used initially are on the medial side of the antecubital fossa of the non-dominant arm. Damage to veins can occur for a number of reasons, including repeated local infections, scarring associated with repeated injections in the same site, use of blunt or barbed needles, and severe chemical irritation associated with additives found in some drugs. Sometimes, veins become thrombosed. As a consequence it is common for drug users to use other veins on the forearms and hands. As venous access in these areas becomes more difficult, veins on the feet, ankles, and groin are used, and then the large and deep veins in the neck.

Cutting compounds and insoluble agents

The drugs injected are often diluted (cut) by dealers with additives such as sugars, corn starch, cellulose, and talc. Cutting the drugs helps to create the appearance that more drug is present. At other times, insoluble binding agents such as talc are injected when drug users grind up tablets intended for oral use, attempt to dissolve the resulting powder in water, and inject the solution intravenously.

Embolic occlusion of small blood vessels of both arteriole and capillary size can result following intravenous injection of insoluble binding agents or from foreign materials such as filters or other contaminants. This embolised material occludes the lumen of vessels, resulting in severe tissue ischaemia, or may migrate through the vessel wall into the perivascular space and act as a focus for an inflammatory reaction that produces both intravascular and extravascular granulomas.

In addition to the adverse effects of the drugs themselves, health complications associated with injecting illicit drugs can result from several factors:
- contaminants in the drugs, including microorganisms and compounds such as talc used to cut the drugs
- use of non-sterile injecting equipment, including needle, syringe, spoon, filter, glass, and rinsing water
- blood-to-blood contact with contaminated blood from another injecting drug user (for example HIV, hepatitis, or any other blood-borne infection), often through injecting equipment
- failure to inject in a sterile site, or injection into inappropriate body locations.

Drug-specific injecting risks

Specific risks of heroin and morphine injection are largely those associated with their depressant effects on the central nervous system. While the most recognised of these is respiratory depression, its anaesthetic and sedative properties increase the risk of other morbidity and mortality while under its influence. These range from accidental drowning following heroin use near water, to severe burns associated with heaters or fires. Heroin is commonly cut with powdered codeine-based tablets that also contain talc, resulting in vascular and tissue morbidity. Talc injection is also likely to be associated with the use of homebake, a form of heroin derived from oral codeine phosphate tablets. Manufacturing agents such as hydrochloric and acetic acids, chloroform and pyridine, are also often left in homebake, and cause localised skin rashes and abscesses.

Cocaine injection is commonly associated with more localised tissue damage than heroin or amphetamine. This is likely to be caused by its local anaesthetic and vasoconstrictive properties. The anaesthetic properties mean that the injector is less aware of any local injury he or she may be causing, and subsequent vasoconstriction delays healing.

Some benzodiazepines such as temazepam are highly irritant to the skin and veins, and regular use quickly causes local vein and tissue irritation, thrombosis, and abscess. A common cause of arterial thrombosis in Australia at present is gel capsule formulations of temazepam. Arterial injection of these formulations (which are sometimes heated to increase fluidity of the gel) is extremely dangerous, and can lead to partial or whole limb amputation.

Steroid injectors rarely see themselves as injecting drug users, but rather as pursuers of body excellence. They are nevertheless similar to other injectors in their exposure to an increased risk of blood-borne viral disease and infection. The common practice of steroid users drawing up from the same vial increases these risks.

Why are drugs injected?

Intravenous injection is the most common form of injecting drug use in most countries, including Australia and New Zealand. This is because there is a widespread belief among drug users that intravenous administration is by far the most effective way of maximising the intoxicating effects of drugs for minimum expenditure. This is, however, not always true, with, for example, inhalation of some drugs (such as heroin or cocaine) in vapour form also being an efficient mode of administration.

The ritual of all forms of drug administration plays an important role in the impact of drug use. Administration of drugs by injection is considered to be highly reinforcing, because a powerful effect is delivered soon after the drug is consumed. Many drug users derive considerable satisfaction from the injecting ritual (needle fixation) in just the same way that many pipe or cigar smokers derive satisfaction from their elaborate ritual.

IDENTIFICATION AND MANAGEMENT OF INFECTION

Infections related to injecting

Infections associated with unhygienic injecting practices account for much of the morbidity associated with injecting drug use. The two most common forms of infection are non-communicable infections and communicable blood-borne viral infections. Non-communicable infections, such as thrombophlebitis, bacteraemia, septicaemia, and bacterial endocarditis, are associated with the use of unsterile injecting equipment or unhygienic injecting procedures. Communicable blood-borne viral infections, such as hepatitis B (HBV), hepatitis C (HCV), and human immunodeficiency virus (HIV), result from the sharing of injecting equipment previously used by an infected person and involve the transfer of microbial agents from one injecting drug user to another.

Non-communicable infections

Thrombophlebitis

Superficial thrombophlebitis, a common complication of injecting drug use, occurs when there is an inflammation of a superficial vein. Thrombophlebitis results from venous stasis, endothelial damage, and hyper-coagulability. Commonly, an injecting drug user complains of localised tenderness close to a thrombosed vein, and the area is often red and warm.

To prevent further damage, injecting drug users are strongly advised to desist from injecting anywhere in the vicinity of the inflammation. Treatment is directed towards reduction of inflammation, and antibiotics may be required. Sometimes surgery is required to allow pus to drain as antibiotics are less effective in the presence of frank pus. Topical agents that reduce inflammation should be avoided if there is any suspicion of possible infection.

The patient who is an injecting drug user should be advised about methods of avoiding thrombophlebitis in the future. This primarily involves advice to avoid injecting, to use sterile equipment, and practise safer injecting. Similar advice is also given for prevention of septicaemia and endocarditis.

Bacteraemia and septicaemia

Bacterial skin flora are sometimes introduced into the body during unsterile drug injecting. Commonly introduced organisms include streptococci and staphylococci. This bacterial invasion of the vascular system (bacteraemia) is often referred to as blood poisoning. Septicaemia is a bacterial infection of tissue and organs which results from the entry of these bacteria into the vascular system. Bacteraemia is commonly asymptomatic, and is not life-threatening. In contrast, the resulting septicaemia is often a life-threatening condition, and is commonly marked by fever, chills, tachycardia, tachypnoea, and a high white blood cell count.

Bacteraemia requires observation to ensure that more serious conditions do not develop. Septicaemia requires hospital admission, intravenous antibiotics, and careful monitoring. Antibiotics should preferably only commence after blood samples have been taken for bacterial and fungal culture and sensitivity. Investigations are ordered to exclude other conditions such as bacterial endocarditis. The drug-injecting

245

patient should be advised about methods of avoiding bacteraemia and septicaemia in the future.

> Apart from the usual advice about trying to avoid future injecting, only using sterile injecting equipment if injecting, and safer injecting practices, opioid-using patients are encouraged to enrol in a maintenance treatment program as a way of reducing drug use and injecting frequency (see chapter 6).

Endocarditis

Endocarditis involves inflammation of the endocardium that lines the chambers of the heart and heart valves. This occurs when infective organisms, such as bacteria and fungi, are introduced into the bloodstream during unsterile drug injecting. The organisms then colonise the endocardium, causing inflammation and tissue damage. The clusters of infected organisms can impair valve function or detach from the endocardium and travel in the circulatory system to lodge (embolise) in distal organs, such as the kidney and brain, or in small vessels. This can then lead to occlusion or localised infection.

Infective endocarditis carries a high risk of morbidity and mortality. As a consequence, rapid diagnosis and effective and aggressive treatment is essential. Hospitalisation, intravenous antibiotics, and careful monitoring are required. As with septicaemia, antibiotics should preferably only commence after blood samples have been taken for bacterial and fungal culture. Intravenous antibiotics should be continued for at least several weeks. Investigations should be ordered to exclude other conditions, such as lung or brain abscess. Wherever possible, valve replacement is avoided during the acute illness. Often the tricuspid valve recovers even after developing incompetence during the acute illness. Renal impairment sometimes complicates severe bacterial endocarditis. Although patients with this condition can be gravely ill during the acute phase, long-term results can still be very gratifying.

Communicable infections: blood-borne viral disease

Human immunodeficiency virus

The incidence and prevalence of human immunodeficiency virus (HIV) infection among injecting drug users in Australia and New Zealand has remained very low, unlike the situation in many other countries such as the United States, the South Americas, Italy, Spain, Portugal, Thailand, China, and Malaysia. The prevalence of HIV infection among injecting drug users in Australia and New Zealand has remained 2% or less.

Control of HIV among injecting drug users in Australia and New Zealand has been a victory for the public health measures designed to prevent this problem. Success was due to the adoption of harm minimisation as Australia's official national drug policy in 1985. This enabled the rapid deployment of public health orientated policies that prevented HIV prevalence among injecting drug users from increasing to the critical threshold levels necessary for rapid transmission. Needle and syringe programs were established early and vigorously. These programs made sterile injecting equipment readily available, and reduced the re-use of injecting equipment. Injecting drug users became increasingly knowledgeable about infection control and the importance of using only sterile injecting paraphernalia. Education campaigns and the establishment of organisations of injecting drug users helped to disseminate this knowledge and reduce high-risk behaviour. The expansion and improvement in drug treatment also helped to reduce high-risk behaviour.

HIV is relatively vulnerable to heat, light, and drying but may sometimes, under the right conditions, still be detected for several weeks in dried plasma.

Hepatitis B

There is some indication that the prevalence of hepatitis B has also declined since the introduction of needle exchange programs in the late 1980s. However, hepatitis B is still more common among injecting drug users than in the general community. Hepatitis B vaccination of injecting drug users has only been carried out sporadically, even though the vaccine is inexpensive, safe, and effective. There is now renewed interest in hepatitis B vaccination of injecting drug users because co-infection increases the progression of hepatitis C infection. Hepatitis D infection can occur either at the same time as hepatitis B infection or after hepatitis B has become chronic. Hepatitis D infection has been very rare among injecting drug users in Australia since the introduction of needle exchange programs.

Hepatitis C

Hepatitis C was already widespread among injecting drug users in Australia by the early 1970s. It is estimated that approximately 200 000 Australians had been exposed to hepatitis C, with more than 150 000 chronically infected by the late 1990s. More than 85% of the prevalent (old) and incident (new) infections have been attributed to injecting drug use. As a consequence of the large number of people with chronic hepatitis C, the number of people with cirrhosis and new cases of hepatocellular carcinoma attributed to hepatitis C is expected to double in the 2000s. It is estimated that there are more than 11 000 new hepatitis C infections occurring in Australia each year attributed to the sharing of drug injecting equipment. Allowing for differences in population size, these numbers are likely to be smaller in New Zealand than Australia because the prevalence of injecting drug use appears to be less; however evidence suggests that a high prevalence of hepatitis C also exists among New Zealand injectors.

In contrast to HIV, the hepatitis C virus is quite robust and may, under the right conditions, remain infective for up to four months in dried blood. The infectiousness of hepatitis C through blood–blood contact is greater than HIV by an order of magnitude (although sexual spread of hepatitis C is minimal in comparison with HIV). The prevalence among injecting drug users of hepatitis C was already 80–90% while HIV prevalence was less than 1% when harm minimisation policies were introduced. As a consequence there is a greater likelihood of hepatitis C than HIV transmission despite the presence of risk reduction programs.

Risk factors

In Australia and New Zealand, injecting drug use is the most important risk factor for hepatitis C infection. The factors primarily responsible for transmission are the sharing of needles, syringes and other injecting equipment (such as spoons, filters, and water) used previously by others who are already infected. The major factors predictive of hepatitis C infection are age (or duration of injecting), a history of sharing injecting equipment, and previous imprisonment.

There is also a greater risk of hepatitis C exposure for regular dependent heroin use as compared to non-regular use. This means that heroin users who have, for example, injected for two years, but spent a longer period in regular (daily) use, have an increased relative risk of hepatitis C exposure compared with heroin users who have injected for two years but spent less of their injecting life as a regular (daily) user.

Evidence also suggests that compared to males, females may have a greater risk of hepatitis C exposure over the initial early years of injecting drug use. One possible explanation for this gender difference is that females may more frequently commence injecting drug use with male partners who are experienced injectors and therefore have a significant risk of prior hepatitis C exposure. If females share injecting equipment with these partners it provides a mode of early female hepatitis C infection. Consequently, strategies which aim to reduce the risk of hepatitis C exposure in females may need to differ from those used with their male counterparts (see chapter 16).

BLOOD-BORNE VIRAL TESTING

What does the test involve?

While testing for blood-borne viruses involves a simple blood test, it should always follow a discussion of the meanings of positive and negative results. Because of the very significant ramifications of a positive result, all testing should occur with the informed consent of the individual. Results are usually provided within a week, and should always be given in person and not over the telephone or through an intermediary person.

Interpreting pathology test results

Interpretation of pathology test results requires an understanding of the limitations of testing as well as of the likely presence of antibodies or viral protein in blood or plasma.

Antibodies to viral infections commonly develop quickly. In the vast majority of individuals, antibodies can be detected within three months of exposure. The interval period between infection and the development of a sufficient viral load to allow antibody detection is referred to as the window period. During this period, tests may be negative (false negative), but the individual may still be at risk of passing infection on to others.

It follows that a negative antibody test result indicates that either (a) infection has not occurred, or (b) that infection is so recent that insufficient quantities of antibodies are present to generate a positive result. A repeat HIV, HBV or HCV test after the window period (considered to be six months) can be very helpful. For both HIV and HCV, positive antibody results indicate that a viral antigen test on the same blood may be required. For HIV and HCV, a confirmed positive viral antigen result indicates current infection. These tests do not indicate the progression of infection or any resulting disease in that patient.

Problems of viral detection in blood

The HIV viral confirmatory test is both very robust and specific for HIV. This is not the case for the HCV viral polymerase chain reaction (PCR) test where a positive antibody and negative PCR may indicate that infection has occurred but resolved, or that insufficient viral levels are present in the blood to allow detection. For this reason the PCR test is often repeated.

249

Positive test and patient reactions

A positive result to any blood-borne viral test is often a great psychological shock to the individual, and can result in considerable distress. Patients' reaction to a positive result may manifest as withdrawal, sadness, anger, or humour. This may be partly reduced by ensuring that a patient has a comprehensive understanding of the significance of test results before they learn of their own result.

However, regardless of their external presentation, the patient will not be in an optimal condition to absorb new and important information on a range of important issues, including their prognosis, need for self care, access to support services, options for treatment, counselling, referral, or prevention of transmission to others. It is therefore extremely important that these issues are openly discussed at the time that testing is agreed to.

Prior to testing, individuals should also be canvassed on how they might deal with a positive result, the availability of support from significant others, and, importantly, who they would inform of their status. This latter consideration is very relevant because some individuals in a state of shock divulge information to inappropriate people such as neighbours and work colleagues. There may also be implications for future health insurance.

Delivering test findings

There is no set formula for providing test results. However, consideration of a number of significant issues will help the practitioner to develop an appropriate framework.

Advice associated with a negative test result

One unfortunate outcome of a patient repeatedly receiving negative antibody test results may be an inadvertent reinforcement that the behaviours the patient has engaged in to date are low risk 'I haven't been infected yet, so I must be doing the right thing.' It is important that the medical practitioner corrects this myth. Having identified that a patient engages in injecting risk activities, it is important to stress that, despite a negative antibody result, the patient is extremely lucky not to have been infected to date. This is particularly the case with HCV where very high prevalence levels within the injecting drug-use community make likelihood of contact sooner or later extremely high.

Delivering a positive test result

At the time of presenting a positive test result, the patient may need to be reminded of previous discussions about disclosure, and guided through the discussion. They should be encouraged to ask questions, with simple answers provided, making it clear that greater detail can be provided at a future time if necessary.

The occurrence of a positive result signals the need to ensure that the patient comprehensively understands the information that has previously been provided.

Assuming pre-test discussions have taken place, the vast majority of patients will have some understanding of general infection control and transmission information. What is commonly lacking are the finer details, such as transmission associated with the use of injecting equipment other than needles and syringes, and risks associated with everyday life activities. Transmission through household contact, such as the sharing of cooking utensils and other household activities where blood exchange does not occur, is extremely low for HIV, HBV and HCV. To be on the safe side, the sharing of common domestic items that could transfer small quantities of blood, such as razors, toothbrushes, and other utensils, should be avoided. Sexual transmission is high for both HIV and HBV, but extremely low for HCV. For women, information should be given on the possible risk of vertical transmission of HCV, HIV, and HBV, and the risk to the mother during pregnancy.

Importantly, the false belief that there is no risk associated with sharing injecting equipment with others similarly infected with HIV, HBV, or HCV needs to

Table 13.1 A safer injecting hierarchy: desirability and feasibility

Option	Desirability	Feasibility
Abstinence	Very high	Very low (in the short-term; may be a long-term goal)
Drug use without injection	High (lowest risk of major adverse health consequences)	Moderately low (unlikely to be sustained over time)
Injection only with new sterile equipment	Moderate (low risk of blood-borne viral infection)	Moderate (assumes availability of sterile equipment)
Disinfecting injecting equipment	Moderately low (concern that this is not always performed adequately)	Moderately high

be corrected. Infections with a different genotype (strain) of HIV or HCV will speed the progression of disease. Similarly, reinfection with the same strain of HCV results in an increase in viral activity, reflected by an elevated viral load and associated liver damage.

Reducing or eliminating alcohol consumption appears to reduce progression of hepatitis B and C.

Provide information and other support

There is abundant literature on blood-borne viruses, with new material appearing frequently. Those newly infected should be encouraged to read this literature. They should also be strongly encouraged to join a support group, as these commonly disseminate new information regarding diagnosis, prognosis, and treatment options, as well as providing the opportunity to meet others with the same condition and to discuss personal questions.

Further investigations

Patients with blood-borne viral infections are investigated using a variety of serological, biochemical, haematological, immunological, and imaging techniques. A liver biopsy is usually performed before treating hepatitis B or C because this is still the most effective way of assessing the severity of liver disease and excluding other causes of liver disease, and also because the presence of cirrhosis restricts treatment options considerably.

PREVENTING MORBIDITY AND MORTALITY ASSOCIATED WITH INJECTING

Advising your patient

In a harm-reduction framework, injecting drug users are provided with a hierarchy of options to reduce the risk of blood-borne viral and other morbidity and mortality related to injecting.

The safest option, but also the most difficult to achieve and sustain for the injecting drug user, is enduring abstinence from all mood-altering drugs. The next option, which is also quite difficult, is to use drugs without injecting, instead using by sniffing, snorting, or smoking. These alternative modes of administration should be promoted as resulting in a satisfactory delivery of the drug, with a lower risk of major adverse health consequences compared with injecting. Next in the hierarchy is injecting, but only ever using new sterile injecting equipment on each injecting occasion. Many users can adhere to this, but some will occasionally inject with used equipment (for example during dependent or withdrawal periods). Use of disinfected, previously used injecting equipment is the next, but much poorer, option. Use of previously used injecting equipment without disinfecting should be discouraged as an option for consideration, although it clearly needs to be discussed. The desirability and feasibility of these options are shown in table 13.1.

To reduce health risks, patients who inject drugs should be provided with the basic advice given below.

Figure 13.1 Injecting drug users should be advised to use a clean spoon, needle, syringe and filter, and sterile water and elastic tourniquet to reduce injecting-related morbidity.

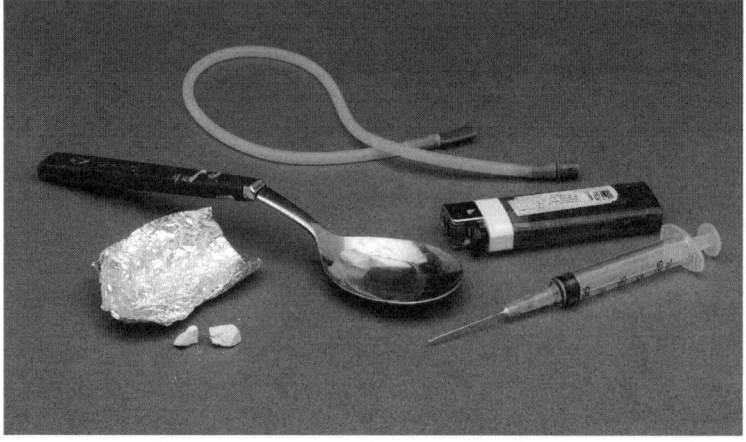

Courtesy Australian Drug Foundation

Injecting equipment

Sterile water for injecting

Sterile water should always be used for injecting, cleaning, or rinsing injecting equipment. Tap water is rich in microorganisms and should never be mixed with drugs or used for cleaning and rinsing injecting paraphernalia. Optimally sterile water ampoules that are readily available from pharmacies should be used for each injection. In reality, however, few injectors regularly use sterile ampoules. As an alternative, non-carbonated mineral water from a sealed bottle can be used. Boiling water for approximately six to eight minutes will also provide a significant level of sterilisation. All water should be discarded after each use, and newly sterilised water used for each subsequent injecting episode and for cleaning of injecting equipment.

Drug additives and filters

Users should be warned about injecting drugs cut with talc, cornstarch, cellulose, or other insoluble agents. They should also be warned to avoid drugs cut with sugars as these provide a fertile environment for the growth of microorganisms, especially when moisture is present.

A sterile filter should be used with each hit to prevent solid components (such as talc) being drawn up into the syringe and injected. In practice, sterile filter paper, cotton wool, cotton buds, or part of a tampon often provide the best filters. Filters should be used only once, since there is no simple and effective way to clean used filters and they become contaminated easily. For example, fungi can grow in the cotton of the filter, especially where cutting compounds from previous injections, such as sugar base, provide a rich nutrient source. Sterile micro-filters (Acrodisks) can be obtained from some pharmacists or needle exchange programs. These filters are more expensive, but they are the best way of reducing insoluble adulterants and bacteria in the drug solution.

253

Needles, syringes, and spoons

Ideally, new, sterile injecting equipment (for example needles, syringes, and spoons) should be used for each injecting episode by each individual injector. This ideal is difficult to achieve in practice. Even when attempts are made to use sterile needles and syringes, sharing of spoons is commonplace. All equipment should be cleaned prior to each person's use, optimally using sterile alcohol, disinfectant (for example bleach), or detergent. Each item is then rinsed thoroughly with clean water (preferably sterile water or mineral water in a sealed container), and dried before use. Failure to rinse and dry equipment adequately can lead to the injection of detergents and bleach or contaminants in tap water.

Of all injecting equipment, it is most difficult to prevent re-use of filters and communal use of spoons.

Injecting drug users should be strongly encouraged to wash their hands carefully before handling injecting equipment. Old silver spoons with residues of silver oxide should not be used, as the silver oxide dissolves during the mixing process. Once injected, the silver oxide causes skin or blood contamination.

Tourniquet

Tourniquets made from materials such as leather or belts abrade and bruise the skin and underlying tissue. Elastic tourniquets are much more effective and less damaging to the skin and tissues. To avoid damage to tissue and blood vessels, injecting drug users should be advised not to leave tourniquets on for longer than 60 seconds. If a vein cannot be located in that time, the tourniquet should be released and reapplied a few minutes later.

The site of injection

Skin injection and skin abscess

The skin area should be prepared for injecting with a sterile swab or other disinfectant. Injecting should not be carried out into skin abscess. Injecting drug users should also be informed about the early signs of an abscess (redness, swelling, warmth, pain, hard pus core) to speed up identification of the problem, and they should be made aware of the need for urgent medical attention. Following withdrawal of the needle after injecting drugs into the vein, gentle but firm pressure should be maintained over the injection site for 30 or 40 seconds to reduce bruising. The use of sharp needles reduces the degree of bruising, scarring, and formation of track marks.

Research indicates that risk behaviours of injectors are significantly reduced when they are made aware of the risks of their behaviours and have access to sterile injecting equipment.

Vascular care

Injecting drug users should be informed of the importance of rotating injection sites, use of only sterile injecting equipment, and use of safer injection sites such as the antecubital fossae. Also of importance are avoidance of blunt and barbed needles, and not injecting contents of gel capsules or crushed tablets. Use of sterile swabs to clean each skin site prior to injection will all help to reduce vascular damage.

Where not to inject

Serious health complications can arise from injection into arteries or close to nerves and tendons. Intravenous drug users should be informed about differentiating veins from arteries, advised to inject only into visible surface veins, and encouraged to avoid injecting into the groin, neck, breasts, or veins below the waist. Due to the small size of veins in the hands and feet and their close proximity to nerves and tendons, injection in these areas should be discouraged. Practical techniques to improve the location of veins include use of a hot bath, shower, or hot water bottle, running hot water over the skin, using a sterile swab, or hanging the arm lower than the waist.

→ Intravenous injection is the most common form of injecting drug use.
→ The most common forms of infection associated with injecting drug use are non-communicable infections (for example thrombophlebitis, septicaemia, endocarditis) resulting from unhygienic injecting practices, and communicable blood-borne viral infections resulting from the sharing of injecting equipment previously used by an infected person.
→ Septicaemia and endocarditis both carry a high risk of morbidity and mortality and should be treated aggressively.
→ All blood viral testing should occur with informed consent and be preceded by a frank discussion of the role and meaning of test results.
→ Drug injectors require clear information on how infections occur so that they can identify high-risk situations and develop strategies to protect themselves.

Case study

You are a GP who has recently moved to an outer suburban practice. Ruth, a 25-year-old primary teacher, comes in complaining of arm pain, and requests opiate-based analgesics. She also says that due to her pain she has difficulty sleeping and would like some benzodiazepines. She seems somewhat confused and has impaired psychomotor performance. Her pupils are constricted. Examination of her arm indicates vasculitis. While examining her you also notice a deep abscess in her forearm.

You suspect that Ruth is an injecting heroin user. You let her know that she has vasculitis and that this is often associated with injecting drugs. You explain that while other professionals might be concerned about the legality of this, you are concerned with her health. She visibly relaxes and says she'd heard that you were an OK doctor who tried to help people.

You ask her if she has ever injected, and she tells you that she is a regular heroin user currently involved in heroin use three times a day, and that she treats herself with other opiate-based medication, benzodiazepines, and alcohol, to assist her during the withdrawal phases. Benzodiazepines are commonly crushed and injected.

She first used heroin two years ago at the insistence of her former boyfriend, who convinced her that it was a once-in-a-lifetime experience, and that the stories about heroin and its grip on people were propaganda. On the first use her boyfriend injected her. Although she only used every couple of months during the following 18 months, this increased dramatically six months ago with regular weekly use progressing to daily use. Where she had originally viewed heroin as something that added to the tapestry of her life, she now finds her life driven and dictated to by heroin use.

Ruth states that she has become estranged from her family and is involved with a range of criminal activities to support her heroin use. She has in the last six months spent her life's savings of $25 000 and has recently taken to buying in bulk and selling small quantities to others to finance her use. She says that she cannot stop using, although she knows it is ruining her life and is concerned that the financial cost associated with her current pattern of heroin use is forcing her deeper and deeper in criminal activity and from her teaching vocation. She asks you to assist her to decrease her level of use. She says she is scared of withdrawal, but would like to do so at home.

You are concerned that Ruth may not have a good knowledge about her poly-pharmacy and infection control associated with injecting drug use, and ask her to outline her injecting process and techniques. You provide her with information to reduce the likelihood of damage associated with subsequent injecting and to prevent future infection, as well as information on reducing risk associated with accidental overdose. You discuss with her the risks of blood–borne viral infection, and viral testing, and she agrees to undertake tests to assess her blood–borne viral status.

While you are keen to assist Ruth to withdraw from heroin at home, you are concerned that there will be a lack of supervision and that medication prescribed may not be used as directed. Following discussion, she agrees to involve her sister and withdraw at her sister's home. You also explore the likelihood that Ruth will remain heroin free, and suggest that she might like to consider long-term treatment following withdrawal. You make an appointment for her to see you in fourteen days to discuss outcomes from her blood tests.

Ruth attends your surgery two hours late for her appointment. You see her between patients, and find out that she has used heroin twice since completing her withdrawal six days ago. Her pathology test reports have been received and were all negative. Issues associated with a negative test result are discussed, and you reinforce the need for safe injecting practices. You raise your concern that if she continues to dabble she will return to dependent heroin use, and discuss a management strategy to move her once again towards abstinence. A further appointment is made for re-testing for blood–borne virus, as her last test may have occurred during the window period.

Case points

Ruth's case illustrates:

- communicable and non-communicable morbidities associated with injecting drug use
- the common association between injecting and poly-drug use
- that prescription medications meant for oral use are not uncommonly injected
- that medical practitioners are required to advise patients on risks and prevention of morbidity and mortality associated with injecting, especially infection control and overdose
- the role of blood-borne viral testing.

REFERENCES AND FURTHER READING

Australasian Society for HIV Medicine 2001, *HIV/Viral Hepatitis: A Guide for Primary Care*, Australasian Society for HIV Medicine (ASHM), http://www.ashm.org.au/

Canadian Medical Association 1995, *Counselling Guidelines for HIV Testing*, Canadian Medical Association, Ottawa; http://www.hivpositive.com/f-TestingHIV/CanadaGuidelines/prelim.htm

Derricott, J., Preston, A. & Hunt, N. 1999, *The Safe Injecting Briefing*. Published HIT. http://www.drugtest.org/books/needle/

Morrison, A., Elliott, L. & Gruer, L. 1997, 'Injecting-related harm and treatment seeking behaviour amongst injecting drug users', *Addiction*, vol. 92, pp. 1349–52.

257

14

The Poly-Drug User

Ken Curry & Stan Theodorou

DEFINING POLY-DRUG USE AND USERS

What is poly-drug use?

The use of more than one type of drug by sectors of the community is becoming commonplace. Within Western society, experimentation and recreational (non-problematic) use of various drugs, for example cannabis, alcohol, stimulants, and hallucinogens, is common as part of the adolescent and young adult exploration of life. Similarly, the elderly commonly use a variety of drugs for medicinal and social reasons. For some people the concurrent or successive use of more than one drug can, however, become problematic, each one adding to the risks and harms.

Poly-drug abuse is commonly defined as the hazardous or harmful use of more than one drug. Usually tobacco and caffeine are excluded from the definition. People who use a number of drugs, and especially those who are poly-drug dependent, are more likely to have multiple social and medical problems, psychiatric comorbidity, and chaotic lifestyles. They will often present as difficult patients needing careful and detailed assessment and management.

Types of poly-drug users

Although there are many patterns of use by poly-drug users, some common patterns do emerge:

- Those who take a mixture or cocktail of drugs within a short space of time for the purposes of exaggerating intoxication and 'getting out of it'. For example, especially in the younger age groups and those with coexisting psychiatric disorders, a person may ingest several benzodiazepine tablets and mix this with alcohol and cannabis.
- Those who use various substances sequentially to regulate their mood or consciousness throughout the day. For example, a person may take a stimulant to start the day, an opioid to help cope and diminish stress, and a sedative/depressant to enhance a dreamless sleep.
- Those who take a cocktail of drugs for their individual and combined effect. For example, dance party/rave drug takers in particular may take alcohol or a benzodiazepine for disinhibition or a sense of detachment, plus amphetamines to attenuate the sedative effects of the former.
- The hazardous use of a second drug by a person already dependent on another drug. For example, an opioid-dependent person may combine the opioid with concomitant use of other licit or illicit drugs. The use of benzodiazepines in illicit opioid-dependent or methadone-maintained opioid-dependent groups is commonplace, and represents a difficult management problem. The use of sedatives such as benzodiazepines or alcohol in conjunction with opioids significantly increases the risk of overdose in these groups (see chapter 13).
- Those with an established diagnosis of alcohol dependence. This group has a far greater likelihood of being dependent on another drug—this is 11 times more likely than for the rest of the population. Treatment of patients dependent on both drugs is more complicated than dealing with either one alone.
- Those who are prescribed multiple drugs—iatrogenic impairment. Opioids and/or benzodiazepines will usually be the primary drug class. This pattern is more common with chronic pain or other medical disorders, and in the elderly (see chapter 19). Greater disability may result from the various drug interactions. Table 14.1 lists the common pharmacodynamic interactions.

Use patterns may be dependent or non-dependent use of one drug with non-dependent use of other/s, or dependent use of multiple drugs. The sequelae of the use will be as for any other drugs used individually, but with potential risks due to synergistic effects or interactions and the increased intoxication of combined use.

EPIDEMIOLOGY OF POLY-DRUG USE

The epidemiology of poly-drug use is difficult to establish. There are at least two reasons for this. First, estimates will depend on how poly-drug use is defined (see

Table 14.1 Common interactions of drugs of abuse

Drug combination	*Degree of interaction*	*Effects and comments*
Benzodiazepines plus alcohol	+++	Increased sedation, and intoxication. OD risk increased.
Benzodiazepines plus opioids	+++	Increased sedation, impairment and intoxication. OD risk increased. Common in methadone users and the elderly (with increased falls and confusion).
Tobacco plus cannabis	+	Some research indicates greater respiratory impairment than with either drug alone.
Cannabis plus alcohol	+++	Increased intoxication and impairment.
Cannabis plus stimulants	++	Offsets the sedation of cannabis. Greater increase in heart rate than with either alone.
Opioids plus stimulant	++	Increased intoxication and decreased sedation. A mixture of cocaine and heroin is called a 'speedball'.
Opioids plus antihistamines	+++	Increased sedation, intoxication, and impairment.
Opioids plus prescribed drugs	– to +++	Various medications can interact with opioids. Special precautions are needed with those that increase respiratory depression or increase sedation.
Alcohol plus prescribed drugs	– to +++	Various medications can interact with alcohol and alter the metabolism and effects. Some antibiotics have an aversive effect, for example metronidazole.

Note that these are mostly pharmacodynamic interactions. For information on pharmacokinetic interactions (for example altered rate of metabolism of one drug by another), reference should be made to the specific drugs in one of the various handbooks on drug interactions (for example Tatro 1999), or to the relevant product information (see MIMS Annual).

above). Different definitions will lead to different epidemiological findings. Second, the illegality and societal disapproval of illicit and problem licit drug use results in an under-reporting of drug use in general. This under-reporting is likely to be even greater for poly-drug use.

A number of studies have, however, provided consistent information. First, the likelihood of being classified as having an alcohol or other drug-use disorder is greater in those with a separate, pre-existing, alcohol, or other drug-use disorder. The Australian National Survey of Mental Health and Wellbeing (Teesson et al. 2000) provided community-based estimates of psychiatric disorders and alcohol and drug-use disorders in the Australian community. A diagnosis of an alcohol-use disorder (that is, people with harmful use or dependent use) in the preceding 12 months was made for 6.5% of people surveyed. Of these, 17% had a diagnosis of another drug-use disorder. Therefore 1.1% of people surveyed had both an alcohol and another drug-use disorder within the previous 12 months. The most common coexisting disorders were for alcohol and cannabis.

These data are in agreement with those from overseas. The Epidemiological Catchment Area Study, a community-based survey of psychiatric morbidity performed in the USA in the late 1980s (Regier et al. 1990), found that the lifetime prevalence of both alcohol and another drug disorder was 1.1% of the population surveyed.

> Estimating the extent of poly-drug use is difficult, being dependent on people's willingness to disclose their drug use on the one hand and definitional aspects on the other. While higher prevalence drugs such as alcohol and cannabis may inflate the prevalence rates for poly-drug use, the numbers of patients abusing multiple drugs is significant and can present difficult management problems.

➡ The use of more than one drug by sections of the community is becoming common.

➡ Poly-drug abuse is commonly defined as the hazardous or harmful use of more than one drug.

➡ Poly-drug users often present as difficult patients needing careful and detailed assessment and management.

➡ Different definitions of poly-drug use will lead to different epidemiological findings.

➡ The illegal nature and societal disapproval of illicit and problem licit drug use results in an under-reporting of poly-drug use.

➡ Significant levels of benzodiazepines are used by injecting drug users.

SPECIAL NEEDS

Adolescence and poly-drug use

Drug use in adolescence is discussed in chapter 15. This section will address the issue of poly-drug use in this particular group.

The teenage years are associated with experimentation in drug use. High numbers of teenagers have tried both licit and illicit drugs by the time they reach their mid to late teens. Not infrequently there is a particular pattern of drug use, commencing with licit drugs such as tobacco or alcohol, moving on to cannabis use, and then to other drugs. Usually at this point experimentation with multiple drugs commences. There may be simultaneous use of more than one drug at any one time, or different drugs may be used at different times. The increasing numbers of adolescents who are experimenting in this way probably reflect, in part, the increased availability of drugs in our society.

Poly-drug use may also be an attempt to cope with unpleasant emotional experiences and low self-esteem. Drugs are also often used to overcome shyness in social situations. The use of drugs in these situations can lead to disinhibited behaviour and risk taking. The consequences may then lead to further loss of self-esteem and dysphoria, thus maintaining the affective disturbance.

Poly-drug use is also associated with conduct disturbances. In adolescents with significant antisocial behaviour, such as those having a history of illegal activities or involved in prostitution, there is a greater prevalence of poly-drug use than in those who do not exhibit these behaviours. It is important to mention that this subgroup of adolescents often give histories of significant emotional, physical, or sexual abuse, and poly-drug use may also be a means of coping with what would be an otherwise overwhelming experience.

A number of poly-drug using adolescents will present to emergency departments intoxicated. Staff need to consider the possibility of poly-drug use during their assessment to enable an effective management strategy to be developed and implemented. These emergency department admissions are often among poly-drug users from more chaotic psychosocial backgrounds.

Adolescents presenting to drug and alcohol services for treatment are also commonly those with greater psychosocial disruption. They usually have longer histories of drug use, and are much more likely than other adolescents to be dependent on one or more drugs. Their assessment and management is complex, and may involve the need to liaise with other services such as child and family or psychiatric services.

Poly-drug use and psychiatric morbidity

The relationship between drug use and psychiatric morbidity is discussed in chapter 20. This section discusses the relationship between poly-drug use and psychiatric morbidity.

Poly-drug use is found across the range of psychiatric disorders, with abuse not uncommon. Up to 25% of patients with a formal psychiatric diagnosis abuse multiple drugs. This may be for a number of reasons. For example, people with anxiety disorders often use multiple drugs to self-medicate, and it is not uncommon for abuse of multiple sedative drugs to be a presenting feature of these disorders.

Poly-drug users have also been found to have higher levels of mental health disorder than non-drug and single-drug users. Some common findings are:
- Poly-drug use is associated with a higher incidence of depressive disorders.
- A greater degree of personality psychopathology has also been associated with poly-drug abuse.
- There is an increased risk of deliberate self-harm in poly-drug users.

Poly-drug use is not only associated with higher levels of psychopathology, it also predicts a poorer outcome for those with psychiatric morbidity, especially severe mental illness. For example, it is associated with multiple admissions to psychiatric hospitals and may be a significant cause of revolving-door admissions.

There is no definitive or simple answer to the question of how or why comorbidity and poly-drug use are associated. The direction of causality between poly-drug use and psychiatric disorders is complex and often unclear. Three possible theories are commonly espoused:
- Poly-drug use increases psychiatric morbidity.
- Greater psychiatric morbidity leads to attempts to self-medicate with multiple drugs.
- Both psychiatric pathology and poly-drug abuse are part of an underlying disorder.

263

It is probable that all three explanations have some validity, and may be applicable to different situations. The first theory can be related to psychotic disorders such as schizophrenia, where the abuse of anticholinergics (for example benztropine and procyclidine), cannabis, and stimulants increases the likelihood of a relapse and therefore leads to a poorer outcome and increased psychopathology. Theory two finds support where the concurrent use of alcohol and benzodiazepines in anxiety disorders may initially be an attempt to control anxiety, but in the long term may worsen symptoms and lead to greater morbidity. Finally, theory three is supported by the finding that an underlying personality disorder, such as the borderline or antisocial type, has been associated with both poly-drug use and a number of psychiatric disorders such as depression.

Poly-drug users have a greater likelihood of psychiatric comorbidity, and those with a comorbid disorder can expect a poorer outcome. A thorough and comprehensive assessment and management plan addressing their drug use as well as their mental health problem is essential.

Heroin dependence and poly-drug use

Dependent heroin users, including those maintained on pharmacotherapy programs (for example methadone or naltrexone), commonly use a variety of drugs. Cannabis use is common in heroin users, including those in methadone-maintenance programs, but little interaction is observed other than a mild increase in intoxication. Benzodiazepine use/dependence and harmful alcohol use generally proves to be the most problematic among the heroin-using population, and is associated with an increased risk of overdose and death. The most lethal combination of drugs is opioids plus another sedative, usually alcohol and/or benzodiazepines.

A recent Australian study showed that, during patient induction into methadone treatment, benzodiazepines and alcohol used in conjunction with opioids account for 85% of recorded mortality. Benzodiazepines, morphine and alcohol accounted for most of this figure, and only 10% resulted from methadone alone (Sunjic & Zador 1999) (see chapters 6 and 13).

In a significant number of instances benzodiazepines are prescribed by medical practitioners directly to poly-drug users. Doctors should be extremely cautious about prescribing benzodiazepines to opioid users, and should advise them of the significant dangers of overdose when benzodiazepines and/or alcohol are used with opioids (see chapters 6, 13, and 21).

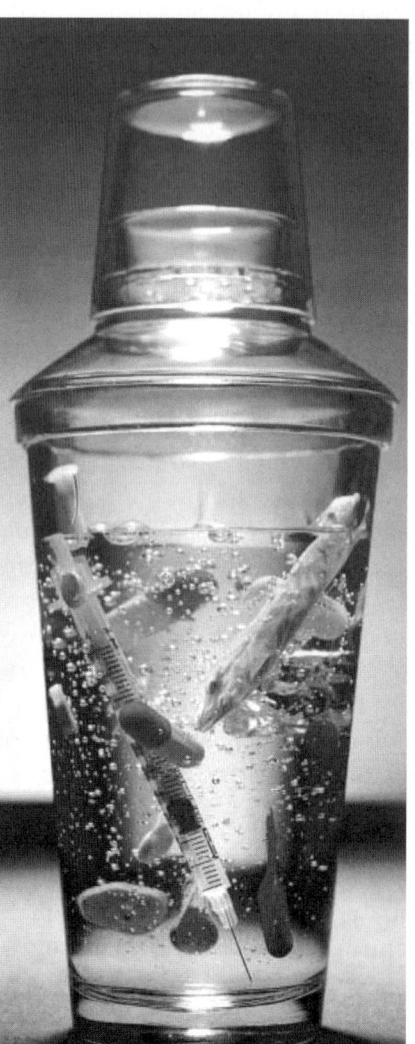

Figure 14.1
Poly-drug use, which is common among some groups of drug users, can be fatal.

Artwork reproduced with permission of the Prevention Branch, Drug and Alcohol Office (Department of Health, Western Australia)

Prescription drug use and doctor shopping

This section should be read in conjunction with chapter 21.

Use of pharmaceuticals, especially prescription drugs, forms a significant proportion of poly-drug abuse behaviour. This may be in the form of prescription drugs only or it may involve mixing pharmaceuticals with illicit drugs. Access to prescription drugs will commonly be in the form of doctor shopping. Doctor shoppers are people who visit multiple general practitioners to obtain multiple prescriptions, giving them access to larger amounts of medication than is clinically necessary.

Medical practitioners and pharmacists can use a central helpline to gain access to information regarding patients they suspect are doctor shoppers (see chapter 21). Doctor shoppers are generally quite specific about the type of drug sought, with most requesting scripts for benzodiazepines, compounds containing codeine, other opioids, or combinations of these. People with chronic pain syndromes or debilitating health conditions are particularly susceptible to poly-drug misuse, either intentionally or iatrogenically (through over-prescription). Problems with chronic pain are frequent, and where this is the case many use benzodiazepines and/or alcohol as well as opioids.

> → For many adolescents who use drugs the dominant pattern is one of poly-drug use.
> → There is a greater prevalence of poly-drug use in adolescents with significant antisocial behaviour, such as those having a significant history of illegal activities or involvement in prostitution.
> → Poly-drug users presenting to hospital emergency departments and drug and alcohol services often come from more chaotic psychosocial backgrounds.
> → Poly-drug users have a higher degree of psychopathology than non-drug and single-drug users.
> → The most lethal combination of drugs is opioids plus other sedatives, usually alcohol and/or benzodiazepines.
> → Medical practitioners can use a central helpline to gain access to information regarding patients who they suspect are doctor shoppers.

265

ASSESSMENT AND MANAGEMENT

Poly-drug use encompasses a great spectrum of use patterns: drugs used sequentially by themselves and in combination, and via various modes of administration. Those with multiple dependencies are likely to have more severe morbidity and therefore likely to come to the attention of medical practitioners. These people need careful assessment and management due to the complexity of their medical, psychological, and social situation.

Ingredients for establishing rapport are those already identified in chapter 4. However, establishing rapport with the poly-drug user may be more challenging and take more time, since this population often has difficulties relating to others, including medical professionals. Nevertheless, the forming of a therapeutic relationship is essential, and, as noted in chapter 4, this will make it more likely that an accurate history is obtained, that any advice given will be considered and followed, and that interventions will be accepted and effective. The patient is also more likely to return for future help with drug or other medical issues.

Drug issues

Patients will view the severity of their drug use and associated harms in a variety of ways. Some may consider that their use is not problematic, even in the face of serious harms and risks. In other instances, patients may acknowledge their drug use and associated problems, but feel that they are too enormous and daunting to do anything about. In such cases, it is important to approach management by negotiating small achievable steps towards an ultimate goal. In both these instances, a motivational interviewing approach can be used to move a person's thinking from the stage of pre-contemplation to contemplation or action (see chapter 5).

Often patients will perceive their use of different drugs with a cascade of concerns. Injecting heroin dependence will usually be seen as an issue of concern, whereas concomitant benzodiazepine use or dependence will not be seen to be significant. Commonly, alcohol or cannabis use or dependence will be of little or no concern to people with other dependencies. Decisions about the management of problems will need to take into consideration the degree of concern the patient has in relation to the drugs used, weighed against the risk assessment made by the medical practitioner.

Where present, heroin dependence will usually be seen by both the patient and medical practitioner to be the issue of most urgent concern, and the priority will be in managing this problem. This is an appropriate priority, as it poses greatest immediate risk to the individual's life and health. Other drug issues will usually only be addressed effectively after some stability is achieved with what is perceived as the primary problem drug.

History and examination

Due to the complexity of poly-drug use, and associated medical and psychosocial problems, assessment needs to cover not only the separate drug effects but also their various interactions.

History-taking is essentially the same as for a comprehensive assessment with users of single problem drugs (see chapter 4), but with particular attention paid to the following issues.

- Past and current consumption of each drug used needs to be determined, including amount, frequency, type, method of administration, context of use, features of dependence, and withdrawal.
- Use of specific drug combinations as described above also needs to be assessed, for example how much alcohol and how much cannabis. Assessing the risk of single and combined drug use is vital to ascertain high-risk behaviours and situations, intoxication, and likelihood of withdrawal.
- Current and past treatments need to be elucidated, especially methadone maintenance or other pharmacotherapies.
- Determine if other medical practitioners are being seen.
- Determine if any other medical practitioners hold an authority to prescribe drugs of addiction or if any addictive drugs been prescribed in the last two months.
  In particular examine for:
- signs of intoxication or withdrawal (which may be complicated because of the poly-drug use)
- other drug-related signs, including pupil size and vein puncture sites.

Urine and blood drug screening may be useful as corroborative evidence or in monitoring progress. Information from other doctors, relevant health authorities, and/or drug and alcohol agencies may also be useful both for initial assessment and in monitoring progress.

> ➡ Establishing a rapport with the poly-drug user may be more challenging and take more time, since this population often has difficulties in relating to others.
> ➡ A therapeutic alliance is important to improve accuracy of information provided and increase the likelihood that advice will be considered and followed.
> ➡ Some poly-drug users consider their use is not problematic, even in the face of serious harms and risks. Motivational interviewing can be used to move a person's thinking from a stage of pre-contemplation to contemplation or action.
> ➡ Poly-drug users will frequently perceive their use of different drugs with a cascade of concern. For example, injecting heroin dependence is considered a concern, but not concomitant benzodiazepine use.
> ➡ Assessment of poly-drug use must include separate drug effects and the various interactions.

267

Management

The management plan can now be developed on the basis of information gained during the assessment. The following areas will guide the formation of the management plan.

- drug issues (see above), and especially whether the person is in withdrawal or dependent, and on which drug/s
- hierarchy of harms or potential harms associated with the particular drugs used and their method/s of use
- the presenting complaint, if that is not a drug issue
- other medical or psychiatric conditions
- social conditions.

> Determining a hierarchy of needs and dangers is essential in working out a management plan. A daily opioid injector will usually require intervention for opioid dependence as a priority over intervention for cannabis, benzodiazepine or alcohol use.

Withdrawal management

Withdrawal from a single drug is covered in each separate drug chapter. This chapter deals with additional considerations for withdrawal of the poly-drug user. As with single drug use, consideration needs to be given to the setting and context of withdrawal with regard to safety, patient preference, and the availability of local services (see chapter 5). However, with the poly-drug user this requires an understanding that the risks are likely to be higher than with single-drug dependence. It is important therefore to identify the most appropriate withdrawal environment for each poly-drug case.

Outpatient setting
The outpatient setting is appropriate for those patients who are motivated, have good social support, and are relatively healthy. Usually it is best to focus on withdrawal from one drug at a time, for example stopping benzodiazepines before addressing cannabis cessation. This can be enhanced with services that offer specialised home-based treatment.

Inpatient setting
The more specialised inpatient services are accustomed to dealing with complicated withdrawal processes, and withdrawal may proceed more rapidly than with outpatient programs. In many instances drugs will need to be withdrawn sequentially because of concerns regarding severity of withdrawal, while in others the two drugs may be withdrawn simultaneously with little risk. The choice of action depends on the drugs used, the doses, and the duration of administration.

The more general wards (usually allied with mental health) may need considerable input from the drug and alcohol specialist. If expertise/experience is lacking, targeting withdrawal from one of the drugs only during admission is indicated. For example, for the person presenting with both an illicit opiate dependence and benzodiazepine dependence, benzodiazepines may be withdrawn on an inpatient basis while the patient is simultaneously stabilised on methadone if that is the best option for the management of their opioid dependence. However, if opioid withdrawal (possibly followed by naltrexone maintenance) is considered appropriate, this can be undertaken on an outpatient basis or during a subsequent inpatient admission.

As stressed in chapter 5, withdrawal from drugs is not an end in itself—it is merely the beginning of a therapeutic process. Counselling, residential rehabilitation programs, and continued support are essential. Attention may need to be given to accommodation needs, social security, or other welfare needs, in addressing the patient's lifestyle issues.

As people with poly-drug dependence are more likely to have a chaotic lifestyle, special attention needs to be given to obtaining psychosocial stability. While this is being achieved, attention may need to be given to issues of child protection where patients have care of children. Referral to a drug and alcohol agency will usually be indicated to assist in the management of poly-drug dependence, and often referral to mental health services will be indicated where there is concomitant psychiatric morbidity.

→ Management decisions must take into consideration the degree of concern the patient has in relation to the drugs used, weighed against a risk assessment made by the medical practitioner.
→ Determining a hierarchy of needs and dangers is essential to working out a treatment plan.
→ An understanding that withdrawal risks associated with poly-drug use are higher than with single drugs is important in determining the most appropriate withdrawal environment.
→ As poly-drug users are more likely to have a chaotic lifestyle, special attention needs to be given to establishing psychosocial stability.

Case studies

Case study 1

Lisa is a 26-year-old single woman who is 10 weeks pregnant. She admits to using a mixture of drugs, including daily heroin injections for the past two years, daily tobacco and cannabis use, and occasionally injecting temazepam tablets. She is concerned that her drug use will affect her baby, but at the same time does not believe that she will be able to just stop injecting, especially the opioids, which she has tried stopping on many previous occasions. Although the pregnancy was unplanned, she intends to keep the baby and move away from the drug scene to live with her parents.

A comprehensive assessment reveals that Lisa has multiple problems but is motivated to address them.

Therapeutic engagement was comparatively successful, and Lisa was maintained on a stable methadone dose throughout her pregnancy, with an increase in the third trimester. She gave birth to a normal baby who had minor opioid withdrawal (managed by a paediatrician), and breast-fed for four months. Her drug use (apart from methadone) diminished greatly. Benzodiazepines and injecting drug use ceased, and although she still occasionally smoked cannabis, the frequency and amount was much lower than pre-treatment. She continued to be maintained on methadone at a year follow-up, with considerable positive change to her health and social environment (also see chapter 16).

Case points

Lisa's case illustrates:
- Her high risk injecting behaviour, including risk of infection and overdose to herself and to her foetus, is initially the greatest concern. Information to reduce these risks should be provided (see chapter 13).
- Stabilisation of the opioid dependency is the next priority. Considering the length of dependent opioid use and previous failed attempts at significantly reducing or stopping illicit opioid use, a regular daily methadone regime is commenced (see chapter 6). This is considered appropriate due to the early stage of pregnancy and maternal motivation.
- Early liaison with an obstetrician and midwives is vital.
- Continuing education and counselling is essential in lessening Lisa's other risky behaviours, including her benzodiazepine, cannabis, and tobacco use.
- Engagement of the patient and significant others (in this case her parents) is considered important to support treatment compliance and improve psychosocial functioning.
- A case-management approach with a key worker coordinating the input from the various agencies is essential.

Case study 2

Dean is a 32-year-old man on a methadone maintenance program. He presents to his general practitioner asking for a prescription of diazepam to help him sleep. He says that he has used diazepam in the past with good effect when he had sleeping problems. Further questioning reveals that he recently ended a long-term relationship, and his insomnia dated from then. He is known to have had benzodiazepine dependence in the past, and in the last two months has been obtaining diazepam tablets off the street to help him cope.

The combination of benzodiazepine use and methadone are difficult to manage. In this case the general practitioner declined the request for diazepam, and, with Dean's consent, conferred with the methadone clinic. Following assessment by a psychiatrist at the clinic, Dean was diagnosed with a depressive disorder, and commenced on an antidepressant. Due to the short length of time he had been taking benzodiazepines and the moderate dosage used, a structured withdrawal regime was not considered necessary. Nevertheless, close follow-up was instituted to monitor for any serious withdrawal symptoms. Monitoring of his urine was also instituted to identify whether benzodiazepine use continued. Dean's mood improved after several weeks and his benzodiazepine use ceased, while the methadone dose remained constant.

Case points

Dean's case illustrates:
- Generally requests for benzodiazepines in drug seekers should be refused.
- Consideration of the possibility of a mood or other psychological disorder associated with life factors, and institution of an appropriate therapy or further assessment by a specialist.
- Alternatives to medication should be considered (see chapter 19).
- The methadone clinic is informed of the patient's predicament (with the patient's consent).
- Assessment of the need for a diazepam reduction and withdrawal regime.
- If necessary, the GP under the guidance of the methadone clinic and in agreement with the patient can initiate a diazepam reduction and withdrawal regime.

Case study 3

Bruce is a 28-year-old professional man who drinks alcohol in moderation during the week and smokes two to three joints of cannabis two to three times per week with friends. He presents to his GP with insomnia. At the weekends he takes a mixture of ecstasy, speed, and cannabis. He frequently takes time off work, particularly at the beginning of the working week. Another GP has been prescribing him temazepam for sleep at usual therapeutic doses for six months, but these are now proving to be ineffective. He is otherwise physically and psychologically well.

Bruce agreed to stop the use of amphetamine-like substances for at least two months as he acknowledged and accepted the link made by the GP regarding his health, including sleep disruptions and drug use. Through a self-monitoring procedure initiated by the GP, he recognised that his sleep had improved and his work functioning increased. The temazepam was increased for a two-week period, then a four-week withdrawal plan was instituted. At follow-up six months later he had returned to occasional use of speed, but suffered none of the health effects he had experienced earlier, being especially aware of the effects of the excessive use of these substances. His cannabis and alcohol use remained at the same level and urine testing revealed no benzodiazepines.

Case points

Bruce's case illustrates:
- Careful assessment reveals a pattern of drug use that, over a period of time, has become particularly severe at the weekends.
- The GP makes a link between the drug use and functional impairment at the beginning of the week.
- The use of amphetamine-like substances (ecstasy and speed) has increased over the last few months, and this was also linked with his insomnia.
- Bruce's recreational use of drugs is rapidly becoming problematic, and there is evidence that there is tolerance to the temazepam.
- A check is made regarding previous prescriptions and the likelihood of drug-seeking behaviour.

REFERENCES AND FURTHER READING

MIMS Annual (Australia) 2002, MediMedia Australia, St Leonards, New South Wales.

Regier, D.A., Farmer, M.E., Rae, D.S. et al. 1990, 'Comorbidity of mental disorders with alcohol and other drug abuse. Results from the Epidemiologic Catchment Area (ECA) Study', *Journal of the American Medical Association*, vol. 264, pp. 2511–18.

Sunjic, S. & Zador, D. 1999, 'Methadone syrup-related deaths in New South Wales, Australia, 1990–95', *Drug and Alcohol Review*, vol. 18, pp. 409–15.

Tatro, D.S. (ed.) 1999, *Drug Interaction Facts. Facts and Comparisons*, Facts and Comparisons, St Louis.

Teesson, M., Hall, W., Lynskey, M. & Degenhardt, L. 2000, 'Alcohol- and drug-use disorders in Australia: Implications of the National Survey of Mental Health and Wellbeing', *Australian and New Zealand Journal of Psychiatry*, vol. 34, pp. 206–13.

15

Adolescence

Doug Sellman & Daryle Deering

Adolescence is a transitional period between childhood and adulthood. It begins biologically with the onset of puberty and ends through the appearance of social independence.

The gap between these two markers is increasing, with puberty gradually beginning earlier in developed countries such as Australia and New Zealand, and the age of social independence becoming delayed in response to growing societal complexity and changing economics. Various definitions of adolescence can be found, inclusive of late childhood and early adulthood and spanning the age range 10 to 25. This chapter will take the pragmatic definition of adolescence commonly used in relation to specialist adolescent treatment services: adolescence is defined as the age range coinciding with secondary education. This normally means people aged 13 to 18, although 12-year-olds and 19-year-olds will also appear in service statistics. One of the reasons for establishing this definition when considering alcohol and drug use and misuse is to highlight the importance of secondary schooling in the treatment of adolescents with alcohol and drug problems. Early adolescence is commonly defined in terms of age as 13–14 years, middle adolescence as 15–16 years, and late adolescence 17–18 years.

EPIDEMIOLOGY

Prevalence of drug use

Alcohol, nicotine, and cannabis are the three drugs most commonly used by adolescents in Australia and New Zealand, with lifetime use by age 19 in the region of 80% for alcohol, 50% for nicotine, and 40% for cannabis. All the other drugs, including stimulants, depressants, hallucinogens, opioids, inhalants, and others, have little significance compared with the big three, with less than 10% of adolescents using any of these drugs even once in their lives, let alone going on to regular use and dependence.

An increasing number of adolescents are using hallucinogens and stimulants as part of the contemporary dance culture, and this is extending into regular street use. Ecstasy (E, XTC, love drug, MDMA; 3,4-methylenedioxymethamphetamine), a stimulant with hallucinogenic properties, is one of the first drugs to have been used widely in the dance scene and to transfer to street use. MDMA is likely to be superseded by similar synthetic drugs designed for recreational use by the young and that combine a number of actions of the traditionally classified drugs.

Although using drugs, including alcohol, is relatively common among Australian and New Zealand adolescents, the rate of significant drug misuse leading to clinically significant problems (drug abuse and dependence) is relatively low. About 5% of adolescents will have had drug dependence and about 10 to 15% will have had additional problems associated with drug use by the time they reach adulthood. It is this 20% of adolescents who are the main concern of treatment services.

> Some experimentation with drugs and other risk behaviours is common and normal in adolescence and needs to be distinguished from problematic use.

Changing patterns of use during adolescence

Nicotine, alcohol, and cannabis are generally the first drugs used experimentally by adolescents and children, although inhalant use can certainly occur in children and early adolescence (see the discussion of solvent use below). Depressants, stimulants and hallucinogens are generally not used before mid adolescence, if indeed they are used at all. The same is true of intravenous drug use, especially of opioid drugs.

Weekly alcohol use in 15-year-olds is less than 10%, but rises to about 30 to 40% by age 18, with the percentage of adolescents drinking 10 or more standard drinks per typical occasion being less than 5% in 15-year-olds but rising to 20 to 30% in 18-year-olds. Similar data can be found for cannabis use, with about 10% of mid adolescents reporting using cannabis at least once a week and about 15% of late adolescents reporting use at least once a week. About 20% of adolescents will have used cannabis 100 times or more by the time they have reached adulthood.

Experimental and regular use of all drugs increases throughout adolescence.

Figure 15.1 Binge drinking and associated morbidity in some adolescents is of major concern.

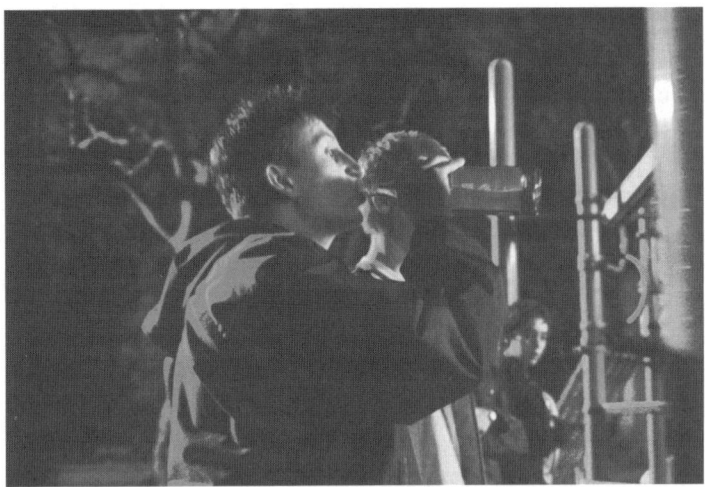

Courtesy of the National Alcohol Campaign,
Commonwealth Department of Health and Ageing.

Solvent use

Inhalants are often referred to as solvents. They are a heterogeneous group of fat-soluble industrial substances breathed in through the mouth or nose to produce a disinhibiting euphoria. This euphoria is not unlike the effect of alcohol, but it is also accompanied by perceptual distortions that may extend into frank hallucinations. They are usually taken intermittently, and often as part of a fad among adolescents in their pre-teens or early teens, or among groups who have limited access to drugs. Those who use regularly tend to abandon use after a year or two, but a small percentage continue to use throughout adolescence and sometimes beyond, normally as part of a multiple drug-use pattern. Death can occasionally occur from respiratory depression, cardiac arrhythmia, asphyxia, or through accidents while intoxicated.

Gender differences

Drug abuse and dependence in females may be greater than in males in early adolescence, but by mid adolescence males have caught up and, by late adolescence, drug abuse and dependence among males is greater than in females. Weight control through the use of nicotine and stimulants has primarily been a female adolescent issue in the past but it is beginning to be relevant for both sexes.

There are important gender differences in drug use, drug problems, and drug dependence among adolescents, and these vary according to the developmental stage.

AETIOLOGY

Adolescent drug abuse and drug dependence is a complex disorder, with its aetiology consisting of multiple genes interacting with multiple environmental influences. Family, twin, and adoption studies indicate that there is a genetic component contributing up to 60% of the variance, and there is evidence for a common addictive genetic factor as well as specific genetic influences for the various substances. Interacting with this genetic vulnerability are a myriad of environmental influences, including early use of licit and illicit drugs and a range of individual, family, and social factors (see chapter 2).

It is important to consider the function of the drug use in each individual. Adolescents frequently report using drugs for fun. In those with past trauma, the key purpose commonly given for their drug taking is to forget or to cope.

Adolescent drug abuse and drug dependence therefore need to be considered in a broader context of problem behaviours that include antisocial peer affiliation and antisocial behaviour, school failure, family disruption and isolation from family, and adolescent pregnancy. There is also a high prevalence of coexisting mental health disorders in adolescents with drug abuse and drug dependence, particularly behavioural and mood disorders.

Certain substances, especially cannabis, have been described as gateway drugs to more socially unacceptable drugs such as heroin and amphetamines. Adolescents who regularly use cannabis are certainly much more likely to use other illicit substances, but otherwise cannabis is no more a gateway drug than is nicotine or alcohol.

Adolescent drug abuse and dependence is strongly associated with other problem high-risk behaviours such as delinquency and early onset sexual activity.

SPECIFIC ADOLESCENT ISSUES

Adolescence is an important developmental period during which critical coping and social competencies are obtained. Australasian society is becoming increasingly complex, necessitating the acquisition of a demanding set of knowledge and skills about how to live as an independent person. Drug abuse and drug dependence can significantly impact on the normal developmental tasks of adolescence, which include individuation and separation from parents/caregivers and the development of a range of coping and social interaction skills.

Regular drug use can interfere directly with brain function underlying learning. Regular drug use with alternating intoxication/detoxification can significantly impede the process of emotional growth and maturation through involvement in a range of normal social interactions, inside and outside of home.

The extent of impact of drug abuse/dependence varies considerably in relation to the quality of premorbid adjustment, the severity of the disorder(s), and the family, social and cultural life context of the individual adolescent.

Addressing adolescent drug abuse/dependence is best undertaken using a broad public health perspective with the goals of minimising the harm associated with drug use and optimising life choices. This broad approach will include health education about the safe use of alcohol and other drugs, as well as a focus on reduction and cessation of problematic and high-risk use and on improving coping and social skills.

Connectedness to school and family have been shown to be particularly important protective factors in adolescents, lessening the association with antisocial peers and decreasing the risk of a range of psychosocial and health problems, including the further development of the alcohol and drug problem.

Fundamental to working with adolescents is involvement with families/caregivers. This is particularly so in the more severe and complex cases. Although consent for treatment can legally be given by adolescents of all ages separate from their parents/caregivers, given that they understand the nature of the treatment, in the majority of cases it is best to attempt to negotiate a treatment plan with parents/caregivers involved. Occasionally a family is so dysfunctional and/or dangerous that treatment begins with finding alternative caregivers and accommodation.

277

ASSESSMENT

Assessment of adolescents can be considered on two main levels:
- screening and brief assessment, which commonly occurs in primary care or non-specialist settings
- comprehensive assessments, which more commonly occur within specialist alcohol and drug or mental health settings.

Establishing rapport and beginning a therapeutic relationship is fundamental to conducting assessments with adolescents in any setting. Experience has led to the identification of a number of ingredients associated with intervening effectively with adolescents:
- showing respect
- being honest, trustworthy, and genuine (not trying to be adolescent)
- demonstrating flexibility

- utilising appropriate humour
- providing confidentiality (but not secrecy).

> It is essential when assessing adolescent drug use to understand the process of behavioural change and to utilise a motivational approach, as ambivalence is often intense and overt.

Screening and brief assessment

Assessment of adolescents begins in a primary-care setting. Adolescents most commonly will present for help within systems they are in daily contact with, or through parents or caregivers expressing concern. Adolescents will therefore generally make first contact with school counsellors, general medical practitioners or practice nurses, youth workers, and staff in dedicated youth health centres.

Assessment in these settings may involve initial screening and then a brief assessment of those who are screened as having a potential problem. There is no evidence that screening instruments in primary-care settings are superior to a brief confidential interview in which information on quantity and frequency of drug use and the nature and extent of problems associated with drug use are briefly explored.

A key aim of a brief clinical assessment is to identify those adolescents who should be referred for more specialist assistance. These adolescents will be those who have moderate to severe dependence and/or additional complicating disorders and problems. Primary-care workers therefore need to undertake a brief diagnostic assessment to explore dependence criteria in relation to those drugs the adolescent is using at least 10 times a month.

The key topics that should be covered in a brief assessment are:
- demographics
- drugs ever used, and when
- pattern and function of drug use, including heaviest six-month use for each drug
- quantity and frequency, problems and dependence features, related to both this heaviest period of use and current use (often this will be the same time period)
- brief history of any alcohol or drug treatment undertaken
- brief psychiatric history
- family history of alcohol and drug use
- other related issues.

There is some debate about the validity of dependence criteria in adolescent drug use. Age-appropriate examples need to be utilised for exploring dyscontrol and salience (increasing dominance of drug use in the adolescent's life). Withdrawal symptoms and relief use can take considerable time to develop, particularly for some substances such as alcohol, and thus these dependence criteria may not be as relevant for adolescents. The challenges in diagnosing adolescent substance dependence are similar to those of other adolescent-onset mental disorders such as major depression, where diagnostic certainty is compromised by the nature of first appearance of symptoms.

> A high index of suspicion for dependence should be exercised in those adolescents showing problematic drug use and who have a family history of addiction.

Whereas three of the seven DSM-IV criteria are normally required for a diagnosis of dependence, moderate to severe dependence in an adolescent can be defined as that level of dependence where most (at least five) of the seven DSM-IV dependence criteria are present and there is overt disruption of the adolescent's life through drug use.

If moderate to severe dependence can be excluded, then a brief intervention is most appropriately undertaken within the primary-care setting in which the adolescent presented, with continuing monitoring and care if necessary. If, on the other hand, moderate to severe dependence is identified, referral to an outpatient specialist adolescent alcohol and drug service is appropriate if available.

Comprehensive assessment

In specialist settings it is probably even more important to gain a deep understanding of the unique individual who is presenting. The first step is a comprehensive assessment. This consists of a similar exploration of the adolescent's drug problem, as in a brief assessment in a primary-care setting, but with two important additions.

An elaboration of the overall history should be undertaken. This should include a more extensive assessment of psychiatric, medical, legal, family, and personal/developmental issues, including early life, schooling, and friendships. This would be supplemented with an examination of mental state, and an appropriate medical examination and investigations where indicated.

A significant other should be interviewed. This may be a parent/caregiver, or another person who is important in the adolescent's life. Where there is significant family breakdown this may be a youth worker, counsellor, or other professional. This interview should be conducted separately from the adolescent's individual, confidential interview.

> There are a number of disorders commonly coexisting in adolescents presenting to specialist services with substance dependence. These are major depression, post-traumatic stress disorder, social phobia, conduct disorder, and attention deficit hyperactivity disorder. Along with a comprehensive screen of medical and psychiatric disorder, these and other disorders need specific attention, and, if present, need to be given appropriate emphasis in an integrated management plan.

A useful model

A model categorising adolescents into four main groups is outlined in figure 15.2.

This model was established by factoring in five common problem areas: early sexual activity, alcohol abuse, cannabis use, conduct disorder, and contact with police. First are 'normal' individuals, comprising 85% of adolescents, who have a low probability for any of these problems. Second are a precocious group of 5% of adolescents, with female predominance, whose main problems have been described as accelerated transition to adult hedonic behaviours, that is, early-onset sexual activity and substance use. Third are 7% of adolescents, male biased, whose main problems relate to antisocial or law-breaking activities, including conduct disorder, police contact, and cannabis use. Finally is a group of 3% of adolescents, those with multiple problems who are at risk of all forms of problem behaviours and of seriously limiting their life choices.

Figure 15.2 Four major groupings of 15-year-old adolescents, based on latent class modelling of five key variables: sexual activity, alcohol abuse, cannabis use, conduct disorder, police contact (Fergusson et al. 1994)

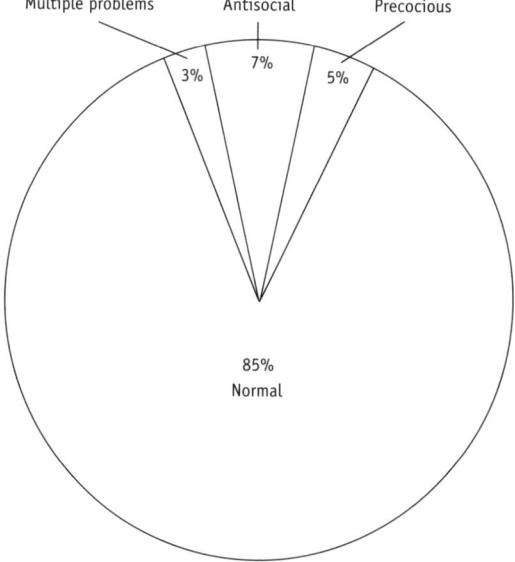

INTERVENTION

The concept of a syndrome of problem behaviours, described above, has implications for the treatment of adolescents presenting with significant alcohol and drug problems. It is important to consider the drug abuse/dependence as part of a larger pattern of problem behaviours and other mental disorders. It is important also to consider protective factors and focus on strengthening resilience.

Interventions with adolescents who have drug and alcohol problems vary considerably, depending on the extent of the substance-use problem along with the presence and extent of coexisting disorders and problems. Interventions may range in length of time from brief (less than an hour) to extended (years), and the settings in which these interventions are undertaken will vary from outpatient, through day-patient, to inpatient/residential programs. In general, the more severe and complicated the problem, the more extensive the intervention is likely to be, and the more likely it is to involve intervention components across the three settings.

For adolescents with complex problems associated with drug abuse/dependence, adequate intervention necessitates a multi-systems approach. This needs to incorporate targeted interventions involving family, close peers, and other significant others, as well as a coordinated response across health, education, social welfare, and justice boundaries. A clinical case-management approach involving a key worker who ensures coordination and continuity of care is critical for adolescents requiring input from a number of services. It also needs to be remembered that for many such adolescents, episodes of care are interrupted by periods of stability and non-problematic drug use. Hence the importance of an attractive, accessible treatment system that is youth friendly.

> Some adolescents have few problems and many strengths, requiring minimal assistance, while others have complex problems and few strengths, requiring intensive assistance, sometimes over a long period of time.

281

Primary-care settings

In primary-care settings where moderate to severe dependence has been excluded and there are no significant complicating factors, a brief intervention involving both motivational and cognitive-behavioural strategies is appropriate. At minimum this would consist of three key components:

- Pertinent information will be provided to the adolescent covering the nature and extent of his or her individual drug problem.
- Therapeutic discussion will be undertaken that leads to the adolescent setting goals for change.
- A mutually convenient date for reviewing these goals will be negotiated.

Involving parents/caregivers is not mandatory for success in many situations of brief assessment and interventions with adolescents.

Specialist settings

In specialist settings an appropriate management plan needs to be formulated following a comprehensive assessment. The first steps in this plan will be negotiated with the adolescent, as far as is possible in close collaboration with their parents/caregivers or other significant others in a feedback session.

Principles for interventions

Below are ten key principles that underpin interventions with adolescents who present in specialist settings with significant drug abuse/dependence. These, considered alongside the key ingredients of working effectively with adolescents described above, provide a guide to an optimal intervention.

1   Engagement and development of a therapeutic relationship. This is critical, and begins from the first contact and during initial assessment. The person who is undertaking the assessment should as far as possible be the same person who continues with interventions.

2   Ensuring safety. This is fundamental to working adequately with adolescents. Sometimes a controlling, caregiving approach is necessary, depending on the imminence of the risk. The typical safety issues include reducing the risks of suicide, pregnancy, blood-borne viral infection, motor-vehicle accident, family violence, and expulsion from school.

3   A motivational, empowering approach. The motivational approach involves a focus on empathy, avoiding argumentation, and 'rolling with resistance'. Strategic and careful confrontation of the adolescent with his or her own volunteered set of negative consequences of drug use (often the crisis that brought about the initial referral) is undertaken, as is inspiring the adolescent with a new vision of him or herself in a future without drug problems. Self-efficacy is strongly supported, and the adolescent is encouraged to set his or her own goals, even if at the beginning they are not as ideal as the clinician and parents/caregivers might wish for.

4   Education about drug abuse and drug dependence. This is a key component of the feedback session following assessment, optimally with both adolescent and parents/caregivers present. This session is a bridge from assessment to treatment during which findings of the assessment are communicated and discussed, including identification of strengths and positive attributes.

5   Involvement of families/caregivers. This should always be attempted with a view to maintaining, improving, or re-establishing relationships in the longer term. Parents/caregivers will commonly need support and assistance in their own right. Another clinician may need to be involved to work with the parents/caregivers to maximise the likelihood of retaining the adolescent in treatment and to ensure that the adolescent's needs remain paramount.

6   Optimising life choices and opportunities. This is a key goal of treatment for adolescents misusing substances, and operates particularly through maintaining or re-establishing schooling or vocational training. This can involve identifying and assisting with specific learning difficulties. For some young women, the avoidance of teenage parenthood can be the most therapeutic endeavour.

7   Promoting and strengthening relationships with at least one positive adult. This can include a parent, relative, teacher, sports coach, church leader, or even the clinician.

8   Attendance at a minimum of three self-help meetings. This could include youth-focused Narcotics Anonymous or Alcoholics Anonymous meetings for all adolescents with severe and complex problems, and/or a re-socialising therapeutic community program lasting at least six to nine months for conduct-disordered adolescents with significant substance use problems and disrupted school and family life. These are two examples of therapeutic interventions that occasionally can bring about dramatic change, but compliance tends to be an issue.

9   Consider possible medications. This is relevant in cases of severe dependence and those involving coexisting disorders. There are no randomised controlled trials for use of medications in adolescents with substance-use disorders, although experience indicates positive outcomes in many cases. A responsible adult, acceptable to the adolescent, needs to hold and administer medications. Medications include naltrexone, acamprosate, clonidine, SSRI antidepressants, mood stabilisers such as lithium and sodium valproate, antipsychotics such as thioridazine, risperidone and olanzepine, psychostimulants such as methylphenidate and dexamphetamine, opioid substitution agents such as methadone and buprenorphine, nicotine substitution products, and bupropion.

10 View treatment as a process rather than a discrete event. In addition, ensure continuity of care and follow-up.

There is a range of services that ideally would be available to adolescents with substance-use problems in any Australasian community. These begin with a broad base of outpatient services supporting an increasingly specialised set of day and inpatient programs. In real life, many communities do not have easy access to a set of services such as these, so clinicians commonly are forced to try to cobble together a management plan for adolescents in their community that utilises those services that do exist and that are frequently overloaded. Outpatient services generally involve adolescents in individual and family work, and sometimes group therapy is available, for instance on a weekly basis. Day-patient and inpatient/residential programs tend to focus on abstaining and are usually group based.

Case studies

Below are four cases of adolescents aged 17, 14, 13, and 16 years respectively. To highlight the breadth of case-mix possible, each of these adolescents has a cannabis problem, but in combination with a variety of coexisting disorders and problems. They have been chosen to illustrate issues related to each of the four categories of adolescents described above, a range of scenarios commonly encountered by clinicians, and the range of developmental issues and problems that arise across the adolescent period. Diagnosis and appropriate intervention is briefly outlined for each adolescent in the event of an ideal set of services being available.

Case study 1: normal

Brett is a 17-year-old apprentice mechanic who lives at home with his two working parents. He and his family are long-term patients. Brett presents requesting information and possible assistance regarding cannabis use. He indicates that he was a passenger in his best friend's car when it was pulled up twice on the same night by police. The smell of cannabis led to the police finding a small supply of cannabis in the glove box, which led to subsequent charges for him and his friend. He realises 'I was stupid' and wants to get help to 'make sure my cannabis use doesn't get out of hand'.

Assessment indicates that he has used cannabis several times at parties last year before he finally left school, but since commencing work he has been using cannabis recreationally most Friday and Saturday nights, and occasionally at work. Although presenting features indicate current cannabis abuse, there are no other drug diagnoses or psychiatric or conduct disorder. There is no background history of behavioural problems or mood difficulties. He is close to both parents, who he says are 'devastated by this court thing'. Assessment also indicates a high level of functioning, consistent with past presentations.

No medications are indicated, and his parents are not involved in the assessment or treatment. You provide brief intervention at the clinic at this presentation in one session. A subsequent follow-up appointment is organised for six weeks' time. Brett presents punctually for this appointment. He reports that he no longer smokes at or before work, and only indulges in mild recreational use on Friday and Saturday nights and on some weekends no use occurs. You provide a booster brief intervention session.

Case study 2: precocious

Sonia is a 14-year-old girl who lives, currently somewhat tenuously, with her middle-class parents. Her mother is a solicitor and her father is an architect. She has been encouraged to attend the clinic (a specialist alcohol and drug outpatient service) by her school counsellor. Her parents have been supportive of this. Referral information from the school indicates that she has been a major worry to her parents since physically maturing at age 11 and beginning to rebel.

You recognise that a major issue during assessment is to ensure Sonia's engagement by allowing her freedom to discuss and talk about issues that she feels are relevant. Sonia tells you that she has an 18-year-old boyfriend with whom she is sexually active. She says that she has been having major arguments about anything and everything with her parents for the past year. She also admits truanting from school on a regular basis, and climbing out of the bedroom window at night to hang out and party with her new-found friends. Enquiry indicates they are all 18 or 19, have left school, are unemployed, and enjoy drinking and drugging most days of the week. Her boyfriend has a car and is 'cool'. Sonia smokes approximately 10 cigarettes a day and has used cannabis most days of the week for the past six months. She binges on alcohol one or two days a week.

Your assessment indicates cannabis dependence, alcohol abuse, nicotine dependence, and oppositional defiant disorder (ODD), but no mood or conduct disorder. Other issues identified include unprotected sexual activity, risk of motor vehicle accident, school deterioration, and rebellion against her perceived high middle-class expectations of parents.

A subsequent appointment is arranged for a separate interview with Sonia's parents, and a separate appointment made for Sonia where you provide the opportunity to involve her boyfriend. Information on the course of intervention and issues is provided to the school counsellor.

During subsequent sessions, Sonia is provided with information about substance use disorders. Issues of safe sex and contraceptive advice are also provided, and you use this as an opportunity to discuss the link between precociousness and ODD. In all sessions you emphasise Sonia's underlying strengths and potential, and encourage her to set her own goals. Bupropion and nicotine replacement are discussed and offered for nicotine dependence.

At the meeting with Sonia's parents you stress the importance of maintaining ongoing communication links with her. Following this a session with Sonia and her parents together is organised. During this session you raise to all the importance of maintaining ongoing communication links, and having already discussed the possibility with her parents, raise the possibility of her staying at a relative's or friend's for a short time, or even long-term, with an emphasis on maintaining schooling.

Overall the intervention with Sonia and her parents took several sessions over a number of months.

Case study 3: antisocial

Zane is a 13-year-old who lives with his single mother and two much younger half-siblings. The family identifies as Māori. Zane's father was killed in an alcohol-related car accident five years ago. Since then his mother has had a number of boyfriends, none of which he has ever got on with. He has particular difficulty with Tony, who is the father of his younger brother and sister, and with whom he has physical altercations when Tony visits.

His presentation to the specialist alcohol and drug service in which you work is precipitated by legal charges. He has to appear in the Youth Court following an incident that he cannot remember, in which he and his mates 'were found inside a local church grossly intoxicated and having caused considerable damage'. His mother is present at the assessment and states that Zane did not adjust well to school following the death of his father. As a result of this he has a poor scholastic record and has often been in trouble for classroom disruption, disobedience, and fighting.

Alcohol and drug assessment indicates that Zane started smoking cigarettes at age eight, and he then had a period of solvent use for a year before he first tried cannabis at 10. This is also when he first got intoxicated with alcohol, supplied by his best friend's older brother. He has recently been expelled from school for a variety of misdemeanours, including using cannabis, but primarily for assaulting other pupils and being insolent and intimidating to teachers. His mother sticks up for him and describes him as 'lovable, but totally unmanageable'.

Assessment indicates conduct disorder (primary diagnosis), but no formal mood disorder, although there may be a chronic grief for his lost father. Alcohol and drug history indicates a past history of solvent abuse, current cannabis and nicotine dependence, and alcohol abuse. Assessment also indicates a high risk of devolving antisocial personality disorder, with possible attention deficit/hyperactivity disorder. Consideration is therefore given to the prescription of methylphenidate. Significant life problems include school failure, inadequate mothering, and antisocial peer group. You believe that the possibility of a specific learning disorder, which may be contributing to a lack of scholastic achievement, needs to be investigated.

You feel that the presence of school breakdown and a home life with a severe complex set of disorders/problems makes the option of attendance at a therapeutic community program ideal. The therapeutic community you consider is one specifically for young people and involves specialist schooling and a multimodel therapeutic program, including therapeutic work on past life events, where issues to do with Zane's loss of his father, living with his mother and her current partner, and cultural issues could be explored.

You present this option to Zane, explaining that after a number of months at the therapeutic community Zane could then be followed up through the outpatient alcohol and drug service, where new skills learned at the community could be reinforced and assistance provided for him to adjust back into real life. Unfortunately, Zane insists he is not keen to enter the therapeutic community.

As an alternative you therefore manage Zane on an outpatient basis at the alcohol and drug service. Sessions involve motivational and educational work related to substance use, and are directed at facilitating Zane to set his own goals. You also arrange for your service to assign a clinical case worker to Zane to coordinate between health, justice, social welfare, and educational service. A separate meeting is arranged where you introduce the case worker and encourage them to form an initial bond.

As part of the management strategy and having engaged Zane in treatments, you prepare a written alcohol drug and cultural assessment for Zane's court appearance. As a result of Zane's involvement in treatment, and your report, he received probation following the Youth Court appearance.

Further assessment indicated no specific learning difficulties or attention deficit/hyperactivity disorder, and so methylphenidate is not prescribed. Endeavours are made to re-establish Zane's schooling. As an initiation to this, Zane is encouraged to attend a specialist day-patient program, with a particular focus on education.

Separate appointments are made for Zane's mother where the importance of Zane having a positive substitute father figure is reinforced. Emphasis is also put into assisting Zane's mother to develop parenting skills where boundaries can be defined and positive behaviours reinforced, and she is encouraged to be actively involved and to attend a parent support group. Issues of cultural connection for Zane's mother are also explored.

Following several sessions (over several months) stability was established in Zane's life.

Case study 4: multiple problem

Maria is a 16-year-old woman who presents to the specialist alcohol and drug treatment service where you work. She indicates that her drug use is 'out of control' and that she has recently begun street prostitution to support her habit. She has never met her father, who was an unknown client of her mother, a former prostitute who is currently in prison for fraud.

Assessment indicates that Maria was sexually abused first by her grandfather and subsequently by several of her mother's boyfriends. She has had a lifelong turbulent relationship with her mother, having suffered multiple beatings from her earlier in her life, until taken into social welfare care at age nine. She has lived in numerous foster homes since this time and began to use alcohol and drugs, with increased frequency, particularly from age 13. She had her first 'taste' of morphine a year ago, and over the past six months has developed a 'habit', now needing to use about 60 mg of morphine sulfate intravenously a day. In addition, she 'mellows out' on cannabis most days, although she tends to take a handful of 'jacks' (benzodiazepines) before beginning work at night. She has been seen at the emergency department of the local hospital three times over the past 12 months; twice for drug overdose and once following the self-infliction of a series of cuts on her forearm.

Your diagnosis is opiate dependence, cannabis dependence, alcohol abuse, nicotine dependence, benzodiazepine abuse, major depression, post traumatic stress disorder (PTSD), and underlying conduct disorder with emerging antisocial/borderline personality disorder. You also recognise that Maria has multiple life problems, including dislocation from mainstream life, living rough, unsafe/unprotected sex, unsafe injecting practices, past physical, emotional, and sexual abuse, criminal household upbringing continuing into criminal lifestyle, and depression with a significant risk of suicide or accidental death.

Your first concern is to give urgent attention to Maria's safety and stabilisation. You immediately arrange for the establishment of a clinical case manager who is a woman, and arrange for opioid substitution treatment (methadone). You prescribe antidepressant and mood stabilising medication, and educate Maria on safe sexual and injecting practices and on reducing her risk of drug overdose.

During the session with Maria you introduce her to her case worker. The case worker identifies a number of issues and indicates she will help arrange social welfare payments. Because there are few (if any) residential rehabilitation options for adolescents undertaking opioid substitution treatments in Australia and New Zealand, the case worker also indicates that she will help arrange suitable interim accommodation.

You and the case worker both recognise that Maria has a complex set of current and past issues, and recognise that many crises will occur over the forthcoming months, perhaps years, until stabilisation is achieved. You recognise the need to identify new positive adult figures, and in time to begin discussions about an alternative occupation and possibly resuming schooling/ education. You also recognise that over the forthcoming years, the intervention will likely involve a number of services and workers, including opiate substitution, detoxification admissions, brief crisis mental health admissions, and periods of residential inpatient rehabilitation. Intervention is likely to be episodic and it could be more than 20 years before complete stabilisation and integration back into the mainstream community occurs.

288

REFERENCES AND FURTHER READING

Fergusson, D.M. & Horwood, L.J. 1997, 'Early onset cannabis use and psychosocial adjustment in young adults', *Addiction*, vol. 92, pp. 279–96.

Fergusson, D.M., Horwood, J. & Lynskey, M.T. 1994, 'The comorbidities of adolescent problem behaviors: A latent class model', *Journal of Abnormal Child Psychology*, vol. 22, pp. 339–54.

Howard, J. 1997, 'Psychoactive substance use and adolescence (Part 1): Treatment', *Journal of Substance Misuse*, vol. 2, pp. 77–84.

Resnick, M.D., Bearman, P.S., Blum, W., Bauman, K.E., Harris, K.M., Jones, J., Tabor, J., Beuhring, T., Sieving, R.E., Shew, M., Ireland, M., Bearinger, L.H. & Udry, R. 1997, 'Protecting adolescents from harm: Findings from the National Longitudinal Study on Adolescent Health', *Journal of the American Medical Association*, vol. 278, pp. 823–32.

Spooner, C. 1999, 'Causes and correlates of adolescent drug abuse and implications for treatment', *Drug and Alcohol Review*, vol. 18, pp. 453–75.

16

Women and Substance Abuse

Glenys Dore

EPIDEMIOLOGY

The 1997 National Survey of Mental Health and Wellbeing (NSMH) of Adults in Australia (Andrews et al. 1999) provided information on the prevalence of a range of major mental disorders for adult Australians. This involved a household survey of 10 641 Australian adults aged 18 years and over. The survey asked questions about the use of alcohol and other drugs, including cannabis, stimulants, sedatives and opioids. The Riverland study in South Australia in 1991 (Clayer et al. 1995), and the 1986 Christchurch Psychiatric Epidemiology Study (Wells et al. 1989) have also provided important information about the epidemiology of substance use disorders in Australia and New Zealand.

The NSMH survey found that alcohol is commonly used by all Australian adults, but more commonly by men: 84% of males and 64% of females had consumed at least 12 drinks in the previous 12 months. In terms of other drug use, 85% of males and 65% of females reported using at least one substance in the past year. Cannabis was the most commonly used drug, with 10.2% of males and 4.3% of females reporting they had used it at least five times in the previous 12 months. With the exception of sedatives, other drugs were used more often by males than females:

stimulants (1.3% of males and 0.6% of females); sedatives (1.9% of males and 2.3% of females); opioids (1.3% of males and 1% of females). More males than females reported injecting drugs in the past 12 months (0.7% of males and 0.3% of females).

Substance use disorders

While men and women had similar overall prevalence rates of mental disorder, there were differences in the type of mental disorder experienced. Women were more likely than men to have anxiety disorders (12% of women and 7.1% of men) and affective disorders (7.4% of women and 4.2% of men). However, men were more than twice as likely than women to experience substance-use disorders: 9.5% of males and 3.6% of females met criteria for an alcohol-use disorder (which includes harmful use or dependence), while 3.2% of males and 1.3% of females had another drug-use disorder. Cannabis was the most commonly used illicit drug, with 1.7% of the sample meeting criteria for a cannabis-use disorder. In total, 11.1% of males and 4.5% of females met the criteria for harmful use or dependence on any substance, including alcohol. Substance-use disorders were more common in the younger age group. People aged 18 to 34 were 6.4 times more likely to have an alcohol-use disorder and 50 times more likely to have a drug-use disorder than people aged 55 or older.

Alcohol-use disorders

The Riverland study found the overall lifetime prevalence of alcohol-use disorders was 18%. As for other major epidemiological studies, men had a much higher rate than women (33% of men and 5% of women). The rate was highest in people aged 18 to 24 for both sexes, with a decline in lifetime rates with increasing age. The Christchurch study found a similar overall rate of alcohol-use disorders, of 19% of the sample. Similarly, in the Christchurch study, men had much higher rates of life-time alcohol-use disorders than women (32% of men and 6% of women).

Drug-use disorders

The Riverland study found an overall lifetime prevalence of drug-use disorders of 3%. As for alcohol, the rates were very different for men and women (6% of men and 1% of women). Rates for both groups were highest in the 25 to 34 year age group. For the Christchurch study, the overall rate of drug use disorders was 6%, with men having a higher rate than women (7% of men and 4% of women).

Tobacco

Smoking in Western cultures increased after World War I, and reached a peak in the mid-1960s. The pattern of women's tobacco consumption has trailed that of men by about three decades, and it was not until after World War II that large numbers of women took up smoking. In the mid–1960s, the health hazards associated with smoking became apparent. This was followed by a drop in the per capita consumption of tobacco, with a marked reduction during the early 1970s that continued into the 1980s. However, while consumption by men has dropped significantly, consumption by women has reduced at a slower rate. In some groups, particularly young women, the incidence of smoking has increased or plateaued. Despite these changes, a review by Bushnell et al. (1994) found that almost a quarter of New Zealanders (23%) were smokers. Young males aged 25 to 34 had the highest rates of smoking (35%), followed by young women aged 15 to 24 (33%). The NSMH found that 25% of the sample reported current use of tobacco, with rates being higher among males than females (27% of males and 23% of females). Smoking was more common in younger age groups: with 33% of 18–34-year-olds being smokers compared with 14% of those aged 55 or more.

A consistent finding across all studies is that:

➡ in most cultures women drink less often and less heavily than men
➡ men are four to five times more likely than women to develop alcohol abuse or dependence
➡ younger women are much more likely to be problem drinkers and drug users than older women

291

Reasons for gender differences

Possible reasons for these different rates of substance use relate to difference in exposure to alcohol and other drug use, differences in social roles, and differences in social attitudes to women and men who use alcohol and other drugs.

The difference in lifetime rates of alcohol abuse and dependence for men and women, and different rates in younger and older individuals, may be explained by the differences in exposure to heavy drinking. Younger men and women have been most exposed to the steep post-war rise in drinking, which may explain their higher rate of problems. This was an era that saw the increased consumption of alcohol in the home, especially wine, and the development of more liberal attitudes towards women drinking alcohol.

Attitudes to women drinking has been changing over time, as have women's drinking patterns. Drinking by women was previously discouraged, and was often confined to those drinks seen as suitable for women on special occasions, for example shandy and sherry. In contrast, young women today tend to see alcohol as a necessary part of many social activities. Alcohol advertising often glamorises the use of alcohol by women, associating it with pleasure, sexuality, and good times. It has also been suggested that women's entry into the workforce and male–dominated careers has coincided with greater acceptance of female drinking.

The social roles traditionally occupied by women provide less access and opportunity for drug use. Women who are at home caring for children or elderly relatives are less likely to be involved in situations where illegal drugs are available, and they generally have fewer opportunities to use drugs with others. They are more likely to have access to pharmaceutical drugs than illegal drugs.

Women are often influenced by others in terms of when and how they use illegal substances. Women start using heroin later than men, and are generally introduced to using it by men. Drug dealing is largely a male domain, and women's access to heroin is mainly through male channels.

Despite changes in attitudes to women who drink, there are very different stereotypes for male and female drinkers. Expressions of approval, such as 'to drink like a man' and 'he can really hold his piss' are familiar to all of us. Heavy drinking among men is seen as normal and desirable. Sports heroes who celebrate their victories with heavy drinking binges are admired by the public and the media. Women who drink heavily and get drunk are more likely to be condemned than praised. Phrases for drunk women include 'she's a lush', 'she's a goer', 'what a slag', 'she's a loose woman'. A drunken woman is seen as sexually promiscuous. This increased level of stigmatisation may make it more likely that women will hide their drinking. Women tend to be more solitary drinkers, drinking less in public, and tend to drink at home, alone or with a spouse.

Similarly, drug-dependent women are seen as sicker, more deviant, and more reprehensible than drug-dependent males. While their treatment outcomes are

Figure 16.1 Intoxication in non-safe environments can put women at increased risk of sexual abuse.

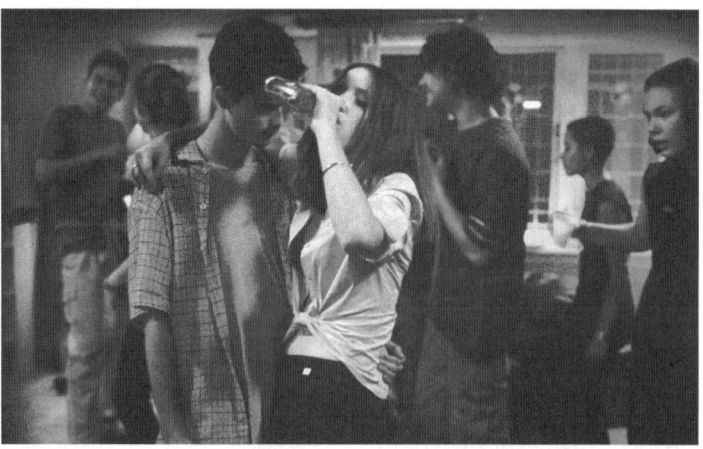

Courtesy of the National Alcohol Campaign,
Commonwealth Department of Health and Ageing

often similar, women who drink and use drugs are generally seen as more untreatable than their male counterparts.

> The taboos against women drinking and using drugs probably surround women's traditional reproductive and parenting roles, which necessitate nurturing and caring for others, particularly children.

WOMEN AND ALCOHOL

Risk factors

Alcohol and other drug-related problems do not have a single aetiology, but are caused by a complex interaction of biological, social, psychological, economic, and other factors. Some of the important factors that have been identified are outlined below.

Genetics

Alcohol abuse is a genetically influenced disorder, with the adopted-out children of alcohol-dependent parents having three to four times the risk of alcohol abuse compared to children with non-alcohol dependent parents (see chapter 2). Most of the earlier research on the genetics of alcohol abuse was carried out on males. However, more recent studies involving women support the findings of earlier studies, showing a stronger genetic contribution to the development of alcohol abuse for males compared with females.

Age

Younger women are more likely to be binge drinkers and to have drinking problems than older women.

Marital status

Women who have never married, or who are divorced or separated, are more likely to drink than married or widowed women. Being in a de facto relationship is strongly associated with problem drinking.

Women are more likely to be influenced by the drinking pattern of their partner than the other way around. A woman who has a partner who is a heavy drinker is more likely to drink heavily than a woman whose partner does not drink heavily. For those alcohol-dependent women who have a partner, their partner is more likely to be alcohol-dependent or to drink heavily, and the two of them often drink together.

Race and ethnicity

Consumption of alcohol by young Māori women is twice as high as consumption among young non-Māori women. At the same time, Māori women are 1.6 times more likely to die from an alcohol-related disease, and 1.7 times more likely to be hospitalised for an alcohol-related problem than non-Māori women. Rates of smoking for all Māori people are twice that of non-Māori (44% for Māori and 23% for non-Māori). While tobacco use among Māori men has been declining, the rates for Māori women have not been declining in parallel with the general population. Prevalent estimates of tobacco use by Māori women in 1981, 1989 and 1992 indicate relatively stable levels of between 57 and 60%. In 1990, around 60% of young Māori women aged 15 to 34 were smokers.

The patterns of alcohol use among both urban and non-urban Aboriginal Australians are similar to those in other indigenous groups, including the Māori. A review by Jenny Davis (Hamilton, Kellehear & Rumbold 1998) summarises recent information about patterns of substance use and misuse in Aboriginal Australians. The pervasive stereotype is that most Aborigines are drunks who drink more than the rest of the community, and who cannot manage their drunkenness. The literature does not support this stereotype. In fact, there is good evidence that most Aboriginal people do not drink at all, or drink in a responsible manner. For example, up to 60% of Aboriginal people have been abstinent for the past six months or more, compared with 26% of the overall population of the Northern Territory. Women are more likely to be non-drinkers than men, with 20 to 70% of women abstinent compared with 10 to 35% of men. Drinking is more prevalent in younger age groups (particularly 21 to 30-year-olds). Young Aboriginal men are more likely to drink alcohol than young Aboriginal women (59 to 83% of men and 12 to 60% of women), although it appears that drinking is becoming more common among young women. Binge drinking and harmful drinking are similarly more common in men than women (for example Kamien (1978) found 31% of men in Bourke were problem drinkers compared with 4% of women). A survey of remote and urban communities (d'Abbs et al. 1994) found 3 to 51% of Aboriginal women were drinking alcohol at harmful levels. This is of particular concern for women of childbearing age.

Employment

Surprisingly, there is no clear relationship between employment and drinking problems in women. Some studies have shown that women in the highest social class, and those in full-time employment, are more likely to describe having an alcohol problem than other women. As well as having access to disposable income that makes alcohol affordable, professional women are also exposed to work-related social situations where alcohol is served. Women in male-dominated professions are particularly vulnerable. Possible reasons for this include the influence of male peers who drink more, and the stress of working in a male-dominated environment.

Rural and urban life

The Otago Women's Health Survey (Romans-Clarkson et al. 1992) found that women living in the country are more likely to report having an alcohol problem than women living in the city. One possible explanation for the higher rates is that rural social life is often based around sports clubs where alcohol is readily available and an integral part of many social interactions.

Poly-drug use

Younger women with alcohol problems often have problems with other drugs, for example benzodiazepines, cocaine, amphetamines, heroin, or marijuana.

Psychiatric problems

Depression, anxiety disorders, sexual dysfunction, and bulimia are all more common in women with alcohol problems than in men with alcohol problems. An Australian study by Copeland and Hall (1992) looked at a group of 160 women attending specialist treatment services. They found that 77% of the group had scores on the Beck Depression Inventory consistent with extremely severe clinical depression. In addition, 50 to 67% of the women had attempted suicide at least once.

Stressful life events

Drinking behaviour can be influenced by a wide range of events, including a relationship break up, unemployment, infertility, children leaving home (empty nest syndrome), bereavement, and physical illness. Negative childhood and adolescent experiences can predispose a woman to use alcohol as a way of dealing with stress.

Women with a history of childhood or adult sexual abuse appear to be over-represented among women who seek treatment for alcohol and drug dependence. Women in community samples and in treatment are much more likely than men to report a history of sexual assault. The psychological sequelae of childhood sexual abuse have been likened to the symptoms of post-traumatic stress disorder. It has been suggested that women who have not had the chance to resolve these symptoms are more prone to relapse.

The Otago Women's Health Survey found higher rates of problem drinking in women physically assaulted as adults (19%) compared with non-assaulted women (5.7%). Similarly, more women who were sexually abused as adults were problem drinkers (23.6%) compared with women who had not been abused (7.3%).

The Copeland and Hall study (1992) found that about 50% of the women in the specialist treatment services reviewed had been sexually abused as adults and 68% had been physically abused as adults. Overall, around 86% of women in specialist treatment services had been sexually and/or physically abused at some time in their lives.

Lesbian women were significantly more likely to report childhood sexual abuse than were heterosexual or bisexual women.

Sex roles

It has been hypothesised that women were more likely to experience problems with alcohol if they were experiencing role strain or role conflict from combining increased care-giving roles (such as being a mother, or caring for a handicapped child or an elderly relative) with other domestic responsibilities as well as with part-time or full-time work. However, the research doesn't always support this. Several studies have found that problem drinking is more related to a lack of significant roles (role loss or deprivation). Combining household and parenting responsibilities with paid employment may be protective against developing alcohol-related problems.

Women and the actions of alcohol

Why do women get drunk more easily than men?

Women become intoxicated after drinking smaller amounts of alcohol than men. Women generally have smaller body weight, smaller liver size, and smaller blood volume than men, so that the concentration of alcohol in their vital organs is higher for a given dose. Their higher levels of body fat and lower body-water content result in a smaller volume of distribution for alcohol; that is they achieve higher blood alcohol concentrations than men after drinking the same amount of alcohol.

Alcohol is mainly metabolised in the liver. However, some alcohol is initially metabolised in the gastrointestinal tissue (first-pass metabolism) by the enzyme gastric alcohol dehydrogenase. Women have lower levels of alcohol dehydrogenase than men, with women having around 50% less gastric metabolism of alcohol than men. Women who are taking the oral contraceptive pill will have delayed metabolism of alcohol due to delayed gastric emptying. This means that in women generally, and women on the pill in particular, less alcohol is metabolised before being absorbed, so for this reason as well women will have higher blood alcohol levels than men who drink the same amount of alcohol.

> Even when differences in weight are taken into account, women are more likely to become drunk at a given dose of alcohol than men, because they achieve a higher blood alcohol level than men. This is particularly likely in the premenstrual phase.

Women are more vulnerable to the effects of alcohol

Women are more vulnerable than men to the adverse health effects of alcohol. Alcohol-dependent women have higher rates of death than do alcohol-dependent men.

The majority of deaths are from pancreatitis, cirrhosis, and other liver disorders, while up to a quarter of deaths may be due to violence and accidents.

Women who drink heavily are more susceptible to liver disease and brain disease than men. They develop severe liver disease with shorter histories of excessive drinking than men, and at much lower daily doses of alcohol. The higher blood alcohol level obtained in women compared with men drinking the same amount of alcohol seems to be one of the key reasons for this. Women may also be more vulnerable to infection and inflammation of the liver, because of the effects of oestrogen. The accelerated development of liver disease in alcohol-dependent women is referred to as 'telescoping'.

Recommended levels of drinking for men and women

These sex differences are reflected in different guidelines for responsible drinking for the normal population.

The upper limits for responsible drinking in New Zealand are:
- On any drinking occasion: six standard drinks for men; four standard drinks for women.
- Weekly upper limits: 21 standard drinks for men; 14 standard drinks for women.

The Australian NH&MRC Alcohol Guidelines are detailed in chapter 10. In summary, these guidelines are:
- For men: no more than four standard drinks daily, and no more than 28 standard drinks over a week.
- For women: no more than two standard drinks daily, and no more than 14 standard drinks over a week.
- At least one or two alcohol-free days each week.

These levels will be too high in high-risk situations, for example driving, flying, operating machinery, in or on the water, skiing, and mountaineering. They will also be too high for vulnerable individuals:
- pregnant women
- the very young and the old (lower tolerance to alcohol)
- people with a history of alcohol or drug dependence
- those with psychiatric illness
- those with other medical disorders (for example epilepsy, diabetes, heart disease)
- those on medications which may interact with alcohol (for example warfarin, gastric irritants, CNS depressants).

WOMEN AND OTHER DRUG USE

Illicit drugs

Drug-dependent females are more likely to be in difficult circumstances than are drug-dependent males. They are more likely to be uneducated, unemployed, and unmarried

297

with dependent children. They may have to rely on other avenues for financial support, such as welfare benefits and prostitution. They have fewer supports than male drug users. They generally have lower self-esteem, are less assertive, and have more symptoms of depression and anxiety than drug-dependent males. Female drug users have more health problems than males, and these are often gynaecologically based.

Women begin using heroin later than men, and are more likely than men to try it in the beginning to relieve personal distress. They are often introduced to the drug by men (such as a boyfriend or partner). The drug subculture is largely male-dominated, with men in prominent positions in large-scale drug dealing. Women are mainly reliant on males for their supplies of heroin.

Substance use in indigenous women

In Australia, while rates of smoking for indigenous males far exceeded those of females in the period from the 1950s to the 1970s, this trend has been changing. In the 1990s, female rates of smoking were almost equivalent to those of males. The 1989–1990 National Health Survey found that around half the adult Aboriginal population were smokers compared with less than 30% of the adult non-indigenous population. More recent surveys indicate the prevalence of smoking among Aboriginal people is declining.

Both the Māori population in New Zealand and the Aboriginal population in Australia have higher rates of mortality and morbidity from substance use than the general population. For example, Aboriginal women are eight times more likely to die of smoking-related diseases than non-Aboriginal women. The death rate for cirrhosis of the liver in Aboriginal women is eleven times greater than that of non-Aboriginal women.

PREGNANCY, BREAST-FEEDING, AND PARENTING

Fertility may be affected by substance use. For example, alcohol use and heroin use disrupt the hypothalamic–pituitary–gonadal axis. Alcohol-dependent women often experience menstrual irregularities, ovulatory failure, and early menopause. Amennorhoea can occur with chronic heroin use. Cocaine and amphetamine use may also cause amenorrhoea because of their-side effects of restricted food intake and increased physical activity. Female substance users have an increased risk of sexually transmitted diseases, which may in turn lead to infertility.

Parenting is a particular concern for drug-dependent women. Women in treatment for drug dependency are more likely than men to have children and to have responsibility for them. While they aspire to be good mothers, they generally feel guilt-ridden about their substance use and fearful about their adequacy as parents. Some will have significant difficulties parenting their children, and an assessment of these issues is an important part of any treatment plan.

Women often avoid treatment agencies because of the fear that their children will be taken from their care if they admit to using drugs. If they do make it into treatment, they find that childcare facilities are often inadequate for their needs.

Alcohol and pregnancy

The developing foetus is particularly vulnerable to the effects of alcohol.

Foetal Alcohol Syndrome (FAS) is one of the most alarming consequences of heavy drinking in pregnancy. Foetal Alcohol Effects occurs when there are some, but not all, of the symptoms required for a diagnosis of FAS. Symptoms commonly include low birth weight, behavioural difficulties and learning difficulties. Women who drink heavily throughout their pregnancy are also vulnerable to other complications, including increased risk of spontaneous abortion and stillbirth, and intrauterine growth retardation.

FAS has been estimated to occur in about one in 1000 births. It is characterised by a cluster of birth defects that include at least one feature from each of the following three categories.
- Characteristic facial malformations, including absent or indistinct philtrum (the groove below the nasal septum), flat midface including maxilla, small head (microcephaly), thin upper lip, small eyes, short upturned nose, shortened palpebral fissures, prominent epicanthic folds, ptosis, low-set ears.
- Prenatal and postnatal growth retardation: babies are typically underweight, with small body length, and they lack catch-up growth.
- Central nervous system dysfunction, including mental retardation, short attention span, hyperactivity, irritability, developmental delays, long-term learning problems, and behavioural problems.

These features may also be associated with cardiac defects, and joint and limb abnormalities.

Drinking six or more standard drinks a day throughout pregnancy may result in a child with fully developed FAS. Binge drinking, particularly in the first trimester, may be particularly harmful because of the effect of high blood alcohol levels on the foetus. An average of two or more standard drinks a day has been linked with low birth weight, behavioural and learning difficulties, and an increased risk of spontaneous abortion.

More research is needed to confirm the safety of light drinking. Currently there is no established safe lower limit for the intake of alcohol during pregnancy.

Given that research to date has been unable to identify what is clearly a safe level of drinking in pregnancy, the best advice for pregnant women and those planning a pregnancy may be to abstain from alcohol during pregnancy.

> Australian 2001 NH&MRC Alcohol Guidelines suggest that if pregnant women or women planning pregnancy choose to drink, consumption should be less than seven standard drinks per week, with no more than two standard drinks per day. Most importantly, they should never become intoxicated. It is noted that the risk is highest in the earlier stages of pregnancy.

Illicit drug use and pregnancy: general comments

Many physical, psychological, and social factors contribute to the risk of obstetrical complications with illicit drug use, including poor nutritional status, lack of prenatal care, infections, states of drug intoxication, and withdrawal.

Drug intoxication and withdrawal

When the pregnant drug user has an irregular supply of drugs, she will alternate between being intoxicated on the drugs, and experiencing withdrawal symptoms when her supply runs out. The foetus is exposed to these same peaks and troughs. For example, opiates are a CNS depressant, and foetal depression can occur if the mother is intoxicated on heroin. If the mother is experiencing withdrawal symptoms from heroin, these can give rise to uterine contractions that result in intermittent obstruction to placental perfusion. Foetal hypoxia and distress can occur, with an increased risk of intrauterine death.

In illicit drug users, an increase in tobacco and alcohol consumption can contribute independently to low birthweight.

The immature liver of the foetus is incapable of effective metabolism of the majority of drugs that cross the placenta. For example the half-life of crack cocaine is increased around six-fold once it enters the neonate.

Infections

Infections associated with injecting drug use include bacterial endocarditis, septi-caemia, cellulitis, hepatitis B, hepatitis C, HIV, and other sexually transmitted diseases.

Problems related to lifestyle

The priority in the drug-dependent mother's life is obtaining drugs and money for drugs. Criminal behaviour and prostitution are common ways of supporting her drug habit. Her nutritional state is often poor because money is spent on drugs rather than food. She may have little interest in home-making and seeking out ante-natal care. She may be fearful of eventually losing her child if she presents for care with an addiction. Her relationships may be unstable and volatile, and she may have major financial difficulties.

Opiates and pregnancy

Complications of opiate use in pregnancy

While uncontrolled use of opiates in pregnancy can result in many obstetrical complications (including abruptio placentae, spontaneous abortion and intrauterine death), the most commonly seen complications are intrauterine growth retardation (with low birthweight) and premature labour.

Methadone maintenance treatment

Methadone is the treatment of choice for women who are dependent on opiates in pregnancy. Methadone maintenance treatment can improve the health of the mother, and improve the chances of a full-term healthy baby. Methadone stops the development of withdrawal symptoms for 24 hours or more, and stops the intense cravings for other opiates. Stable drug levels in utero mean the foetus is not exposed to the extremes of drug intoxication and withdrawal. Other benefits of methadone maintenance treatment include reduced intravenous opiate use, with concomitant reduced risk of transmission of infectious diseases, reduced criminality, and improved health and lifestyle, including improved nutritional state and more engagement in antenatal care.

Women who are already on methadone maintenance treatment prior to becoming pregnant should remain on their pre-pregnancy dose. Withdrawing methadone may increase the risk of relapse into injecting drug use. Methadone withdrawal during the first trimester increases the risk of spontaneous abortion. Methadone withdrawal in the third trimester increases the risk of foetal distress and premature labour. If methadone is being withdrawn, this should be done between 14 to 32 weeks, at a rate of no more than 5 mg every two weeks. Withdrawal should be supervised by a specialist drug treatment service, in association with a perinatal unit with access to foetal monitoring equipment, so that emergency procedure can be instituted and methadone reinstated if there is evidence of foetal distress or premature labour.

Plasma levels of methadone decrease for some women in the third trimester, and they experience withdrawal symptoms. This can be managed with a higher dose or split dosing.

Methadone is only one part of the treatment process. A successful outcome involves a well-coordinated treatment plan incorporating obstetrical services, paediatric services, and methadone services. This should include a planned visit to the neonatal intensive care unit well before the delivery.

301

Neonatal abstinence syndrome

Nearly 60% of infants born to mothers on methadone will develop the clinical features of a withdrawal syndrome, called neonatal abstinence syndrome (NAS). Symptoms usually occur within 72 hours of delivery, but they can occur soon after birth, and may be delayed to two weeks of age (because of the long half-life of methadone). There are no adverse long-term sequelae if managed well.

Signs and symptoms can be remembered with the acronym WITHDRAWALS:
- Wakefulness, wide yawning
- Irritability
- Tremulousness, Temperature variability, Tachypnoea
- Hyperactivity, High-pitched cry, Hyperacusis, Hypertonus, Hiccups
- Diarrhoea and vomiting, Disorganised suck
- Respiratory distress, Rhinorrhoea, Rub marks
- Apnoeic attacks
- Weight loss/failure to gain weight
- Alkalosis—respiratory
- Lacrimation, Light sensitivity
- Seizures, Sneezing, Stuffy nose. Seizures occur in 5 to 7% of babies born to mothers on methadone.

The key principles of management involve the following:
- Monitor the baby for symptoms of NAS. This is best done by using a standardised scale, such as the Finnegan scoring system for NAS.
- Rule out other problems such as hypoglycaemia, infection, and hypocalcaemia, which can look like NAS.
- The baby should be admitted to a neonatal intensive care unit if it develops NAS.
- Mild symptoms of NAS can be managed by providing a quiet environment with not too much stimulation in it. The baby can be swaddled in a dark quiet room. These babies often suck vigorously and dummies can be helpful, as can small, frequent feeds.
- For more severe NAS, medication in the form of an opioid substitute is needed (such as neonatal opium solution). The baby can be gradually withdrawn off this medication once the NAS has resolved.
- Mother–infant bonding may be more difficult for a number of reasons. Babies with NAS are less cuddly and rewarding to be with than normal babies—they are more irritable and restless, and they feed poorly. It is important to educate the mother about this, and to help her to find positive ways of bonding with her child.

Benzodiazepines and pregnancy

Although the results of studies are contradictory, the use of benzodiazepines in the first trimester has been associated with a small increase in the rates of congenital malformations of the urinary tract as well as cleft lip, cleft palate, and neurological malformations. Regular use of benzodiazepines during pregnancy could result in the baby being physically addicted to these drugs, as benzodiazepines cross the placenta readily. This means the baby could experience withdrawal symptoms after delivery. Use of benzodiazepines immediately prior to delivery has been associated with hypotonia, hypothermia, sedation, and respiratory depression in the neonate.

Stimulants and pregnancy

Cocaine causes vasoconstriction and hypertension, which may result in acute or chronic foetal hypoxia. Cocaine use during pregnancy leads to an increased risk of miscarriage, pre-term labour, low birthweight, abruptio placentae, and stillbirth. Babies born to cocaine-using mothers may show behavioural disturbances, such as an increased startle response, and abnormal sleep patterns. It is unclear whether these effects are short-lived or more persistent. The possible teratogenic effects of cocaine are unclear. One study found a statistically significant increase in urogenital malformations in children of cocaine users.

Given their similar pharmacological properties, it seems likely that cocaine and amphetamines would have similar effects in pregnancy. These few studies on amphetamine use in pregnancy found increased rates of congenital malformation, foetal neurological abnormalities, low birthweight babies, and perinatal mortality.

Nicotine and pregnancy

Nicotine and many other substances in tobacco cross the placenta and are also found in breast milk. Smoking leads to a reduction in placental blood flow with reduced oxygenation. Decreased foetal birthweight is directly related to the number of cigarettes smoked per day. Smoking also inhibits foetal breathing, which may relate to the recorded increased incidence of stillbirths, perinatal death, and increased risk of sudden infant death syndrome. Women should be advised to stop smoking before becoming pregnant. For pregnant smokers, stopping at any stage of the pregnancy is beneficial to the foetus. While nicotine patches and gum are generally not recommended in pregnancy, they may be a safer option than smoking cigarettes, as the amount of nicotine absorbed from patches and gum is much less, and the other toxic substances in cigarettes are absent.

Cannabis and pregnancy

One comprehensive study found increased tremors and exaggerated startle reflex in the children of cannabis users, as well as developmental delay in the neonate's visual system. These effects appeared to be transient. A link has been found between cannabis use in pregnancy and acute non-lymphoblastic leukaemia in childhood.

The impact of cannabis on foetal growth and development is unclear. Some authors claim that cannabis causes similar effects to tobacco (such as foetal growth

303

retardation with low birthweight) by reducing oxygenation to the foetus. However, a recent meta-analysis found that, once the confounding variable of tobacco smoking was removed, there was no clear evidence that cannabis at the amount typically consumed by pregnant women causes low birthweight.

Breast-feeding

Australian 2001 NH&MRC Alcohol Guidelines state that women should not drink alcohol prior to breast-feeding as alcohol in the blood passes into breast milk. Even relatively low level-drinking may reduce the amount of milk and cause irritability, poor feeding, and sleep disturbances in the infant.

Contraindications to breast-feeding include ongoing use of illicit drugs, as well as risk of infection. Maternal HIV infection is a contraindication to breast-feeding. Hepatitis C is rarely transmitted by breast-feeding (5% or less), but the mother needs to be informed of the possible risk. Methadone is found in significant amounts in breast milk, and breast-feeding may prevent withdrawal symptoms if the mother is on methadone treatment. Breast-feeding beyond six months is probably not advisable in this situation, because of the increasing amounts of milk the larger child ingests. A mother on high doses of methadone should wean her baby slowly to avoid the baby developing withdrawal symptoms if breast-feeding is stopped suddenly.

TREATMENT ISSUES

Alcohol and other drug services for women

Treatment models for alcohol and drug problems have been largely developed for men, and by men. It has been argued that, because of this male bias, services have often failed to meet the specific needs of women. Effective treatment programs need to be comprehensive and flexible in order to address the diversity of needs for both male and female clients. They also need to be culturally, racially, and ethnically sensitive. Some of the important treatment issues for women are outlined below.

Need for adequate childcare facilities

It is difficult for women to attend treatment services if they don't have accessible, affordable childcare. Many women will not consider using inpatient services that don't allow their children to live in with them. Drug-dependent women often have major concerns about parenting, and these are rarely addressed in traditional mixed-sex treatment settings. Guilt, shame, and feelings of inadequacy about being a parent are significant issues that need to be addressed.

Inappropriate focus on male-orientated interventions

Many treatment programs are designed for males. Men are socialised to be more competitive, independent, and confrontational than women. Substance-dependent women, even more so than men, have very vulnerable self-esteem. They need interventions that help to build self-confidence rather than remind them of their failures.

Women in mixed-sex residential programs often do not feel physically or emotionally safe. Mixed-sex groups are often dominated by the males in the group. Women may find it difficult to be assertive in a male-dominated environment, and they may not wish to discuss anything personal. Many women with substance-use problems have been sexually and physically abused by males, and so feel frightened in a male-dominated environment. Some women have been further abused in such environments. In addition, women rarely discuss issues of abuse in male-dominated groups, and many women will be reluctant to discuss such issues with a male therapist. Some studies have found that women in mixed-sex services had higher rates of relapse after treatment if the primary therapist was male, than if they were in a mixed-sex service with a female primary therapist. Women who have been sexually abused need to have the option of an environment that is women-only, and have access to specialised sexual abuse counselling from female therapists.

305

Treatment of coexisting psychiatric disorders

While substance-use disorders are more common in men, women have higher rates of psychiatric disorders, particularly anxiety and depression. Failure to detect and treat these disorders will result in much less effective treatment outcomes. Some treatment programs have unrealistic expectations that women will be completely drug-free, and this expectation includes coming off any essential psychiatric medications. Treatment programs need to be more flexible in allowing women to continue with such medication while they learn the skills to manage their addiction and other problem areas in their lives.

Developmental delay

It appears that many women use substances to try to medicate and reduce emotional pain. Women who begin abusing substances early in life will have difficulty completing many of the developmental tasks of adolescence. Treatment programs need to address these gaps by providing access to educational services, pre-vocational training, social skills training, self-esteem building, courses on sexuality, and emotional regulation.

Other issues of dependency in women

As well as being dependent on chemicals, women may experience low self-esteem through being economically and financially dependent on others. These areas need to be addressed in treatment programs. Many women do not have access to social supports and have little financial support to allow them to escape abusive situations. They may use drugs as a way to escape the reality of their situation. For some women, basic survival needs (food, clothing, and shelter) must be attended to before effective treatment can begin.

Lesbian women

While there are few studies of substance use among homosexual women, lesbian women are often reported to have higher rates of substance-related problems than heterosexual women. Lesbian women addicted to drugs or alcohol face the triple stigma of being women, being addicted, and being homosexual. Many lesbian women have children, and may be declared unfit mothers. Lesbian women may be reluctant to enter mixed-sex treatment services because of their concern about male sexual harassment, homophobia, and the lack of understanding of their specific treatment needs. Addiction services with trained staff and lesbian-sensitive interventions attract greater numbers of lesbian women.

Gender and cultural issues

Women from different cultural groups need access to services that are well coordinated and appropriate to their needs. More research is needed to identify programs that are successful and involve indigenous people and women from other minorities in program planning and evaluation.

The need for broader outcome criteria

Often the criteria used to define a successful treatment outcome are too narrow for most clients, especially for women. If negative urine drug screens and attendance at appointments are seen as the criteria for successful treatment, many other positive aspects of women's progress in treatment will be ignored. Attending appointments may be difficult for women because of lack of money for transport, homelessness, lack of childcare, hunger, and personal hygiene issues (for example no access to hot running water for showers). A wide range of criteria need to be looked at as a measure of change, including improvements in parenting skills, social skills, financial management, self-esteem, better control of anxiety and depression, practising harm reduction techniques, improved physical health, reduced substance use and criminality, and resolution of homelessness.

How to work with the female substance user

Empathy is essential

Try to understand the patient rather than condemn her, even if her reactions seem irrational to you.

Think of all the possible reasons why she might be in this position.

Spend time with her, and explore the reasons for her behaviour.

Help her to consider the consequences of her actions, and to find alternative ways of dealing with her situation.

Remember that the patient may have the developmental level of someone much younger than her chronological age. This is because most substance users start using drugs in their teenage years, making it difficult to successfully negotiate the usual developmental tasks of adolescence.

Have a realistic perspective on alcohol and drug problems. Remember that these are long-term relapsing disorders, and change takes time.

Watch and manage your own reactions

Accept that it's common to have negative reactions to women who use substances. Fear and anxiety are common (for example you may feel manipulated and fearful of an angry response if you confront the patient about her behaviour; you may be anxious about how to deal with her, particularly if you have little experience in this area). You may feel angry, disgusted, and frustrated because of her lack of commitment to a substance-free lifestyle, particularly if she has children or is pregnant. You may feel guilty because you have little empathy for her, and you see yourself as normally very caring and helpful. You may feel the situation is hopeless, particularly if you have little training in this area, or if you have had a negative personal experience with addiction.

Don't act on your feelings. Share them with a colleague rather than let them affect your work with the patient.

Watch out for over-involvement or withdrawal. Some health professionals deal with their negative reactions to a patient by pulling away and doing as little as possible. Others become over-involved, doing more and more in the belief that they can somehow fix the problem.

If you feel you can't work with the patient in a professional, non-judgmental way, tell your colleague or senior and arrange for someone else to take over your role. In a sole practice this may mean referral to another, more suited practitioner.

➡ While men are four to five times more likely than women to develop alcohol-use disorders, women drinkers are more vulnerable to the health effects of alcohol.

➡ Women are more likely to be stigmatised for drug and alcohol use than are men, presumably because of preconceptions about their traditional reproductive and nurturing/care-taking responsibilities.

➡ Women with substance-use problems, particularly those who have been sexually abused, may find it difficult to seek treatment in a male-dominated environment. While treatment resources available are limited, the ideal is for women to have the option of female therapists and female-only treatment environments.

➡ Parenting is a particular concern for female substance users. They often avoid treatment agencies because of fear that their children will be taken from their care. If they do enter treatment services, childcare facilities are often inadequate for their needs.

➡ Women who are pregnant or planning to get pregnant need to be given clear advice about the likely effects of alcohol, nicotine, and other substances on the foetus.

➡ When treating women with drug and alcohol problems, it is important to watch and manage your own reactions. Try to understand the patient rather than becoming over-involved or over-critical.

Case study

Katrina is now a 30-year-old woman. She was sexually abused by her father in childhood, and began using alcohol and drugs in adolescence to try to ease her emotional pain. She was introduced to heroin by a boyfriend when she was 16, and she was addicted to it by 17. She would also binge drink whenever she felt stressed. She went onto a methadone program in her 20s, but kept using heroin and alcohol as well, because she felt depressed and anxious, and she was homeless. She had a child who was taken from her care because of her drug use. Her use of heroin and alcohol gradually ceased once she had permanent housing and treatment with antidepressants and supportive counselling for her psychiatric problems. She was able to arrange regular contact with her child once she was stable on the methadone program.

Case points

Katrina's case illustrates many typical features of substance-use problems in women:

- sexual assault as a predisposing factor
- introduction to illegal substances by a male partner
- a high rate of anxiety and depression, and use of substances to medicate her symptoms
- childcare as a critical issue
- the treatment options available need to comprehensively address women's need.

REFERENCES AND FURTHER READING

Andrews, G., Hall, W., Teesson, M. & Henderson, S. 1999, *The Mental Health of Australians*, Mental Health Branch, Commonwealth Department of Health and Aged Care, Canberra.

Brady, K.T. & Randall, C. 1999, 'Gender differences in substance use disorders', *Psychiatric Clinics of North America*, vol. 22, pp. 241–52.

Bushnell, J., Carter, H. & Howden-Chapman, P. 1994, 'A review of the epidemiology of substance use disorders in New Zealand', Paper prepared for the Ministry of Health, November 1994.

Clayer, J.R., McFarlane, A.C., Bookless, C.L., Air, T., Wright, G. & Czechowicz, A.S. 1995, 'Prevalence of psychiatric disorders in rural South Australia', *Medical Journal of Australia*, vol. 163, pp. 124–5, 128–9.

Copeland, J. & Hall, W.A. 1992, 'Comparison of women seeking drug and alcohol treatment in a specialist women's and two traditional mixed-sex treatment services', *British Journal of Addiction*, vol. 87, pp. 1293–302.

D'Abbs, P., Hunter, E., Reser, J. & Martin, M. *Alcohol-related Violence in Aboriginal and Torres Strait Islander Communities: A Literature Review*, AGPS, Canberra.

Dore, G.M. 1998, 'Women and substance abuse', in Romans, S.E. (ed.), *Folding Back the Shadows*, University of Otago Press, Dunedin.

Hamilton, M., Kellehear, A. & Rumbold, G. 1998, *Drug Use in Australia: A Harm Minimisation Approach*, Oxford University Press, Melbourne.

Kamien, M. 1978, *The Dark People of Bourke: A Study of Planned Social Change*, Australian Institute of Aboriginal Studies, Canberra.

Romans-Clarkson, S.E., Walton, V.A., Herbison, P. & Mullen, P.E. 1992, 'Alcohol-related problems in New Zealand women', *Australian and New Zealand Journal of Psychiatry*, vol. 26, pp. 175–82.

Thomas, D. 1995, 'Substance abuse in pregnancy', *Modern Medicine of Australia*, October, pp. 118–27.

Wells, J.E., Bushnell, J.A., Hornblow, A.R., Joyce, P.R. & Oakley-Browne, M.A. 1989, 'Christchurch Psychiatric Epidemiology Study, Part I: Methodology and lifetime prevalence for specific psychiatric disorders', *Australian and New Zealand Journal of Psychiatry*, vol. 23, pp. 315–26.

17

An Approach to Substance Misuse Problems among Indigenous Australians

Denis Gray, Sherry Saggers, Gary Hulse & David Atkinson

Indigenous affairs are a source of contention, and when discussion also involves alcohol and other drugs feelings run particularly high—especially as the stereotype of 'the drunken Aborigine' is widely held by non-indigenous Australians.

In this chapter, we aim to assist the clinician with limited familiarity with indigenous affairs to confront this stereotype. To that end, we provide a basic epidemiology of alcohol and other drug use among indigenous Australians, put such use in its social context, and discuss some strategies that can enable doctors to assist indigenous people to address problems of substance misuse.

SUBSTANCE MISUSE AND ITS CONSEQUENCES AMONG INDIGENOUS AUSTRALIANS

Accurately determining levels of substance use and its consequences is difficult for any population. It is even more so for indigenous populations due to problems in clearly identifying indigenous people in various data collections, the small size of the populations being studied, and the extent of variation between different indigenous populations. Thus the figures presented below, while providing a reasonable general description, need to be treated with some caution.

Alcohol

Although there is considerable regional variation, the percentages of indigenous and non-indigenous Australians who have never drunk alcohol (15% and 13%), or who drink occasionally (29% and 27%), are about the same. However, among indigenous people, the percentage that no longer drinks is higher (22% versus 9%), and the percentage that drinks regularly is less (33% versus 45%). Nevertheless, among regular drinkers, 68% of indigenous people, compared with 11% of non-indigenous people, consume alcohol at hazardous levels.

> Those who consume alcohol in a hazardous—though not necessarily a socially disruptive—manner are a minority (22%) of the indigenous population.

As a consequence of the relatively higher frequency of hazardous consumption, alcohol contributes to a greater proportion of Indigenous than non-indigenous health problems. Thus approximately 10% of deaths and 4.5% of hospital bed-days for indigenous people are recorded as being due to alcohol, compared with 3% of deaths and 3% of hospital bed-days for non-indigenous people. These are most commonly injury-related problems but also include specific alcohol-related conditions such as cirrhosis and alcohol toxicity and dependence. Unfortunately this is only part of the picture of alcohol-related illness and death. Alcohol is also a direct or indirect contributor to many other health problems; for example by increasing susceptibility to infections, contributing to delays in accessing appropriate care, and also contributing to many problems that do not result in hospitalisation.

Tobacco

Levels of tobacco use are approximately twice as high among indigenous people than among non-indigenous people (56% and 46% of indigenous men and women compared to 27% and 20% of non-indigenous men and women). As among non-indigenous people, at least 20% of both indigenous men and women are ex-smokers. While smoking accounts for about 13% of all deaths among indigenous people and 15% among non-indigenous people because of differences in population structure, age-standardised tobacco-caused mortality rates among both indigenous men and women are over twice those among non-indigenous people. Among indigenous Australians the most common tobacco-caused deaths are ischaemic heart disease, lung cancer, and chronic bronchitis, and the most common causes of hospitalisation due to tobacco smoking are chronic bronchitis, pneumonia, and ischaemic heart disease.

> While tobacco smoking is the single most preventable cause of death among indigenous Australians, indigenous people themselves often consider it less of a problem than other drug misuse because, unlike alcohol, it is not associated with social disruption.

Illicit drugs

Among those aged 15 years or older, about 50% of indigenous Australians, and 40% of non-indigenous Australians, report ever having used cannabis, although data on comparative frequency of use are not available. The percentages of indigenous people who have used other substances such as amphetamines (6%) and heroin (3%) are similar to those in the non-indigenous population. However, there is evidence that use of illicit drugs is spreading both within and beyond major urban areas.

Illicit drugs account for a little less than 1% of deaths in both the indigenous and non-indigenous populations. However, among indigenous people, there has been an increase in first-time hospital admissions for problems such as cannabis misuse, amphetamine misuse, and drug psychosis. As many illicit drugs are injected, there is considerable concern about the potential for spread of blood-borne viruses, such as hepatitis C, as a result of sharing injecting equipment, particularly among people in urban populations and those in prisons.

Volatile substances

In some, though by no means all, small communities in central and northern Australia, inhalation of petrol fumes is a serious problem. 'Petrol sniffing' has an analogue in the sniffing of other volatile substances by young people in urban areas, although in urban areas sniffing is often part of experimentation with a range of other widely available substances. Prior to the introduction of unleaded petrol and aviation fuel in remote communities, lead poisoning was a major health problem among petrol sniffers. While this has been alleviated, petrol sniffing and the inhalation of other solvents remains a significant cause of a variety of psychosocial problems.

THE SOCIAL CONTEXT

The colonial legacy

Within 150 years of British settlement, indigenous Australians had largely been dispossessed of their traditional lands, and the original population of about 750 000 had been reduced by at least 75% as a result of violence, introduced disease, and diseases related to the poverty that was the consequence of colonialism. Few indigenous people were included in the new economy, and those who did find employment were paid either in kind or at extremely low wages. Those excluded were institutionalised in missions or government settlements for their so-called 'protection'. In addition, as a result of government policy that sought to assimilate indigenous people, many children were forcibly taken from their families and institutionalised or fostered out to non-indigenous families, with emotional trauma for the children themselves and for their families.

Today, as a consequence of this continuing legacy, indigenous Australians have the lowest levels of employment, income, and education, and the poorest housing, of any group in the country. Since the 1970s, various government programs have been implemented to ameliorate these conditions. However, none of these programs have been of sufficient magnitude to transform the economic status of indigenous people, and many have simply been substitutes for the services provided to other Australians. Nevertheless, indigenous cultures—based on strong attachment to land and reciprocal kinship obligations within a strongly spiritual framework—though transformed, have remained resilient. It is participation in these cultures and acceptance by other members of their communities that is of central importance to the self-definition of indigenous people.

The prohibition of alcohol

Prior to British settlement, substance use among indigenous Australians was largely confined to native tobaccos. However, British settlers provided alcohol to indigenous people for sexual favours, labour, and their own (that is, the colonists') amusement. In the early nineteenth century, concern about public order led colonial governments to enact laws prohibiting the consumption of alcohol by, and the supply of alcohol to, indigenous Australians. Nevertheless, even under prohibition, alcohol was supplied to some indigenous people by private citizens, and governments granted exemptions that allowed some employers to pay indigenous employees in alcohol and permitted those few indigenous people who were granted citizenship to drink.

Prohibitions on indigenous drinking were repealed between the mid-1950s and the late 1960s. During this period, citizenship was also extended to indigenous Australians. The coincidence of these events led at least some indigenous people to regard drinking as an expression of equality with non-indigenous Australians. Though this was not the major factor, it was one of several that led to a dramatic increase in alcohol consumption and related problems among indigenous Australians.

Reasons for indigenous substance misuse

Indigenous people use and misuse psychoactive substances for many of the same reasons as non-indigenous people, including enjoyment, as a response to social and emotional problems, through an inability to control their levels of consumption, and in response to the availability and promotion of such substances. There is no evidence that indigenous people are genetically susceptible to higher rates of misuse. There is evidence that, among some, sharing psychoactive substances is a positively valued activity that helps to cement important social relationships.

Additionally, higher levels of substance misuse among indigenous Australians may be attributed to a response to a variety of social stresses that particularly affect indigenous people, among them dispossession from country and culture, discrimination, impoverishment, under-employment and lack of alternative valued activities, unresolved levels of grief associated with high death rates, and, among the stolen generations, the traumas of separation from family.

Indigenous action

Nationally there are more than two hundred substance-misuse intervention programs developed and run by indigenous community organisations. These programs include night patrols, sobering-up centres, residential and non-residential treatment, after-care, and health promotion and prevention. In addition, many communities are restricting the availability of alcohol, either by declaring their communities alcohol-free, or by applying to liquor licensing authorities to tighten regulations on the sale of alcohol.

> ➡ indigenous people have acknowledged the problems of substance misuse within their communities, and it is they who have taken the greatest initiative in dealing with it.

INTERACTING WITH INDIGENOUS PEOPLE

Confronting stereotypes

The interactions of non-indigenous people with indigenous people are frequently based on stereotypes. Indigenous people are often stereotyped as dirty, drunken, unemployed, shiftless people, unwilling and unable to participate in the wider society. A particularly insidious form of stereotyping is the use of skin colour to judge whether individuals are or are not Aboriginal, or the degree to which they are perceived as being Aboriginal. However, as stated previously, indigenous Australians identify themselves in terms of shared cultural and social relationships, not on the basis of skin colouring. Even people who avoid the more extreme stereotypes often make stereotypical assumptions such as 'young indigenous people are good at sport but not at school work'.

Such stereotypes neither consider the causes of the social problems confronting many indigenous people, nor acknowledge the achievements of indigenous people who, as well as being successful and active participants in their own communities, have also succeeded against significant obstacles in non-indigenous society. Many indigenous people competently lead or work in community-based organisations, government departments, or local businesses, own their own homes, mix easily with indigenous and non-indigenous people, and contribute significantly to Australia's economic and social development.

Medical practitioners are likely to stereotype indigenous living circumstances, the expected cause of signs and symptoms, the likelihood of attendance at follow-up appointments, of compliance with medical treatment, and the extent and circumstances of substance use. One of the more extreme examples of these types of assumptions by people working in the medical system is the case of a Perth ambulance team taking a person, who had been deliberately run over and who subsequently died of his injuries, home, instead of to hospital, because they assumed he was intoxicated. The assumptions that epileptic fits must be alcohol related, that an altered conscious state is due to alcohol, or that failure to take medication must be the reason a condition has worsened, have all frequently compromised medical care for indigenous people. At the least, failure by medical practitioners to recognise their use of stereotypes will result in interactions that many indigenous people will find condescending and hurtful, and that will prevent doctors from developing appropriate relationships with their indigenous patients.

Apart from confronting their own stereotypes, doctors need to be aware of how their patients may see them. Patients' opinions and expectations of doctors will be influenced by general relationships with non-indigenous people in which they have been subject to prejudice and discrimination. In the past doctors have been privileged representatives of a hostile society who have provided justification for, and participated in, the removal by the state of indigenous people from their families and communities. Thus, while most doctors today have a more positive and sympathetic approach, it is understandable that some indigenous people will not automatically view doctors as benign practitioners who always have the best interests of their patients at heart. Doctors may have to overcome the mistrust engendered by previous culturally inappropriate interactions their patients have had with misguided health practitioners, and will often need to adapt their usual approaches to gain the respect and trust of their indigenous patients.

> ➡ To assist indigenous people to address substance misuse problems, doctors must recognise the commonly held stereotypes and expectations they and their patients have of each other.

315

Culturally appropriate communication

Good communication is essential to the provision of high-quality care, and doctors need to have an understanding of appropriate ways of communicating with indigenous patients. This entails recognition of the diverse range of changing indigenous cultures, the fact that indigenous people have ways of communicating that they regard as appropriate among themselves but which they may modify, or not expect to be adhered to, in their interactions with non-indigenous people, and the idiosyncratic ways individuals have of communicating with others.

Culturally appropriate communication cannot be based on a detailed, prescriptive list of rules, such as avoiding prolonged eye contact and not mentioning the names of deceased people. While such rules may be important in some communities, they are not applicable to all. It should also be recognised that, while culture is important, each encounter requires situationally specific responses. Nevertheless, there are some general principles that can facilitate the opening of communication with indigenous patients.

First, it is important to recognise that, throughout Australia, many indigenous people speak a non-standard variety of English known as 'Aboriginal English', which is recognised by linguists as a distinct language. Given this, doctors need to assess the extent to which their indigenous patients are proficient in standard English, and to modify their communications accordingly. It is important not to make assumptions about patients' knowledge or intelligence based on ethnocentric views about Aboriginal English.

> It is important to take the time to become familiar with local indigenous forms of verbal and non-verbal communication. Careful listening, observation of body language, and patience are the keys to better communication with indigenous people.

When talking to those indigenous patients who use non-standard English, medical practitioners should speak slowly and clearly. While it is sometimes important to use local terminology and modes of speech to be understood, it is important not to mimic indigenous ways of speaking as this can be seen as patronising and offensive. As in speaking to non-indigenous patients, jargon and complex vocabulary and syntax should be avoided. This includes the avoidance of double negatives, and of asking multiple questions without allowing patients adequate time to consider and respond to each question. As with all patients, sensitively asking patients to repeat important pieces of information in their own words may help to ensure they understand what has been said.

A non-judgmental communication style is essential. One of the greatest barriers to cross-cultural communication is an authoritarian manner. Patients will be reluctant to speak openly if doctors convey the impression that they believe their views on a subject are the only correct ones. Confronted with such a manner, patients are likely to disagree passively and resist. Doctors must appear open and listen attentively to what is being said.

Whether from a desire to appear either all knowledgeable or particularly sympathetic, it is important that doctors not attempt to display their 'knowledge' of indigenous people to their patients. Given the heterogeneity of indigenous cultures, more often than not such 'knowledge' will not be applicable locally, and this strategy is likely to undermine rather than facilitate the communicative process.

Despite paying attention to these issues, doctors cannot simply assume that communication between them and their patients has been effective. The provision of high-quality health care requires teamwork, particularly when the cultural distance between providers and clients is large. Local indigenous people, or indigenous people with local connections, are essential members of any team attempting to provide appropriate health services to an indigenous community. Such people are extremely important in facilitating culturally appropriate communication. Local community-controlled health services or government-run community health services will, in most areas with a significant indigenous population, employ trained indigenous health workers, interpreters, or liaison officers. Even where patients appear to speak and understand standard Australian English well, communication can be improved dramatically by involving these workers.

Doctors need to both improve their own communication skills and make greater use of local resources if they wish to improve the effectiveness of health care services for indigenous people.

THE ROLE OF THE DOCTOR IN THE CLINICAL SETTING

Institutional barriers

The treatment setting itself can be a source of significant barriers to effective therapeutic relationships. Among the barriers indigenous people face are the formality of hushed waiting rooms, concerns about the negative attitudes of other patients and staff towards them, and requirements to fill out forms when they may have only limited levels of literacy. Barriers such as these were among the reasons that led to the establishment of indigenous community-controlled health services. Accordingly, it is important to ensure that indigenous patients are made to feel welcome and comfortable.

Assessment

A number of factors are relevant for eliciting the accurate case histories on which effective patient care depends. Meeting a new person in an unfamiliar environment can be a daunting experience for some indigenous people. Once dialogue has been established by an exchange of greetings, doctors should offer their names in full— without use of the title 'doctor', which should be used as a description of function, not a term of address. After patients have disclosed their names, doctors should ask them how they would like to be addressed. This is important, because in some communities personal names are not used in general conversation. In indigenous communities, older people are usually held in respect and it may be appropriate to acknowledge this by addressing them as 'Mr …' or 'Mrs …'—even though these same patients may call doctors by their first names.

It is important to ascertain whether patients have been accompanied by family members, and, if so, whether or not they would like them to be present during the consultation. In indigenous cultures, relatives have important roles of support. They may give patients confidence in potentially stressful encounters, assist doctors in obtaining more accurate and comprehensive histories, and patient management plans may be negotiated with them.

Where patients are not accompanied by others—particularly if their proficiency in standard English is limited—indigenous health workers or liaison officers can play a valuable role in the clinical setting. However, it is important to ask patients whether they are comfortable with this. It is also important to be aware that one health worker is not inter-changeable with another, and that, because of issues such as gender or kin relationships, it may not be appropriate for a particular health worker to be involved.

Indigenous patients expect doctors to talk honestly and openly about health problems, often, but not always, including substance use. However, while some may expect doctors to get straight to the point, others may perceive questioning in a formalised fixed-time session as inappropriate and discourteous. It is important, therefore, to take the time to ask about patients' activities and general well-being before asking about substance-use issues. It is also important to let patients tell their own stories, in their own time.

Within local indigenous cultures there are realms of belief and behaviour that are gender specific—explicitly or implicitly designated as 'men's business' or 'women's business'. It is inappropriate to broach such matters with persons of the opposite sex. Doctors need to be sensitive to this, and to the fact that some patients may be particularly uncomfortable or unwilling to discuss matters of a sexual nature with a doctor of the opposite sex. If this occurs, it is advisable to ask patients whether they would prefer to be referred to another doctor of the same sex as them, or whether they would like to have a trusted person of the same sex assist in the interview.

> Given the heterogeneity of local indigenous cultures and the diversity of expectations among individual patients, the key to effective patient assessment is to make no assumptions and to take the lead from patients themselves.

Management

Many indigenous people with alcohol or other drug problems present for other reasons. In such situations, it may be best to focus on the presenting problem and use management of that problem as a means of building rapport with the patient before openly addressing underlying substance misuse problems. Nevertheless, given the higher rates of hazardous drinking among indigenous people and the role of alcohol in exacerbating a wide range of medical problems, it is important that doctors routinely, but sensitively, ask patients who attend for other problems about their levels of alcohol and other drug use. Doctors may be particularly influential in prompting indigenous patients to contemplate reducing their consumption of alcohol and other drugs. In fact, many indigenous people consider it the responsibility of the doctor to do so.

Putting contemplation into practice is difficult. Within indigenous communities there are many pressures to continue high levels of substance use, including a dearth of alternative activities, the positive aspects of sharing substances with others and the social pressure to continue to be part of a substance-using group, and the stresses of unemployment and poverty. Many doctors understandably feel overwhelmed by the serious issues with which substance-dependent indigenous patients may present. However, while treatment cannot solve the social problems faced by indigenous patients, it can provide an alternative way of dealing with them.

A potentially important strategy is brief intervention, in which the doctor simply counsels patients about their level of consumption and related harm, and advises them to either abstain or reduce their use to safe levels. Case studies of indigenous people who have ceased drinking include frequent reference to the life-changing impact of doctors' warnings about its health consequences. Such warnings can legitimise patients' desires to reduce their alcohol or other drug use within the broader social group.

> Where patients are reluctant to discuss their consumption of alcohol or other drugs directly, a useful strategy is to focus on the problems that arise as a consequence of substance misuse and to allow patients to raise issues of consumption in their own time and in the context of addressing the associated problems.

Given the social pressures on patients to continue using, enlisting family members to support them should be an important element of any strategy to help patients quit or reduce their substance use. Such people can both provide direct support for patients, and facilitate broader social acceptance of patients' attempts to reduce substance use. The possible involvement of such persons should be discussed with patients and, wherever possible, negotiated as part of a management plan. However, it must also be recognised that many families are burnt-out by a range of factors, and may be unwilling or unable to assist. It is also important to provide patients with the opportunity to get involved in alternative activities.

For a variety of reasons, including communication difficulties, low literacy levels, complexity of the social security system, and lack of awareness, many indigenous people do not access, or are not aware of, the health and welfare benefits to which they are entitled. Access to such services can facilitate the efforts of patients to address their substance misuse problems, and doctors should explore these issues with them and, where necessary, assist them to access any requisite services.

> As substance misuse by indigenous people is embedded in a wider social context, it is important that management not focus solely on patients themselves. Careful consideration must also be given to whether the circumstances of patients are such that they can realistically be expected to comply with treatment recommendations and whether it is possible to modify the environments in which substance use occurs.

Follow-up and referrals

Consultations in which indigenous patients express a clear desire to stop drinking or using other substances are common. Although a single visit may sometimes make a difference, an ongoing therapeutic relationship is more likely to achieve a positive outcome. Doctors and other health service staff often act as if they believe that simply by making future appointments patients will automatically return, and then become negative when such appointments are not kept. Appointments are not attended for a wide range of reasons, from issues as relatively straightforward as transport problems, to issues related to the intricate social fabric of indigenous life. Some family or community commitments are more important than commitments outside the community, including medical appointments. Having failed to keep an initial or subsequent appointment, some indigenous patients may feel reluctant to attend a service, either because of their embarrassment at having to explain why they did not attend ('shame'), or their fear (often justified) of being told off for not being compliant. The likelihood of this occurring needs to be discussed to encourage patients to feel comfortable about attending services following missed appointments. However, by itself verbal reassurance is not enough—a non-judgmental approach also has to be demonstrated by the health service as a whole.

It is important to ensure that all health service staff are welcoming to patients, especially when they have not been compliant. Receptionists and nurses frequently make patients who have missed appointments or who are late feel unwelcome. This can undo the efforts of a doctor who may understand how difficult it is for some patients to attend. Working with indigenous health workers or other indigenous workers to try to arrange follow-up consultations is an important part of the process of making patients feel welcome and hence feel comfortable about returning.

> Building trust with the local indigenous community is essential to improving care for individuals from that community. Doctors who are accepting and non-judgmental, and who also ensure the health service in which they work is not judgmental, will gradually gain the trust of the local indigenous community and will be more effective over time.

Doctors can sometimes manage patients with substance-use problems with little or no assistance from others, and patients may sometimes wish for their problems to be addressed in this way. However, the chances of success are often slim. Individual counselling or agencies or groups established for non-indigenous people, such as Alcoholics and Narcotics Anonymous, are often ineffective in assisting indigenous patients to deal with substance-misuse problems. As a consequence of this lack of success, numerous indigenous community-controlled organisations have been established to provide specialised alcohol and drug treatment services. In addition, most indigenous community-controlled health services also provide some level of counselling and/or support services for indigenous people with alcohol or other drug problems.

For a variety of social reasons, some indigenous patients may be extremely mobile. In such cases, collaborative case management on a regional basis can be crucial in achieving successful outcomes. As multi-agency case management requires information disclosure to other health services, this should be discussed openly with indigenous patients; any concerns about confidentiality should be addressed, and their approval obtained prior to embarking upon such arrangements.

> Whenever possible it is recommended that, with the agreement of the patients themselves, some arrangement for collaborative case management be entered into with indigenous health agencies.

For many indigenous patients, especially those from remote areas, referral to a hospital is a bewildering experience. The size of hospitals, the number of wards and patients, the presence of unfamiliar medical equipment, and the lack of relevant information from medical staff, are ingredients for intimidation and alienation. For many indigenous people, hospitals represent an environment where they have lost control and everyday logic is discarded. The requirements to wear a medical gown day and night when one is capable of dressing, or to be moved about in a wheelchair or stay in bed during the day when one has mobility, may seem incomprehensible.

Two steps can be taken to reduce the distress and disassociation of indigenous patients referred to hospital, and make hospital contact more positive. First, frank discussions about the hospital environment are needed so that patients are prepared and have realistic expectations. Second, call ward staff, the hospital social-work department, and treating consultants, to alert them to, and advise them of, the needs of indigenous patients. Indigenous liaison officers are employed in some hospitals to facilitate these processes, and if indigenous staff are not available at the hospital there are often local indigenous agencies that will assist.

> Detailed, culturally sensitive, information provided by referring doctors is invaluable in ensuring that patient hospital stays are positive and beneficial.

THE ROLE OF THE DOCTOR IN THE COMMUNITY

As well as addressing the needs of individual patients, doctors are well placed to take action to assist indigenous people to change the environment in which substance misuse takes place. Importantly, this includes advocacy on behalf of indigenous communities. Those wishing to make a broader contribution first need to contact relevant indigenous community-controlled organisations. Many of these organisations are chronically short-staffed, and the skills that doctors can bring—some only indirectly related to their medical training—will usually be greatly appreciated, providing the doctor genuinely accepts indigenous community control. Unfortunately sometimes doctors find it difficult to avoid 'knowing what is best', and attempt to take over the agendas of the community organisations with which they work, to the long-term detriment of the doctor, the organisation, and the local indigenous community.

Working with a community-based agency requires acknowledgment that the primary qualifications to work in this area are the life experiences and knowledge of indigenous people themselves. It also requires that doctors seek to understand, and work within, the aspirations and priorities of indigenous people, and work collaboratively with them to build consensus on what needs to be done.

> Working effectively with indigenous community-based agencies requires doctors to play a role with which they are not usually familiar—playing second fiddle.

Doctors can also play an important role through their professional organisations. For example, in the Northern Territory, members of the Central Australian Rural Practitioners Association—in consultation with indigenous community-controlled organisations—have played an important role in drawing attention to health problems, lobbying for measures to address them, and developing appropriate treatment procedures.

➡ To assist indigenous people to address substance-misuse problems, doctors must recognise the commonly held stereotypes and expectations they and their patients have of each other.

➡ It is important to take the time to become familiar with local indigenous forms of verbal and non-verbal communication. Careful listening, observation of body language, and patience are the keys to better communication with indigenous people.

➡ Building trust with the local indigenous community is essential to improving care for individuals from that community. Doctors who are accepting and non-judgmental, and who also ensure the health service in which they work is not judgmental, will gradually gain the trust of the local indigenous community and will be more effective over time.

➡ Where patients are reluctant to discuss their consumption of alcohol or other drugs directly, a useful strategy is to focus on the problems that arise as a consequence of substance misuse and allow patients to raise issues of consumption in their own time and in the context of addressing the associated problems.

➡ As substance misuse by indigenous people is embedded in a wider social context, it is important that management not focus solely on individual patients. Careful consideration must also be given to whether the circumstances of patients are such that they can realistically be expected to comply with treatment recommendations, and whether it is possible to modify the environments in which substance misuse occurs.

➡ Whenever possible it is recommended that, with the agreement of patients themselves, some arrangement for collaborative case management be entered into with indigenous health agencies.

Case studies

Case study 1: communication between organisations

George, a 35-year-old Aboriginal male, attends your outer-suburban practice because he has a sore elbow. He is not sure how he injured it, but it has bothered him for several weeks. He has seen you on three occasions over the past six years, but only for minor acute problems. You ask him how things are going for him and for his wife and children, who attend your practice somewhat more often than he does. He says they are all 'good'. You examine his elbow, find he has a slightly tender olecranon bursa, and briefly discuss the condition with him.

You then ask George if there is anything else you can do for him. He says 'not really' but that perhaps he might need a bit of a check up. You have previously noted that George is a smoker and that he drinks alcohol, although you have not previously recorded how much he drinks and he has declined offers of other check ups—except for his blood pressure, which was in the normal range two years ago.

You ask him about his current alcohol and tobacco consumption. He tells you he is still smoking. He also says that he has been drinking a bit lately, since he was laid off from his job doing maintenance for a government-housing agency because the work had been contracted out to private firms. You ask how much he is drinking, and he says he used to drink only on weekends when he was working but lately he has been drinking nearly every day. He shares a 'block' (30 cans) of full-strength beer between himself and his brothers and cousins. (It is not clear how many people share the block, but you get the impression it may be as few as three or four on any one day).

His blood pressure is elevated at 155/105, he is obviously somewhat overweight (BMI 29.5), an office glucometer reading is 9 mmol/L (non-fasting), and urinalysis shows a trace of protein. The remainder of his examination is unremarkable. You tell him that his blood pressure is up today and that you want to carry out some more tests for diabetes and other routine tests. You explain that alcohol can increase blood pressure, and that smoking increases his risk of heart disease and stroke, especially if he has high blood pressure. He tells you his older brother had a heart attack last year and also has diabetes, and that his father died aged 52. His family thinks it was probably a heart attack. He admits his wife has been asking him to have a check up for some time.

You collect blood for FBC, Hb_{A1C}, LFTs including gamma GT, UEC, and request an ACR (Albumin Creatinine Ratio) on his urine. You also give him a form for fasting lipid and blood glucose levels, and ask him to have this test at the local laboratory one morning before he has anything to eat. You make an appointment for the following week but he does not attend, and he also does not attend for his fasting tests. His Hb_{A1C} from the previous week is 8.5% (poorly controlled diabetes), ACR is 4.5 (slightly raised), and Gamma GT and ALT are moderately raised. Other results are normal.

You ring George; however his telephone is disconnected. You therefore send him a letter but he does not respond. You contact the Aboriginal Community Controlled Health (ACCHS) Service in the city and ask if there is anyone who can get a message to him. An Aboriginal health worker (AHW) who lives in the same area as George agrees to contact him and see if she can get him to come back for follow-up. About two weeks later the AHW gives George a lift to the surgery and asks if she can see you before you see George. She tells you that she is George's cousin, that his family situation is much more complex than you may have been aware, and also that he has been having some medical care at the ACCHS which included a referral to an Aboriginal Alcohol and Substance Misuse Service (AASMS). You then see George and tell him the results of his tests. You ask him if he would be interested in working with the ACCHS and the AASMS as well as with you. He is enthusiastic and pleased that you are interested in working with Aboriginal organisations, and gives you permission to talk to staff at these two organisations about him. He says he did not tell you he had also been seeing a doctor at ACCHS as he felt you may not have liked him going to another doctor.

You contact his doctor at the ACCHS and agree to work with her on finding the most appropriate supports for George as he tries to address his health problems. The AHW you met, who is part of the ACCHS diabetes team, agrees to liaise with you to ensure services are better coordinated, since George and his family often find it more convenient to see you close to home than travel to ACCHS in the city.

Over the following year George makes some significant improvements. He quits smoking except when drinking, he drinks less often (although still to excess on occasions), his weight has gone down and up again but he has lost a net 5 kg, and he does some regular walking. His diet is improved but still variable as he finds it difficult to eat a separate diet from other family members, he takes an ACE inhibitor and Metformin regularly, and his diabetes is better controlled but not ideal (Hb_{A1C} of 7.5%). You have only seen him four times since, but he has had contact with the ACCHS and AASMS staff on a fairly regular basis and they have kept you informed of his medical follow-ups and test results. George still has a long way to go and will continue to have ups and downs, but he has taken some important steps. The chances of a better outcome have improved because the agencies working with him are communicating with each other.

Case points

George's case illustrates:
- the high level of morbidity and early mortality among indigenous Australians
- the benefits of involving an Aboriginal Health Worker in case management (for example increased patient information, appointment attendance, compliance with treatment regimens)
- that indigenous people are often more comfortable attending indigenous health services
- that non-indigenous doctors can work collaboratively with indigenous health services to improve health outcomes for indigenous patients.

Case study 2: the potential for doctors to influence changes over time

Walter, aged 26, is in a remote-area district hospital with pneumonia. He has had asthma since childhood, and is a smoker. He had a period of heavy drinking prior to this admission to hospital, and this probably contributed to his illness. He was initially very unwell and quite weak, but after a couple of days he is in better spirits, and, for the first time you, his GP, are able to get to know him a little.

He tells you he worked as an apprentice motor mechanic for a couple of years, but that it was very difficult to remain employed when none of his mates had jobs—the town has very high levels of unemployment. He had also worked for the local Aboriginal resource agency. He has been on CDEP (Community Development Employment Program, a 'work for the dole' scheme) for the last couple of years. He is obviously intelligent and has a good grasp of issues relevant to the town; this surprises you a little as previously you had only met him when he had been intoxicated.

You discuss his health with him and the importance of quitting smoking to his health, especially because of his quite severe asthma. You also point out the consequences, both short- and long-term, of excessive alcohol consumption. You suggest a referral to an Aboriginal alcohol treatment service in the next town, 100 km away.

Walter does not seem very enthusiastic about any of your suggestions. He explains that there is not much to do as a young man in town if you do not drink. He has tried not drinking on a couple of occasions, but people just gave him 'humbug' and he went back to drinking. He says he could try to give up smoking, but he doesn't really smoke much anyway—he just smokes when he is drinking and someone else has cigarettes. He also says he is not worried about what might happen in 10 or 20 years—he is not sure he is going to live that long.

You discuss education, suggesting that he is smart and could probably do some university study. Maybe he would make a good lawyer since he is pretty good at speaking up for himself. He says he has thought about going back to school and that his sister has been to university in the city and trained as a nurse. She does not come back to the town very often, and he is not sure that he wants to leave town and lose his mates. You discharge him from hospital the next day and he returns to CDEP work and occasional heavy drinking. You see him from time to time and have a chat. At first he seems to be drunk less often and looks healthier than he did, but this does not last and you sadly form the view that nothing is likely to change in his life.

You leave town about a year later and return to work in the city. You do not see Walter for the next five years, then one day you bump into him at a suburban shopping centre. He is looking healthy, and tells you he started a university bridging course and wants to study law. When he is finished with study he plans to go back out bush and work with the Aboriginal Legal Service. He says he remembers you talking to him and telling him he was smart and should study. He said that the next year he got sick again. He was told that he nearly died, and his sister got stuck into him. After that he decided to move to the city to stay with his sister. About a year later he decided to give education a go, and after not taking it seriously at first he got right into it. He says he only drinks occasionally these days and has slowed down a bit. He also says he very rarely smokes now—just at parties.

You think about this meeting while working in your suburban practice, realising how much people can change and that it is important to be positive with all patients. The effect is not always immediate, but you can sometimes contribute to significant improvements in people's lives.

Case points

Walter's case illustrates:
- that problem substance use is often embedded in a wider social context
- that the sharing of psychoactive substances may be important in maintaining social relationships
- that lack of social opportunity is often an impediment to reducing psychoactive substance use
- that medical practitioners are seen as authoritative, important figures who can have a significant impact on lifestyle with minimal input.

REFERENCES AND FURTHER READING

Gray, D., Saggers, S., Sputore, B. & Bourbon, D. 2000, 'What works? A review of evaluated alcohol misuse interventions among Aboriginal Australians', *Addiction*, vol. 95, pp. 31–42.

Hunter, E., Brady, M. & Hall, W. (eds) 2000, *National Recommendations for the Clinical Management of Alcohol-Related Problems in Indigenous Primary Care Settings*. Department of Health & Aged Care, Canberra. http://www.health.gov.au/oatsih/pubs/pdf/rec.pdf

Saggers, S. & Gray, D. 1998, *Dealing with Alcohol: Indigenous Usage in Australia, New Zealand and Canada*. Cambridge University Press, Melbourne.

18

Working with Māori who have Alcohol and Drug-related Problems

Paul Robertson, Terry Huriwai, Tuari Potiki, Rosemary Friend & Mason Durie

The aim of this chapter is to facilitate more effective clinical interaction with Māori who have substance-use problems. A primary focus is to help readers to develop a basic understanding of key issues and broad principles relevant to this area, such as the need for a holistic approach and cultural consultation, as well as awareness of the diversity of contemporary Māori identity and the centrality of the collective. 'Collective' in this sense relates to sense of community and the individual's place within it, where community is defined both in terms of traditional social structures and via reference to other areas of commonality. While the focus is on what may be considered more fundamental issues, this chapter is also likely to be useful for those who already have some experience in this area, in terms of consolidating their knowledge and practice.

In the chapter, we first consider sociohistorical factors, including patterns of substance use, before discussing more explicitly clinical issues. The information presented here can be applied to the specific content areas outlined in other chapters.

WHO IS MĀORI?

Following settlement of Aotearoa by Māori, around 800–1000 AD, a unique culture developed in which whānau (extended family), hapu (subtribe), and iwi (tribe or clan) (also see glossary for definitions) constituted the primary cultural units. Today Māori are a highly heterogeneous group, with some affiliating primarily with hapu and/or iwi, while many identify simply as Māori. Others identify as 'New Zealanders', and have no significant affiliation with Māori. This reflects a continuum of Māori identity shaped by a range of social, historic, economic, and cultural factors. Despite differences, there are commonalities that distinguish Māori from other New Zealanders. They have inherited a distinctive world-view, made broadly similar life journeys, and have relatives in common.

> Māori today experience and participate in an array of diverse realities.

These diverse realities have implications for treatment, for example, those who identify as 'sole Māori' suffer from the highest levels of ill health as a group, and are more likely to present with severe problems. Rejection of Māori identity may also be linked to substance-use problems. However, it is important to remember that identity changes over time, both individually and collectively, such that a 'snap-shot' is unlikely to provide sufficient account of the longer-term search for a balanced and secure identity.

> Assertion and maintenance of a secure cultural identity is central to Māori well-being (Durie 1994).

While there is no simple answer to the question of who is Māori, it clearly extends beyond blood quantum. Several factors are salient, with individual choice being a primary variable; however, possession of whakapapa (genealogy) determines whether or not such a choice can be made. Participation in and acceptance by 'the Māori community' is also important, with knowledge of te reo (language) being cited as critical by some. Ultimately, being Māori is a function of belonging to Te Ao Māori—the Māori world—and its networks. Current place of residence is less important than access to and participation in whānau and other institutions.

PATTERNS OF SUBSTANCE USE

Alcohol

Historical records provide no indication of systematic use of psychoactive substances prior to the arrival of Europeans, and suggest Māori responded to the introduction of alcohol in a variety of ways. Although problems developed later, initial introduction did not lead to the widespread ruination of the 'natives'. In fact, Augustus Earle (1827, cited in Mancall et al. 2000) noted Māori 'have the utmost aversion to wine or strong drink, very often severely taking us to task for such an extraordinary and debasing propensity, or, as they call it, of making ourselves mad'.

Seamen and missionaries were a significant influence on the development of norms related to alcohol use, as were laws enacted in the mid-nineteenth century restricting Māori access to alcohol, its production, and distribution. These restrictions are likely to have impeded the development of structures and practices to facilitate safe consumption and problem resolution, with alcohol abuse becoming more prevalent in Māori communities towards the end of the nineteenth century.

Many Māori with substance abuse problems adopted the philosophy and treatment modality of Alcoholics Anonymous (AA) despite the lack of acknowledgement of cultural differences by AA. Reasons for this affinity include AA's focus on spirituality (wairuatanga) and fellowship (whānaungatanga), and alignment of abstinence with absence of alcohol in 'traditional' Māori societies. A historical lack of treatment options is also likely to have been an important factor. A significant proportion of the Māori workforce have themselves utilised '12-step' programs, contributing to a strong abstinence focus. Approaches currently taken by Māori services, however, are becoming broader.

A recent survey (Dacey 1997) indicated that, compared to the general population, fewer Māori than non-Māori drink. Those who do drink tend to do so less frequently, but consume more per occasion, compared with non-Māori. There are potential clinical implications of this binge type of drinking. Individuals taking part in this drinking pattern may not perceive or report problems, even when drinking bouts have a negative impact.

➡ Although binge drinking appears to be prevalent, not all Māori who drink have a major problem—brief intervention may suffice.

330

Cannabis and other illicit drugs

Since the 1970s, cannabis use has increased markedly in New Zealand. Some suggest is it is more problematic for Māori, especially where cultivation conditions are favourable and socioeconomic conditions are not. There is little research on the prevalence of cannabis use among Māori or the nature of related problems. A recent survey of Māori revealed 60% used marijuana some time during their lives, 18% were regular users, and 4% used heavily (Dacey & Moewaka Barnes, 2000). A clinically focused sample indicated that Māori cannabis users are over-represented in alcohol and drug services (Adamson et al., 2000). Both studies suggested cannabis users are younger than alcohol users and users of other illicit drugs. This has implications for both prevention and intervention, given the relative youth of the Māori population.

There is some evidence of opioid and benzodiazepine use becoming problematic, with increasing numbers of Māori on methadone programs throughout New Zealand (Potiki, 2000). Notably, nearly 18% of Christchurch Methadone Programme clients are Māori, despite only making up approximately 9% of the city's population. This is occurring despite limited acceptance of drug substitution therapy by many Māori. Additionally, anecdotal evidence suggests increasing numbers of Māori youth are indulging in so-called party drugs such as ecstasy and ketamine; however, there is little data on the nature and extent of use of these and similar drugs.

Inhalants

The highly visible, but relatively low prevalence, use of solvents continues to be a characteristic of some younger, usually male, sections of the Māori population. Although solvent use appears to have a relatively low base rate, it was cited by respondents in a recent community survey on substance use as being second only to the problem of illicit drug use (excluding cannabis) and equal in seriousness to alcohol-related problems (Dacey & Moewaka Barnes, 2000).

Nicotine

After alcohol, nicotine is the drug most commonly used by Māori. Nearly 50% of women and 35% of men smoke; however, men tend to smoke more heavily. Older smokers tend to smoke more heavily, but a considerable number of 15 to 29-year-olds smoke up to 10 cigarettes per day. The health impact of smoking is well recognised, and interventions are detailed elsewhere in this book. Application of the principles outlined below are strongly recommended for ensuring that treatment for smoking is culturally responsive.

The impact of alcohol and other drugs

There is clear evidence that substance use has a negative impact in a range of mental health related areas for Māori, including psychiatric admissions. Significant associations with physical health problems are also well recognised, for example in relation to heart disease. Much research has focused on alcohol use, but there are obvious links between other drugs and health problems, for example cannabis use and cancer/respiratory diseases, and intravenous drug use and hepatitis. Additionally, research indicates a comparatively high rate of accidents related to substance use for Māori. While other social problems have also been associated with substance use, for example criminal offending and unemployment, the exact nature of such associations has yet to be clearly elucidated.

331

CLINICAL ISSUES

Māori health and well-being

This section provides a starting point for understanding some key concepts in Māori health. A holistic view, including spiritual aspects and connection with natural phenomena, is central to well-being. Kin ties, the centrality of the collective, and appropriate ceremonial protocols are also important. Such fundamental values are enduring; however, their expression may alter over time and content. Many Māori health frameworks draw on customary concepts, for example Te Whare Tapa Whā, the four-sided house (Durie, 1994). This model represents health as four interdependent domains: taha wairua, taha hinengaro, taha tinana and taha whānau.

These approximate to the spiritual, the mental, the physical, and family/collective domains. Other models, for example Te Wheke and powhin models, incorporate similar elements and all emphasise the need to restore/maintain the balance of the various interactive constituents of well-being.

None of the above represent *the* definitive model of Māori health, but all take health beyond conventional Western medical conceptualisations. Reference to such frameworks should be tempered by awareness of the diverse realities of Māori, however, even for those who have limited contact with Te Ao Māori these concepts and values are relevant. Patients may not be willing or able to articulate the impact of customary beliefs on their lives, so clinicians need to exercise sensitivity when exploring the potential role of such factors. It is also prudent to remember that like other frameworks, such as DSM IV, Māori models are more complex than they may initially appear.

Engagement

Engaging Māori with substance-use problems is in many ways similar to engaging non-Māori, that is, with empathy, respect, and professionalism. There are however, important, albeit subtle, differences when attempting to engage with Māori. A frequent trap is making assumptions about people who look Māori, for example, by greeting them with 'kia ora'. In some cases it may be more appropriate not to greet Māori in this way, lest they are embarrassed by a lack of knowledge of te reo, or by the interviewer's poor pronunciation.

A single Māori greeting is not enough on its own to ensure a culturally responsive service. A minimum requirement is possession of fundamental skills and knowledge, such as being able to pronounce Māori names and words correctly. Awareness of potential areas of sensitivity is also important, for example in relation to the tapu or restricted nature of some parts/functions of the body. A clinician may facilitate engagement by how he or she asks questions, the areas he or she chooses to focus on, or by conveying acceptance of factors important to the patient, even if they seem irrelevant. It is important to err on the side of giving Māori clients time and space before attempting to elicit information directly. This enables the patient to assess the clinician's motivation, awareness, and trustworthiness. Rushing things can be seen as a precipitous intrusion and disrespectful of personal and interpersonal boundaries.

Assessment of cultural variables

Understanding the potential impact of cultural variables on patients' substance use is crucial. An obvious example is labelling cultural/spiritual experiences as psychotic. The influence of cultural variables is often more subtle, however, reflecting under-lying beliefs and expectations. Many examples relate to the importance of collectivity and spiritual elements, as well as negative experiences associated with being Māori in New Zealand society. The latter may contribute to rejection of Māori identity.

It is useful to differentiate between the various types of cultural assessment. Some assessments focus on the degree to which a person is connected and comfortable with Te Ao Māori, with items referring to knowledge of tikanga—cultural practice—and te reo, as well as participation in Māori networks. Assessments of this type are usually sought from Māori workers to provide a 'Māori perspective'. The degree to which the cultural assessments are integrated with clinical assessments depends on a number of factors, including clinicians' knowledge and willingness to accept the relevance of cultural variables.

A second type of cultural assessment attempts to link cultural variables directly with patient's symptomatology, for example, as outlined in DSM-IV (Appendix 1, p. 843). This represents an attempt to improve diagnostic systems, but characteristically such assessments are relatively unsophisticated. This type of cultural assessment is usually undertaken by non-Māori clinicians with little understanding of specific issues for Māori, thus limiting the degree to which cultural information can be integrated into case formulation and management.

A third variation, cultural screening, is most appropriate for non-Māori clinicians with limited knowledge of the culture. Such a screen contributes to identifying options for intervention (for example whether or not to refer a patient to a Māori service), as well as giving a broad idea of whether cultural variables may contribute to substance-use problems. Identification of the latter ideally leads to referral to appropriately qualified Māori to clarify the nature of the interaction between cultural and other variables related to substance use. Basic knowledge of key Māori concepts and values is crucial in enabling identification of possible cultural variables. Recognition of the limits of one's knowledge is also vital. This approach parallels screening for any issues outside one's area of expertise (for example GP screening for an eating disorder).

333

Engaging Māori patients

These following hints are not definitive rules, but rather broad guidelines to assist further development and integration of your skills and knowledge.

- Be aware of the impact of your own cultural beliefs/assumptions, including how you define 'being Māori', especially if you are non-Māori.
- Establish and maintain reciprocal relationships with appropriately experienced Māori who can provide advice, post-screening assessment, and/or appropriate cultural intervention.
- Maintain awareness of the limits of your knowledge of Māori concepts and concerns.
- Develop awareness of the diverse realities of Māori.
- Increase understanding of key Māori processes, concepts and values, especially taking a holistic approach to health.
- Increase knowledge of how cultural and clinical variables might interact.
- Convey the fact that you consider cultural variables important and relevant.

Cultural screen

The following are general guidelines. The details of a cultural screen, including what questions to ask, need to be developed *in consultation with appropriately experienced Māori* and with reference to fuller information on Māori processes, concepts, and concerns, as well as specific alcohol and drug related issues.

1 Ensure you are attending to the issues outlined in the section above on engaging Māori patients.
2 Develop screening questions to ascertain information in the following areas:
   - the patient's willingness to discuss cultural issues with you or Māori workers
   - Māori values and beliefs held by the patient that may have implications for assessment and treatment of alcohol and drug problems (for example whanaungatanga, wairuatanga)
   - whether the patient thinks there are Māori issues implicated in his/her substance-use problems
   - what being Māori means to the patient, both historically and currently, for example in terms of participation in Māori groups and organisations
   - the patient's experience of whānau, particularly in relation to alcohol and drug use
   - whether the patient wants to utilise Māori resources, including preferences for culturally-focused treatment options, for example working with a Māori clinician, attending a kaupapa Māori residential service, receiving collabora-tive input from a Māori service/expert
3 Take action on the basis of the information gathered, for example refer on to an appropriate service or individual, consult with an appropriate person, arrange to meet with the whānau, or at the very least record relevant information.

Notes

- As with any other patients, Māori patients may not be able to articulate or be aware of all the issues impacting on their substance use.
- Refusal to discuss, or denial of the impact of, cultural variables should not be taken at face value, but do not insist on continuing if the patient declines to participate in this line of enquiry.
- The screening suggested above may involve either direct or indirect questioning.
- Information may be gained from various sources, for example the clinical file or, with consent, other workers, whānau, and so on.

Working with Māori in conventional services/practices

Assessing appropriate options for patients requires knowledge of the services and workers available. In the alcohol and drug area a number of options exist, from Māori residential programs, to single Māori workers in 'mainstream' services.

When assessing whether a person would benefit from a dedicated Māori service or a more conventional service, it may be useful to consider salient issues within a 'stages of change' framework. A patient may not identify strongly as Māori (pre-contemplation), but referral may increase his or her ability to connect with (contemplation) or utilise the resources of Te Ao Māori (preparation/action). Additionally, some Māori expect conventional services or individuals to be unable to respond to their needs. Resistance to engaging in a 'Māori way' may be a defensive stance against perceived invasion of personal space, rather than a rejection of Māori identity. More positive engagement may occur with time if empathy and understanding are demonstrated.

Unfortunately referral options are limited as many 'mainstream' services/practices lack facilities or frameworks for working within patients' own setting or with whānau. Thus, even if clinicians can screen competently for cultural needs, their choices may be limited. Shared care, with clinical and cultural input being provided by different agencies, may be possible. To ensure success, this arrangement requires significant collaboration and mutual respect.

Increasing responsivity to Māori within mainstream services and practices

- Identify and address culturally unsafe practices and processes within your service/practice.
- Make the environment more user-friendly, for example with Māori posters, signage, and the provision of space (both physical and conceptual) for whānau to be involved.
- As a team or practice, identify and address reasons for Māori accessing or not accessing services.
- Develop relationship or partnership with appropriate Māori organisations, services and individuals.
- Identify service/practice development and training needs in this area.

Working with whānau and beyond

Considering the reciprocal relationship with family members is crucial in the alcohol and drug area, and is especially relevant for Māori (Huriwai et al., 2001). Defining whānau and its role is not clear-cut, as it exists in a variety of forms in contemporary New Zealand. Despite this, fundamental values of collectivism continue to provide a framework for cooperation and collective identity. For a significant number of Māori, non-kin-based whānau replace or take precedence, which contributes to diversity in the experience of and participation in whānau. This diversity notwithstanding, most Māori cite the importance of belonging to and being accepted by a close-knit group of people. This represents more than the usual affiliative needs of humans, and reflects the primacy of the collective for Māori in terms of identity, functioning, and shared aspirations.

The centrality of the whānau is well recognised in alcohol and drug services, however approaches have often been simplistic and have not necessarily alleviated difficulties. Consideration of many factors needs to be taken into account before assuming the whānau approach is appropriate. Assessment of the patients' relationship with whānau is often neglected, and little rationale provided beyond 'involving whānau is what one does with Māori'. The above notwithstanding, affiliation with a 'recovery whānau' is important for some Māori addressing substance-use problems. This allows those alienated from kin-based whānau to experience the essence of a positive whānau.

In recent years a number of culturally relevant health promotion resources have been developed for working more widely with whānau/hapu/iwi. Posters encouraging safer alcohol use, such as the one in figure 18.1 have drawn on important

Figure 18.1 Kai Wai Manaaki poster. Designed by Nikora Ngaropo with Jason Fox of Mataaho Limited. Reprinted with permission of the Alcohol Advisory Council (ALAC).

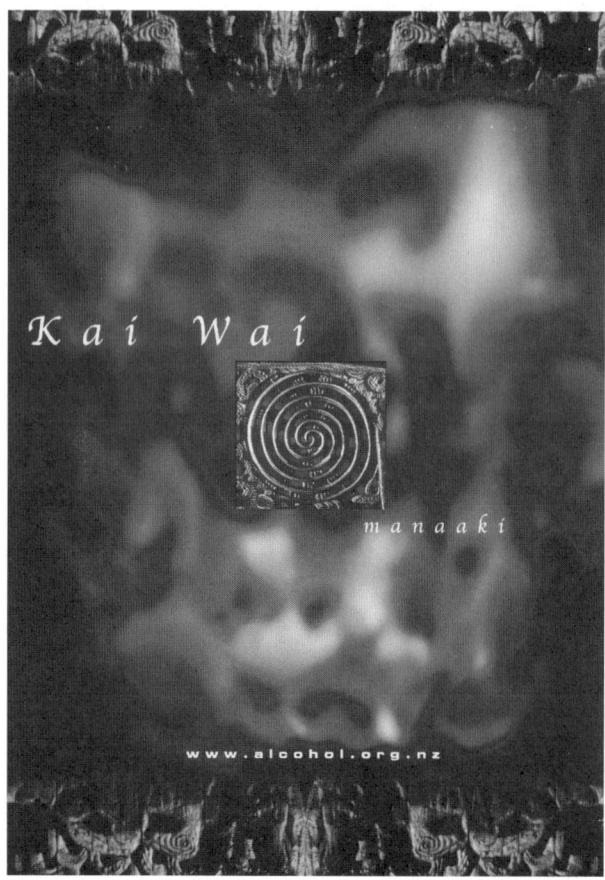

Māori concepts. In this case these are related to whanaungatanga, social links and responsibilities, especially caring for members of the collective (that is, manaakitanga). (For further information see 'Te Roopu Maori' at www.waipiro.org.nz.) This poster incorporates general safe-drinking practices, namely ensuring that food is available and alternating alcoholic with non-alcoholic drinks (in this case wai—water). A recent campaign promoting safer drinking (SIP—Stay In Play; see 'Te Roopu Maori' cited above) via a youth focused Māori radio station appears to have impacted positively on some young Māori. Both of these safer drinking campaigns seem to have had some influence, despite a traditional abstinence focus of many Māori. Campaigns to reduce smoking, such as 'Auahi Kore', have also had some success, as have interventions providing nicotine replacement therapy through Māori health organisations.

Involving whānau/hapu/iwi

- Develop strategies, with a Māori worker/service, for approaching and involving whānau.
- Be mindful of the diversity of whānau and people's experience within them.
- Clarify patients' past experience of whānau and who they currently identify as whānau.
- Clarify the nature of patients' relationships with their various whānau and their willingness to be involved.
- Make use of culturally relevant alcohol and drug health promotion material when working with whānau/hapu/iwi.

Working with Māori agencies and organisations

Engagement of Māori clients in mainstream services is aided by collaboration with Māori agencies and organisations. This will increase options and patients' confidence in a clinician/service. Māori will not necessarily be eager to support services perceived as well resourced, and could be wary of exploitation. Attempts to make contact may not be welcomed, but input may be provided for the sake of the patient. Developing and maintaining reciprocal relationships (whakawhanaungatanga) is vital when interacting with Māori workers. Sharing knowledge is one option, as many Māori working in the alcohol and drug field appreciate the skills possessed by medical staff.

Challenges may arise when working with Māori services and consultants because of potential differences between conventional clinical models and approaches taken by many Māori. Clinicians may have difficulty working with an explicit spiritual focus, while a primarily medical focus may create difficulty for some Māori. In addition, as noted above, many Māori adopt an abstinence-based approach, which may challenge clinicians focused on harm reduction.

With regard to cultural interventions, you need to identify what options are available and have realistic expectations of what can be provided. Services may run primarily under a Māori kaupapa or philosophy, incorporating Māori content throughout, or they may use conventional interventions in a Māori context. Some services are based entirely on AA tenets, while others incorporate interventions such as motivational interviewing and person-centred therapy.

Developing a relationship with Māori workers/services

• Develop knowledge of Māori alcohol and drug services in your area and nationally.
• Develop relationships with appropriate workers and/or services.
• Identify what workers/services can and cannot provide.
• Identify how you could develop more responsive services for Māori patients in your area.

Coexisting psychiatric disorders

The interaction between psychiatric and substance use disorders confuses presentation for all patients (see chapter 20). However, the situation can be further complicated when working with Māori because of unfamiliar values and beliefs held by a patient or their whānau. Such values and beliefs are likely to impact on presentation and management.

Important issues can arise from differing conceptualisations of comorbidity. A Māori perspective may utilise a framework connecting whānau, wairua and other core aspects of well-being. A more conventional Western model is likely to focus on what are considered the primary elements, or dual diagnosis, with less consideration of other key variables. Clinicians also need to be aware that cultural resources are likely to be required to address some issues related to coexisting disorders fully, for example, stabilisation of whānau relationships or development of culturally safe treatment environments.

Working with Māori who have coexisting psychiatric disorders

• Attend to safety, especially cultural safety, to increase patient comfort and participation in treatment.
• Stabilise areas inhibiting assessment and intervention, including spiritual issues and whānau relationships.
• Undertake a comprehensive assessment, including a cultural screen, and identify relevant cultural resources.
• Clinical case management involves active attention to salient cultural variables, necessitating collaboration with appropriately skilled Māori.

• Integration of care involves conceptualisation of culture as a thread that runs through treatment, rather than just an add-on.

SUMMARY

Working effectively with Māori who have substance-use problems is a significant challenge, not least because of the diversity of experience of Māori patients. Understanding of the influence of one's own culture and basic grasp of key Māori concepts, notably related to the centrality of the collective, is crucial. This knowledge, along with a willingness to take a holistic approach and work in a collaborative manner with Māori, provides a starting point from which to meet this challenge.

→ Understanding one's own cultural assumptions provides the basis for understanding and engaging with Māori.

→ Knowing and working within one's limits is vital, as is developing relationships with appropriately skilled Māori to facilitate intervention beyond those limits.

→ Although Māori culture, like others, is dynamic, key principles and institutions endure, and a basic knowledge of these is essential.

→ Māori in contemporary Aotearoa (and Australia) are not a homogeneous population; diversity is the rule.

→ Problematic substance use is currently a contributing factor in a number of areas of health, as well as being implicated in other social problems.

→ Problems related to substance use need to be located in a broader socio-historical context to enable assessment to be accurate, and effective intervention to be developed.

→ Working with whānau and Māori workers, in a shared-care arrangement, will facilitate progress with a significant number of Māori patients.

Case study

Rose, a 35-year-old woman, presents to your medical centre reporting symptoms indicative of diabetes. Despite her physical appearance suggesting that she is Māori, Rose describes herself as 'a New Zealander first and foremost'. She was brought up in a 'traditional' setting, but she wants nothing to do with her family, or any 'Māori stuff'. Assessment reveals that she suffers from depression and ultimately she acknowledges heavy alcohol use. She states that after drinking heavily she frequently has dreams in which she is visited by a dead uncle. She also reports having seen him in the street several times when she was sober. Her statement does not appear to be indicative of psychiatric disturbance. In relation to her low mood she reports strong feelings of shame related to being identified as Māori.

Case points

Rose's initial presentation illustrates:
- the need to avoid assumptions about cultural identity based on appearance
- that it is useful to understand patients' ethno-history, but also important to establish how they feel currently, that is, what does being Māori mean to them at this point in time
- the need to clarify Rose's beliefs/attributions about the nightmares and sightings of her uncle
- the need to clarify the relationship between low mood, drinking, and shame about being identified as Māori
- the importance of seeking cultural advice to clarify the nature of 'hallucinations' and other phenomena that may have a culture-based explanation or component.

Case study continued

After a number of appointments it becomes apparent that alienation from whānau and Te Ao Māori are implicated in Rose's drinking and low mood. As Rose maintains resistance to responding to or discussing 'Māori stuff' with you, at this stage you seek advice from [...]. (This space and those following have been left blank as you will need to identify and develop relationships with the Māori workers and/or services who will most appropriately fill them.) After you develop a better understanding of the potential impact of cultural factors as a result of cultural consultation, you develop a stronger alliance with Rose, despite her missing two appointments after you suggested that sessions begin with a karakia! She becomes more open about her childhood, describing some positive experiences, but also traumatic events. She purposely moved away from her whānau, but since reconnecting with a sister has begun to miss them. However, she does not want to re-contact them for reasons she will not discuss and remains wary of, but is not so resistant to things Māori. Her sister is supportive, but is unable to take a primary role in treatment because of the demands of her own whānau and work.

Case points

The subsequent contacts illustrate:
- being Māori does not just 'go away'

- unwillingness to discuss cultural issues may persist for some time
- whānau members may be supportive, but could have difficulty playing an ongoing and consistent part in treatment for a range of reasons
- the value of developing a relationship with and seeking advice from appropriately knowledgeable consultants
- that you cannot expect that a person will suddenly just embrace all things Māori
- the need to avoid forcing what you think it is to be Māori on the patient (for example saying karakia)
- the need to be wary of patronising or becoming an instant expert on things Māori
- incorporating Māori words or ideas may (or may not) be useful in strengthening the therapeutic alliance
- the importance of developing an ability to convey knowledge and understanding of important Māori concepts in a low-key manner.

Case study continued

Ultimately Rose decides she does want to see her family, but she experiences considerable anxiety about having contact with them. She is concerned about not being a 'proper Māori', as she is not a fluent speaker and cannot remember much about marae protocol. To help her with these issues and to develop a better understanding of the impact of cultural variables on her drinking and related problems, you arrange for her to have some sessions with [...]. A referral to a Māori residential program following these sessions is mooted. Ultimately Rose does not attend this program, but she does work with her sister and [...] on reconnecting with some of her whānau living locally. She also becomes involved with a 'recovery whānau' which she is introduced to by [...], and she works with an alcohol and drug counsellor to further address issues related to substance use. Throughout this process she continues to have contact with you, and you continue to monitor her medication for her mood and diabetes.

Case points

The care of Rose's health beyond the immediate problems of diabetes and alcohol use illustrates:
- facilitating contact with whānau may be a complicated process
- re-contacting or even suggesting reconnection with estranged whānau is likely to elicit a range of responses, not all positive
- expertise is likely to be required to facilitate the process of re-contacting whānau and addressing related issues

- shared care involving a number of experts will facilitate optimal intervention
- it cannot be taken for granted that all Māori will want or need to attend a Māori program
- reconnection with all members of whānau of origin may not be possible, or desirable
- non-kin-based whānau may provide important support and positive experiences of whānau, as well as increasing a patient's confidence in his or her ability to function in Te Ao Māori.

Case study continued

A crisis occurs after Rose spends time on her whānau marae, re-establishing contact with her extended family. She becomes seriously depressed and suicidal in response to frequent 'visits' by her dead uncle. After initial management by the crisis team, consultation with [...] leads you to refer her to [...], who has expertise in the spiritual realm and can work with issues related to the 'visitation'. (This person may have expertise in wairuatanga and Māori concepts of spirituality or could be a minister, depending on the needs and beliefs of the patient.) After consultation with Māori staff the crisis team recommend referral to an appropriate counsellor to address abuse-related issues that have become salient following increased contact with whānau. Because you are acting as primary case manager, you continue to coordinate her treatment, as well as monitoring her diabetes and the antidepressant medication previously prescribed, to which she has responded positively.

Case points

Rose's ongoing problems illustrate:
- facilitating reconnection with Te Ao Māori, including re-contacting whānau, may initially exacerbate coexisting conditions or precipitate emergence of new problems
- culture-related issues rarely arise in a pure form and are likely to be interwoven with other problems
- not all Māori have the necessary expertise or knowledge to deal with all 'cultural' issues
- ideally one person will take responsibility for overseeing and coordination of care, although it is unlikely that one person would be able to provide all of the treatment required
- addressing presenting problems optimally requires flexibility, relationships with, and/or knowledge of a range of service providers, and an eclectic approach.

ACKNOWLEDGMENT

The authors wish to thank Jillian Larsen and Meg Harvey for their assistance in the preparation of this chapter.

REFERENCES AND FURTHER READING

Adamson, S.J., Sellman, J.D., Futterman-Collier, A., Huriwai, T.T., Deering, D.E., Todd, F.C. & Robertson, P.J. 2000, 'A profile of alcohol and drug clients in New Zealand: results from the 1998 national telephone survey', *New Zealand Medical Journal*, vol. 113, pp. 414–16.

Dacey, B. 1997, *Te Ao Waipiro: Māori and Alcohol in 1995*. Whariki Research Group/Alcohol and Public Health Research Group, University of Auckland, Auckland.

Dacey, B. & Moewaka Barnes, H. 2000, *Te Ao Taru Kino: Drug use among Māori, 1998*, Whariki Public Health Research Group, University of Auckland.

Durie, M.H. 1994, *Whaiora: Māori Health Development*, Oxford University Press, Auckland.

Huriwai, T.T., Sellman, J.D., Sullivan, P. & Potiki, T. 2000, 'Optimal treatment for Māori with alcohol and drug-use related problems: the importance of cultural factors in treatment', *Substance Use and Misuse*, vol. 35, pp. 17–35.

Huriwai, T.T., Robertson, P.J., Armstrong, P., Kingi, J. & Huata, P. 2001, 'Whakawhanaungatanga: a process in the treatment of Māori with alcohol and drug use related problems', *Substance Use and Misuse*, vol. 36, 1033–51.

Mancall, P.C., Robertson, P.J. & Huriwai, T.T. 2000, 'Māori and alcohol: a reconsidered history', *Australian New Zealand Journal of Psychiatry*, vol. 34, pp. 129–34.

Metge, J. 1995, *New Growth From Old: The Whānau in the Modern World*, Victoria Press, Wellington.

Pere, R.R. 1984, 'The health of the family', *New Zealand Health Review*, vol. 14, p. 17

Potiki, P. 2000, 'Māori and methadone', Paper presented to the National Māori Alcohol and Drug Summit, Manu Ariki, Taumaranui.

343

GLOSSARY

These are basic translations. Readers seeking more understanding should refer to the references cited above.

Aotearoa	New Zealand
hapu	subtribe
iwi	tribe/clan
kai	food
karakia	'prayer'
kaupapa	purpose, principles
manaakitanga	practices for ensuring the care of others

marae	gathering place
noa	profane, not 'restricted'
powhiri	ritual of encounter
taha wairua	spiritual dimension, includes both esoteric and everyday/more mundane aspects
taha hinengaro	mental dimension, includes both cognitive and affective aspects
taha tinana	physical dimension
taha whānau	literally extended family, but refers more broadly to collectivity, belonging, and so on
tapu	'restricted', can also refer to aspects of the 'sacred' realm
Te Ao Māori	the Māori world
te reo	the language (characteristically Māori)
Te Whare Tapa Whā	the four-sided house—a model of health and well-being
Te Wheke	the octopus
tika	right action
tikanga	cultural practices or, more specifically, practices for ensuring right action in a particular context
wai	water
waipiro	alcohol—literally, stinking water
wairuatanga	spirituality
whakapapa	genealogy, including links to land
whakawhanaungatanga	making connections with others
whānau	extended family
whanaungatanga	connection, traditionally based on whakapapa

19

The Elderly

Moira Sim, Mary Surveyor & Gary Hulse

EPIDEMIOLOGY OF DRUG USE AND RELATED MORTALITY

Drug use in the elderly is often equated with pharmaceutical drug use only. However, drug use is influenced by practices of younger days, and so it extends to alcohol and a range of other drugs. It should therefore not be assumed that drug use in the older person follows patterns set by preceding cohorts (Rosenberg 1995).

Figure 19.1 Drug use in persons aged 60+ and at all other ages

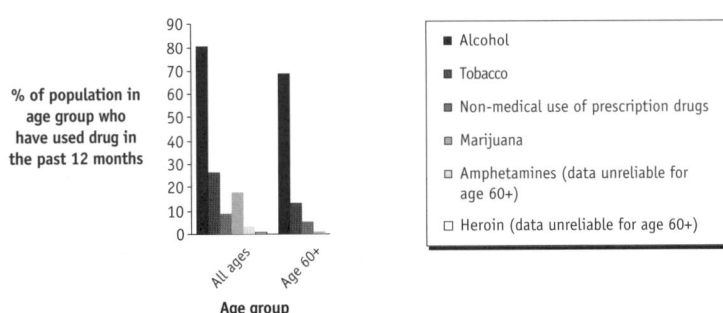

There have traditionally been sex differences in the use of various drugs. However, given that younger generations display less sex difference in consumption patterns, this effect is likely to decrease over time.

Tobacco

Tobacco is the major cause of drug-related mortality in the elderly. Male smokers outnumber female smokers; however, this difference is decreasing. Tobacco-related morbidity tends to impact most substantially in elderly men. For example, tobacco-related cancers and cardiovascular disease occur commonly after the age of 50.

Alcohol

Although total alcohol consumption is lower in the elderly than in the general population, daily drinking occurs more frequently. Alcohol use in the elderly results in falls and diseases of the gastrointestinal, cardiovascular, and central nervous systems. Harmful and hazardous alcohol use is more common in males than in females.

Prescribed medication

The use of multiple prescribed medications increases with age. Benzodiazepines and other sedative drugs are frequently prescribed to the elderly, especially to women. These are associated with considerable morbidity, with one quarter of all hospital admissions in the elderly being due to problems related to medication. Benzodiazepines, alone and in interaction with alcohol and other medications, are a major cause of falls that can lead to considerable morbidity and loss of independence.

Illicit drugs

While the use of illicit drugs is generally considered to be low in the elderly, past drug use influences drug-using behaviour in later life. Particularly in groups such as alcohol-dependent and psychiatric populations, some illicit drug use, particularly cannabis, may continue and impact on current health status. For example, cannabis use is often unsuspected in the elderly, and may cause chronic bronchitis or exacerbate existing psychiatric morbidity. In addition, past injecting drug use may emerge as talcosis or complications of blood-borne viral infections, such as cirrhosis from hepatitis C, many years after cessation of use.

Misuse of other categories of drugs

Pharmaceutical drugs are sometimes used in greater quantities than prescribed or for reasons other than as prescribed. Some elderly people misuse analgesics, and especially preparations containing codeine, which may lead to problems such as confusion and constipation. The latter may then result in laxative abuse. Other drugs sometimes misused include appetite suppressants and other weight-reducing modalities, such as diuretics and thyroxine. All the above carry significant risks, especially for those with coexisting medical problems.

Poly-drug use

The risk of poly-drug use and interactions between prescribed medications, alcohol, and other drugs increases with age. Older people commonly hoard medications, and use over-the-counter (OTC) drugs, alternative health products, or other people's medications. Many of these medications may not be considered by the elderly to be drugs and are therefore not mentioned to medical practitioners.

> Drug use in early life is a strong predictor of later use of drugs.
>
> Morbidity and mortality associated with alcohol and tobacco use become common after age 50.
>
> Interactions between multiple medications, alcohol, and other drugs are more common in the elderly.

For up-to-date information on medications that may interact with alcohol, see the MIMS website, http://www.mims.hcn.net.au

347

THE EFFECTS OF AGEING

As the body ages, the effect of drugs can change in the following ways.

Absorption, metabolism, and distribution of drugs

A reduction of gastric alcohol dehydrogenase (which metabolises alcohol prior to absorption), so that higher blood alcohol levels occur for the same amount consumed.

An increase in body fat prolongs half-lives for fat-soluble drugs such as benzodiazepines, and a decrease in lean body mass results in a smaller volume of distribution for water-soluble drugs such as alcohol. This leads to higher plasma/tissue levels of both water- and fat-soluble drugs.

- Prescribe smaller doses.
  Renal impairment is common and often clinically important in the elderly.
  Changes in hepatic metabolism may be clinically important (although there is no clear link between age and hepatic alcohol metabolism).
- Consider checking renal and hepatic function.

Vulnerability to illness caused by drugs

Smoking and alcohol tend to cause disease in later years.

The acute consequences of smoking and alcohol use (such as myocardial infarction, cerebrovascular events, internal bleeding, falls, and mental confusion) are frequently key events which result in the loss of independent living and the need for institutional care.

Age-related loss of mobility and bone density together with excessive alcohol consumption result in falls and fractures. The elderly person with poor diet is particularly vulnerable to nutritional deficiencies associated with heavy drinking.

Organic mental syndromes related to substance use (such as Wernicke's encephalopathy, chronic alcoholic dementia) are more common.

- Because of increased vulnerability to illness, quitting smoking and reducing alcohol can have substantial effects on mortality.
- There is an increased risk of complications and mortality associated with drug withdrawal (for example dehydration in alcohol withdrawal). Consider admission to monitor withdrawal.

The effect of multiple drug combinations

The interaction between benzodiazepines and alcohol results in sedation, postural hypotension, and injury.

Alcohol interferes with the metabolism of drugs such as warfarin, phenytoin, and benzodiazepines, all common medications in the elderly. Psychoactive drugs or drugs that interfere with hepatic metabolism may lower the level at which alcohol becomes hazardous.

Aspirin and other NSAIDs that can cause gastrointestinal bleeding are frequently prescribed to, or purchased over the counter by, older people. The risk of mortality associated with gastrointestinal bleeding increases with age and alcohol consumption.

A number of medications used in the elderly (for example H_2 blockers and aspirin) further reduce gastric alcohol dehydrogenase, with potential increases in blood alcohol level.

Drugs that cause disulfiram-like aversive reactions (for example sulfonamides, metronidazole) may cause severe cardiovascular consequences when mixed with alcohol.

> ➡ Alcohol interacts with many prescribed medications.
> ➡ Problems related to alcohol and other drug use can occur at lower consumption levels in the elderly compared with the younger population.
> ➡ Consider the high level of poly-drug use in the elderly when prescribing any additional drug.
> ➡ The elderly are more susceptible to complications in drug withdrawal.

ASSESSMENT

Maintaining an index of suspicion

Remembering alcohol and other drugs

Clinicians generally underestimate alcohol and other drug use in older people, as those who misuse drugs do not usually fit the stereotype of the 'alcoholic' or the 'drug addict'. The effects of drug use may mimic depression, dementia, cerebrovascular disease, and other common illnesses in older people. However, it must not be automatically assumed that symptoms and signs are related to alcohol or drug use, as the elderly are more likely to have other medical problems, such as Alzheimer's disease and cerebrovascular disease.

Many of the negative effects of drugs, such as chronic liver disease and cancer following alcohol or injecting drug use, are long-term or delayed. While health outcomes may improve on drug cessation, relative risk may remain higher than in those who have never used the drug.

> Consider not only alcohol, tobacco, and prescribed drugs in the elderly person, but also past/current use of illicit drugs, over-the-counter, and 'alternative' drugs, as well as drugs obtained from family and other prescribers.

Noting the clues

Suspect harmful use of alcohol and other psychoactive drugs in the patient with frequent falls, bruises, insomnia, depression, unstable diabetes, and deteriorating hepatic, renal, or cognitive function. In addition, suspect alcohol use with hyperuricaemia, gastrointestinal disturbances, hypertension, and malnutrition. Women with alcohol-related problems are more likely to remain undetected by medical practitioners and have a higher risk of developing alcohol–drug interactions, since they are prescribed more psychoactive drugs. Problem alcohol and other drug use is more likely in those who lack social support or during times of acute stress or depression.

Considering other sources of medication

Where there is no system of patient registration, as in Australia and New Zealand, there is great scope for polypharmacy. Patients may attend a number of different doctors and collect prescriptions. This may result from the appropriate consultation of specialists for different conditions, or it may represent an unmonitored search for other opinions. Although drug-abusing younger people doctor-shop deliberately to obtain extra prescriptions, this is uncommon in the elderly. A regular review and rationalisation of all drugs obtained from various sources reduces polypharmacy and associated morbidity.

Taking a history

Asking the questions

Whenever hazardous drug or alcohol use is suspected, seek disclosure and do not be deterred by fear of embarrassing patients or their family. Various strategies can be used to introduce the subject, such as asking 'Did you find your drinking increased after a significant other's death?', 'Does alcohol make you sleepy so that you often fall asleep in your chair?', 'Do you find that a drink helps you go to sleep?' or 'What do you do to help you cope when you're feeling sad?'

Using screening instruments

Some diagnostic instruments such as MAST and the Alcohol-related Problems Screening Questionnaire include indicators such as work performance and tolerance, and so may be less suitable for the older person. Newer instruments designed specifically for older adults, such as the MAST-Geriatric Version (MAST-G) (Blow et al. 1992) and U-OPEN (DeHart et al. 1997) have been developed with these limitations in mind. Although the CAGE and AUDIT have both been shown to be moderately useful in screening elderly populations, the AUDIT is considered slightly superior. Both are easy to use.

Competence in self-care

Self-care and the competence of the older person to attend to financial matters and make legal decisions may be impaired by alcohol and drug misuse as well as other causes of cognitive impairment, such as Alzheimer's disease, multi-infarct dementia, and electrolyte imbalance. Misuse of drugs can be an unintentional result of errors caused by confusion and poor sight or memory.

Specific issues to check for in elderly persons who are thought to consume alcohol or other psychoactive drugs include the following:
- falls or accidents
- nutritional adequacy
- family problems and social isolation
- medical problems
- ability to attend to activities of daily living
- fitness to drive a car.

> → A full drug history includes alcohol, smoking, prescribed drugs, over-the-counter drugs, 'alternative' drugs, drugs obtained from family and other prescribers, as well as illicit drugs.
>
> → Suspect harmful use of alcohol and other psychoactive drugs in a patient with frequent falls, bruises, insomnia, depression, unstable diabetes, and deteriorating hepatic, renal, or cognitive function. In addition suspect alcohol use with hyperuricaemia, gastrointestinal disturbances, hypertension, and malnutrition. Consider other medical problems, the social situation, and the ability to self-care in the elderly.
>
> → Complications of drug use can lead to considerable loss of function in the elderly.

INTERVENTION

Why treat at all?

Medical practitioners should not be pessimistic about achieving a significant and sustained change in drug use in the elderly patient. There is increasing evidence that in the elderly patient, long-term outcomes associated with attempts to reduce or cease alcohol and other drug use are at least equal if not superior to those of younger people. Perhaps this is because the elderly become increasingly aware of their increased vulnerability to illness and death. In view of the high rates of morbidity in the elderly, any small reduction in drug use can make a very significant contribution to health and well-being.

Smoking

After a lifetime of smoking, older persons may be reluctant to quit because they see the damage as already done. They may represent the 'hard-core' group whose dependence is harder to let go of, and the family may consider smoking to be one of the few pleasures left to them. However, smoking cessation has been shown to lead to substantial improvements in health. Even in the presence of significant disease, cessation may at least slow the rate of disease progression.

Alcohol

Alcohol alone or in combination with other prescribed and non-prescribed drugs contributes considerably to preventable morbidity and mortality in the older population.

Benzodiazepines

Benzodiazepines are a common cause of injury associated with falls, burns and scalds, motor vehicle accidents, as well as urinary incontinence, and confusion. Exploring non–pharmacological alternatives can substantially reduce morbidity.

> Before prescribing, ask if a drug is really needed.

Offering treatment options

Specialist alcohol and drug services tend to focus on younger people, leaving older people to the care of general practitioners in the community. The elderly need slower-paced and less confronting programs that emphasise social relationships and social support, and consider age-appropriate lifestyle issues. Stress the importance of a healthy diet and regular exercise. Encourage the use of community facilities that help with exercise appropriate to the patient's age and health. Deal with social, financial, and relationship issues, using other disciplines where appropriate.

Smoking

It is commonly assumed that older people are not as concerned about body image and pleasure as are the young. However, like younger people, older smokers fear weight gain, loss of pleasure, failure, and boredom in smoking cessation.

Although encouragement to quit smoking should generally be given regardless of age, common sense should prevail in special circumstances such as terminal disease. It is important to be optimistic and to encourage the patient to quit by providing the following information.

Following tobacco cessation (Quit: South Australian Smoking and Health Report 1992–5):

- within one month, improvements in blood pressure and lung function occur
- within three months, there are further improvements in lung function and blood flow to the limbs
- within one year cardiovascular mortality is reduced and the risk continues to fall over ensuing years
- within five years the risk of oral and oesophageal cancers is halved
- within ten years the risk of lung and pancreatic cancers is halved.

Advise the patient that continued smoking is associated with reduced mobility and physical function. Ex-smokers report better quality of life than continuing smokers. Offer advice and assistance, but respect the patient's right to follow or reject that advice.

Offer information and support, discuss alternative activities, and give positive reinforcement to offset the sense of loss and depression that may be associated with quitting. Discuss the management of insomnia during withdrawal, since this is already a common symptom in the elderly, reminding the patient that symptoms are temporary and that health improvements will occur.

Older smokers should be considered for nicotine replacement therapy and anti-craving pharmacotherapy as long as contraindications are considered, such as unstable angina, recent myocardial infarction, or cerebrovascular events.

Alcohol

Many elderly people who drink in a hazardous manner are not aware of the potential for harm. The clinician should explain the effects of alcohol, personalising its effects where possible. The knowledge of personal effects (for example increased risk of strokes in a patient known to be hypertensive) is a stronger stimulus to change behaviour than general information. In the elderly it is easier to find illnesses that can be attributable to alcohol and other drug use.

Many older adults may consider alcohol use to be beneficial; however the possible cardiovascular benefits of moderate alcohol consumption have not been established for the elderly. The optimal level of consumption is uncertain, and any levels set are likely to be overestimates for the elderly population.

Even moderate alcohol consumption may aggravate problems such as depression, domestic violence, and falls. Informing an older person who drinks at hazardous or harmful levels that moderate consumption is beneficial is likely to reinforce hazardous behaviour. In spite of these considerations, reduction of consumption may be a more realistic goal than abstinence in some patients, and may need to be negotiated.

353

> Australian NHMRC Guidelines advise older persons that if they consume alcohol, to consider drinking less than the levels set for the general population (see chapter 10). In view of the increased vulnerability of the elderly to alcohol, it may be safer with older persons to advise drinking no more than one standard drink per day in women and two standard drinks per day in men.

Complications of alcohol withdrawal are more common, and admission for monitoring and treatment of withdrawal may be advisable in the elderly.

Disulfiram is not recommended in the elderly because of severe aversive reactions if taken with alcohol, and it is contraindicated in patients with cardiovascular disease. Poor renal and poor hepatic function are contraindications to other drugs used to treat alcohol dependence, such as acamprosate and naltrexone respectively.

> Older people with problems related to drinking are more likely to live alone, experience loneliness, and to lack social support and satisfying leisure activities.

Benzodiazepines

Compared with other age groups, the elderly experience more sleep disturbance. While other treatment options are often employed for younger persons, hypnotics are commonly used as the first line of management in the elderly. While the use of benzodiazepines is a much easier and more rapid solution to the problem of insomnia, it is no more effective than the use of good sleep management techniques. However, unlike benzodiazepines, such techniques do not cause falls or confusion, and do not result in tolerance and rebound insomnia on drug cessation.

Benzodiazepines should not be used as the first line treatment of insomnia in the elderly. Alternative strategies should be offered.

*   It is essential to destroy the myth of the eight-hour sleep. Explain the normal decrease in sleep time that occurs over a lifetime.
*   Encourage exercise during the day (since this promotes deeper sleep), a regular wake-up time, and the use of bed for sleep only (not for worrying, reading, watching television, or keeping warm).
*   Reduce caffeine, alcohol, drugs, and environmental stimuli that interfere with REM sleep.
*   Discourage naps during the day, and encourage relaxation techniques in place of worrying.
*   Adequate pain management techniques are also important to reduce insomnia and early waking, which is often related to pain from osteoarthritis. In many instances, all that is required to promote a good night's sleep is use of a simple analgesic such as paracetamol before retiring or when awoken by pain.

Especially in residential care, boredom often results in early bedtimes, so that six or more hours' sleep may be completed by 2 a.m., at which time the patient believes that he/she should be asleep, and so complains of insomnia. Strategies to address this include later evening meal times, a late snack, and activities to delay retiring time. Availability of staff during the night can combat loneliness and fear and discourage sedation.

The older person is more likely to have experienced stressful life events, such as death and illness of loved ones, loss of health, loss of important relationships, and other significant life changes such as retirement. Alcohol, other sedatives, and tobacco are often used to block out loneliness, to cheer up, to help with sleep and relaxation, to relieve pain and boredom, or to give self-confidence. This may lead to overuse of these drugs.

Benzodiazepines are often first prescribed as a short-term aid during a significant stressful life event, such as bereavement or an episode of acute anxiety. However the high rate of consequent regular use suggests it is better avoided or better used for only one or two days. Consider the causes of anxiety and other ways of managing the stress associated with acute life events, for example by changing the environment. Furthermore, prescribed sedative drugs with or without alcohol are common methods of suicide in the elderly. Routine hospital use because of noisy surroundings is inappropriate. Where benzodiazepine use is unavoidable, use short–acting drugs that are less likely to result in morbidity.

> Suicide attempts in the elderly are much more likely to result in death.

During the withdrawal from drugs such as antidepressants, alcohol, benzodiazepines, and opiates, the elderly are more susceptible to sleep disturbances. As a general rule, withdrawal from medications should be more gradual than in a younger person.

Medical problems

If alcohol or drug misuse is related to ongoing medical problems, such as lack of sleep due to pain or social isolation due to mobility or other health problems, seek to optimise the management of medical problems while minimising polypharmacy.

→ Drug use in the older person may be related to loneliness, depression, and stressful life events.
→ The elderly respond better to supportive programs that are slower-paced, non–confrontational, and that focus on age-specific issues such as dealing with loneliness, learning to build social networks, and bereavement.
→ Emphasise that quitting smoking reduces illness and the progression of many common conditions, and increases mobility and general physical function.
→ Insomnia is commonly treated with inappropriate sedative prescribing in the elderly. Offer other treatment options.

355

Case studies

Case study 1

Michael is 65 years old. He retired six months ago, and is divorced. His daughter makes an appointment and accompanies him to your general practice because she is concerned that he has had a number of falls and may eventually seriously injure himself. You are not his usual GP, but Michael and his daughter are able to explain that he is diabetic with high blood pressure, and that until recent months his blood pressure and sugar had been well controlled.

Michael has taken 5 mg of nitrazepam every night for 15 years, and he appears to have been compliant with his hypoglycaemic and antihypertensive medications, but his blood pressure is now elevated and his blood sugar levels somewhat erratic. He has a few bruises of varying ages on his limbs.

He explains the falls as carelessness and says he has had no other symptoms of concern. But he admits to some difficulty with coping with not working, and to drinking more in the last six months (currently about six cans of beer a day), since he ceased work. After you explain about normal sleep patterns with age and the effect of alcohol and benzodiazepines, Michael agrees to changing from nitrazepam to temazepam at night, and to limit his alcohol intake to a maximum of two cans of mid-strength beer daily. With his daughter's help, he somewhat reluctantly agrees to trial attendance at a senior citizens' centre twice a week.

After two weeks, his blood sugar levels have stabilised and his blood pressure is improved. Although he feels that he slept better with nitrazepam, he is sleeping with temazepam and is drinking within agreed limits. To his surprise he has enjoyed the social contact at the centre.

Six months later, he is doing well and agrees to trial occasional nights off temazepam.

Case points

Michael's case illustrates:
- alcohol use often increases in response to specific life events
- alcohol and benzodiazepines interact to increase sedation, frequently causing injury
- alcohol and other drugs can exacerbate existing illness
- considering the social situation is important in the management of alcohol use in the elderly
- short-acting benzodiazepines are less likely to cause daytime sedation than long-acting counterparts.

Case study 2

You regularly attend the residents in a hostel for the frail aged. You become increasingly concerned with the large number of scripts for night sedation that you are asked to write. Further investigation indicates that many residents retire at 7 p.m. and wake up at 2 a.m., feeling lonely, and convinced that they should remain asleep until daylight, despite having had seven hours' sleep already. You discuss the problem with the hostel manager, who voices her concerns at the number of falls and fractures experienced by the residents. Over the next few weeks a number of strategies are developed and implemented.

The manager invites both residents and their relatives to attend an open meeting with you. At the meeting, you explain your concerns about the regular use of night sedation, and provide evidence of the increased risk of falls and fractures associated with this. You then invite all those present to work with you in reviewing each resident's complete list of medications with the aim of reducing dependence on sedation. It is emphasised that no one would be refused continuing sedation, but that it should be a cooperative effort. The manager suggests changing tea-time from 5 p.m. to 6 p.m., and this is agreed to by a large majority of the residents.

Subsequently a regular activities program, including organised walks, other physical programs, and concerts, is instituted on most afternoons, thus discouraging afternoon naps. The evening staff take an evening trolley to each wing at 8.30 p.m., offering a warm drink and a small sandwich to encourage later retiring.

Three months later the number of residents using regular night sedation has been reduced by 30%, and several others have substituted temazepam for nitrazepam. The residents are extremely happy with the later tea-time, the increased afternoon activities, and the late snack trolley. The number of falls recorded is also significantly reduced.

The manager and her staff ask you to hold another information evening for residents and families to discuss medication issues in general.

Case points

This study illustrates:
- the need for institution managers to assist elderly people to adjust their bedtimes to avoid lengthy early morning wakefulness
- the value of working with elderly people and their families so a program of medication management can be agreed
- the need for a slow approach to sedation reduction
- reduction of sedation leading to a significant reduction in falls.

357

Case study 3

Joe is a 75-year-old man with hypertension and heart failure, living in a nursing home, who has smoked 30 cigarettes a day since he was 17. He has tried to quit on numerous occasions, but has never managed more than a week without smoking. He is becoming increasingly short of breath and you have been encouraging him to try to quit again, but Joe is very reluctant.

Eventually Joe admits that he is fearful that he will gain a lot of weight if he stops smoking, and that that may aggravate the problems of his painful knees and hips. You then arrange for Joe to have a restricted calorie diet and offer him nicotine patches, which Joe has never tried before. Joe agrees to have a try, so you arrange to see him each week to support him. After two weeks you are able to congratulate Joe, who has stuck to his plan. The staff at the home organise a special cake for Joe to celebrate his achievement. After three months, Joe, although having relapsed to smoking at smaller quantities, feels confident of his ability to cease and is comfortable with his weight gain of 2 kg.

Case points

Joe's case illustrates:
- the difficulties associated with quitting smoking, and the need for continuous support and encouragement
- concerns such as weight gain are often common to both young and old.

REFERENCES AND FURTHER READING

Australian Institute of Health and Welfare 2000, *1998 National Drug Strategy Household Survey: Detailed findings*, AIHW, AIHW cat. no. PHE 27, Canberra.

Barry, K.L. & Blow, F.C. 2001, 'Brief alcohol interventions for older adults'. *Alcoscope International Review of Alcoholism Management*, vol. 3, pp. 8–11.

Blow, F., Brower, K., Schulenberg, J., Demo-Dananberg, L., Young, J., Beresford, T. 1992, 'The Michigan alcoholism screening test. Geriatric version (MAST-G): A new elderly-specific screening instrument', *Alcohol Clinical Experimental Research*, vol. 16, pp. 372.

DeHart, S.S. & Hoffmann, N.G. 1997, 'Screening and diagnosis: alcohol use disorders in older adults', in Gurnack, A.M. (ed.) *Older Adults' Misuse Of Alcohol, Medicines, and Other Drugs: Research and Practice Issues*, Springer Publishing Co, New York, pp. 25–53.

Rosenberg, H. 1995, 'The elderly and the use of illicit drugs: sociological and epidemiological considerations', *International Journal of the Addictions*, vol. 30, pp. 1925–51.

20

Coexisting Alcohol and Drug Use and Mental Health Disorders

Fraser Todd

OVERVIEW

Drug use and mental health disorders occur together more often than chance would predict and, when they do, they present significant problems for the patient and the treatment service. Patients with coexisting disorders tend to fall through the gaps between existing treatment services, are less likely to respond well to traditional treatments when they do engage in them, and are more likely to drop out of treatment. Many of these treatment issues arise as a result of the historical differences in culture between the mental health and alcohol and drug services, with many of the current approaches to treatment attempting to overcome these differences.

Terms and definitions

There are several terms in common usage that all mean much the same thing, none of which has met with universal acceptance. 'Dual diagnosis' is currently used by many working in the field, though many people argue that patients with dual diagnosis often have far more than two diagnoses. Another commonly used term is comorbitidy. This as well as other terms such as MICA (mental illness with chemical abuse), and coexisting drug use and mental health disorders, are, however, considered by some in the field to be either cumbersome or imprecise. However, regardless of the label given to them, there is an emerging consensus regarding the nature and treatment of coexisting disorders.

What are coexisting mental health and drug use disorders?

Coexisting drug use and mental health disorders are said to be present when mental health and drug use disorders coexist independently in the same person. While drug use (including alcohol) is often associated with psychological phenomena characteristic of mental disorders, many of these are due to the drug use itself and abate when it is no longer used. These secondary symptoms are usually considered part of the alcohol or drug disorder, and it is only when they persist independently, or when they are prominent in the face of ongoing drug use, that they can be considered a coexisting disorder.

The heterogeneity of coexisting disorders

The area of coexisting drug use and mental health disorders encompasses a wide range of mental health disorders, and several drugs of abuse, and as such is heterogeneous. The range of combinations is as wide as the number of drugs used and the variety of mental disorders suffered in a society. It is important therefore that the general principles of assessing and treating coexisting disorders must be informed by knowledge of the unique interactions between specific drugs and certain mental disorders. For example, the nature of the interaction between alcohol and social phobia, opiate use and mania, and cannabis use and schizophrenia, is quite different in many respects, not least in aetiology, course, and treatment.

➞ Coexisting disorders are common.
➞ Coexisting disorders show considerable heterogeneity, and different combinations of problems differ in their nature.
➞ Coexisting disorders are associated with poor outcomes with standard treatment approaches.
➞ Multiple problems frequently involve a range of different services with differing approaches to treatment.
➞ Coexisting disorders highlight the gaps and poor coordination between services that is inherent within the health system.
➞ Coexisting disorders respond well to integrated and comprehensive treatment approaches.

EPIDEMIOLOGY

The prevalence rates of coexisting disorders vary significantly, depending on the definition used and the population studied. Most surveys report on the prevalence of drug-use disorders without recognising that the level of drug(s) use and associated characteristics may impact significantly on the mental disorder but not meet diagnostic criteria for abuse or dependence. The majority of studies continue to exclude nicotine dependence as a drug-use disorder, despite evidence that nicotine use or withdrawal complicates a number of mental disorders. In general, however, evidence is emerging to give us a reasonable picture of the prevalence of coexisting disorders in a range of settings.

Surveys of the prevalence of mental disorder and alcohol and drug disorders in the general population have been undertaken in a number of countries, making it possible to estimate the prevalence of coexisting disorders. Most of these studies report a lifetime prevalence of coexisting disorders in the general population of between 20 and 30%.

Most studies of the prevalence of mental disorders in patients presenting to alcohol and drug services indicate that rates of coexisting disorders are higher than in the general population, but the actual prevalence rates vary markedly between studies.

The prevalence of drug use disorders among mental health patients has consistently been shown to be much higher than in the general population. Most studies suggest that for most mental health disorders, between 30 and 50% also experience a drug use disorder. The highest rates are reported in people with antisocial personality disorder, followed by bipolar disorder and schizophrenia.

361

Most of the studies performed in Australia and New Zealand indicate that the prevalence rates are largely similar to those in other countries with similar cultures. It is important to remember, however, that the differing patterns of drug use, especially the low levels of cocaine and amphetamine use in New Zealand, mean that the specific combinations of mental health and drug-use disorders are likely to be different.

AETIOLOGY

Numerous hypotheses have been proposed to explain the high rates of co-occurrence of drug use and mental health disorders. The heterogeneity and complexity of coexisting disorders is such that no simple aetiological explanation is likely to be adequate.

While it is important to understand how a person has developed the problems they present with, and future therapeutic developments often stem from increased knowledge about the causes of disorders, an understanding of how coexisting disorders have arisen in a given patient has limited impact on treatment. More important as targets for intervention are the factors that maintain and reinforce the patient's current patterns of drug use and mental dysfunction.

Theories of the aetiology of coexisting disorders

There are several theories that attempt to explain the co-occurrence of drug abuse or dependence and mental disorder.

Genetic models

A significant part of the vulnerability to both alcohol dependence and a range of mental health disorders is genetically transmitted. The importance of genetic transmission of drug-use disorders appears to be similar, but has been less well studied. The exact nature of this genetic transmission is still being explored (see chapter 2). While coexisting disorders do appear to run in families for some combinations of disorders, the disorders appear to be inherited independently.

Neurochemical models

Neurochemical theories attempt to explain coexisting disorders in terms of the relationship between a drug's effects on neurotransmitters and the underlying neurochemical changes that accompany many psychiatric disorders. For example, cannabis increases synaptic dopamine levels and this mechanism is postulated to explain its tendency to precipitate psychosis and exacerbate schizophrenia, both of which have been linked with elevated dopamine levels.

Biological reinforcement models

Biological reinforcement models consider the effects of psychoactive drugs on various neurological pathways that are involved with positive and negative reinforcement of behaviour. While presenting plausible explanations of drug abuse or dependence, these models are not necessarily relevant to other mental health problems.

Theories of temperament, character, and personality

Several theories of temperament and personality link mental disorders and drug disorders. It is likely that temperament is associated with problematic drug use, and it may influence the vulnerability to and expression of certain mental health disorders. With respect to personality, there is a strong association between certain personality disorders, especially antisocial personality disorder, and drug abuse or dependence.

The self-medication hypothesis

This popular hypothesis arose from self-reports of psychiatric patients who attribute their drug use to the need to control psychiatric symptoms, especially depression. As mentioned, there is little empirical support for the self-medication hypothesis, and the aetiology of coexisting disorders is likely to be much more complex than allowed for by this hypothesis.

Psychosocial hypotheses

Few psychosocially based theories have been proposed to explain coexisting disorders, but psychosocial factors appear to be important. Certain childhood factors such as sexual abuse, physical abuse, childhood hyperactivity, and a disadvantaged family background clearly predate the onset of drug use and are found at increased rates in those with coexisting disorders, suggesting a role in the aetiology of coexisting disorders.

Comprehensive models

Each of the models mentioned above is either supported by evidence or is clinically useful. They fall short as an explanation of coexisting disorders because they are incomplete. Drug use and mental health disorders are increasingly seen as arising due to a complex interaction of factors acting across all levels of brain organisation, including genes, neurochemicals, temperament, and character, as well as psychological, social, cultural, and spiritual factors (see chapter 2).

ASSESSMENT

It is reasonable to expect that all patients presenting with significant alcohol and drug problems are adequately screened for the presence of key mental disorders such as depression, bipolar disorder, antisocial personality disorder, social phobia, and anxiety disorders. Similarly, any patient presenting with a mental health problem should be asked about alcohol and drug use, and screened for abuse and dependence as part of the routine assessment.

An important function of the assessment interview is to engage the patient and to assess the patient's readiness to change (see chapters 5 and 7). Thus, the aim of the assessment interview, while incorporating the need to obtain information, must include as an integral component the development of rapport with the patient.

A corroborative history obtained from a significant other will make the assessment more complete.

Primary versus secondary

One of the key tasks of the initial assessment when coexisting disorders are suspected is to determine whether the mental health symptoms are a true separate condition or are secondary to the drug-use problem. While the best method of doing this is to observe the course of those symptoms during a period of abstinence from the drugs misused, it is often useful to get an idea of this relationship during the initial assessment.

There are three main lines of questioning which help determine whether the mental health disorder is secondary to the drug use or independent: age of onset, symptoms during periods of abstinence, and family history.

Age of onset

Mental health problems that occur before the onset of drug use are usually primary disorders. Mental health problems that begin in the context of pre-existing drug use may be secondary to the drug use or may represent a separate disorder. Alcohol and drug-use disorders are rarely secondary; that is, they are rarely caused by pre-existing mental health disorders.

Symptoms during periods of abstinence

While secondary mental health symptoms can persist for several weeks after drug use is stopped, symptoms that persist during longer periods of abstinence are usually primary disorders. Usually, a period of abstinence lasting over three months is considered adequate to determine safely that persisting mental health symptoms are the result of an independent mental disorder.

Family history

Most of the drug use and mental health disorders that commonly co-occur have significant genetic components, and are independently inherited. If the patient with a drug-use disorder and mental health symptoms has a family history of the same mental disorder, it is likely that that disorder is primary.

> Drug-use disorders are rarely secondary to mental disorders. To distinguish primary from secondary mental health symptoms, consider:
> - age of onset
> - symptoms during periods of abstinence
> - family history.

INTERVENTION

Interventions for people with coexisting drug use and mental health disorders are based on combining appropriate and effective treatments for both the alcohol and drug disorders, and the mental health problems, in a consistent and comprehensive treatment package that will encourage engagement and retention of patients in care. Five key principles of treatment have been identified that provide a framework for organising treatment. These are: safety, stabilisation, comprehensive assessment and treatment planning, clinical case management, and treatment integration.

Safety

Ensuring the safety of the patient and others who may be at risk takes precedence over all other decisions. This involves the assessment of risk of harm to self and to others, reviewing the patient's physical health and dealing with any urgent medical problems, and assessing the patient's ability to care for themselves safely. In doing so, consideration should be given to whether the patient should be managed as an outpatient or an inpatient, and whether initial treatment should be in a psychiatric, medical, or alcohol and drug setting. Compulsory treatment may be required.

It is relevant at this point to stress the need for cultural safety, and for all clinicians involved in the care of the patient to recognise the limits of their expertise, to take responsibility for increasing their cultural skills, and to involve appropriate health workers to address these issues (see chapters 17 and 18).

Stabilisation

Once safety is ensured, any acute issues that interfere with further treatment need to be stabilised. Such issues include acute intoxication and withdrawal, psychotic symptoms, psychosocial crises, severe anxiety or depressive symptoms, or a combination of these.

365

Comprehensive assessment and treatment planning

A comprehensive assessment and treatment plan is a dynamic process that begins with the patient's first contact, and is reviewed continually throughout the course of treatment. It aims to assess all relevant areas of a patient's life, and sets the direction of further treatment. It should be undertaken by a clinician trained in either mental health or alcohol and drug assessment.

Clinical case management

Care of the patient with a coexisting disorder is usually initially carried out by a specialist mental health team, but as stability is achieved the general practitioner is in a position to be the key worker, usually working with the support of the specialist team in a shared care arrangement.

Once the patient is stable and a comprehensive assessment has given rise to a comprehensive treatment plan, clinical case management becomes the focus for ongoing treatment. In the early stages this is usually part of the duties of the specialist team. Essential features include the following:

* continuity over time
* integration of the case manager within a multidisciplinary team
* skills in a range of interventions, such as comprehensive assessment and treatment planning, motivational interviewing, relapse prevention, monitoring of psychiatric symptoms, and education of the patient and family
* assertive follow-up and active enhancement of compliance with appointments and medication
* mobile community-based services.

The case manager should be responsible for monitoring the patient's mental state, fostering the therapeutic alliance, liaising with all clinicians involved, coordinating the management of crises, and carrying out as much of the treatment as he or she is skilled to do.

Treatment integration

Treatment integration aims to integrate the conceptual models and treatments for drug use and mental health problems into a coherent package that is easy for the patient to access and understand.

Strategies to assist treatment integration:

* arrange a single coordinating point within mental health and alcohol and drug services that delivers 24-hour care;
* consider all persisting alcohol and drug and mental health disorders as primary disorders of multiple aetiology that may follow a chronic, relapsing course;
* use compatible models and conceptual frameworks. Some of the models used in alcohol and drug treatment are compatible with those used in mental health, while others are not. For example, a strong abstinence-based approach to alcohol and drug problems does not always work well alongside a treatment approach focusing on the need for adherence with psychiatric medications;
* concentrate on harm minimisation. This approach encompasses abstinence of alcohol and drug use, and elimination or significant reduction of psychiatric symptoms, as the ultimate goal of treatment, but accepts degrees of improvement as valid goals in their own right;
* a simple framework for integrated care follows the 'Engagement–persuasion model'. This divides treatment into four stages, and is a useful way of integrating and organising the various components of treatment. Each stage has different core tasks that are the focus of treatment.

The engagement–persuasion model

The four stages of this model are: engagement, persuasion, active treatment, and relapse prevention.

- Engagement: The core task is to engage the patient in treatment and to develop the therapeutic relationship. Concentrating on this in the early stages of treatment is associated with significant improvements in retention.
- Persuasion: Once the patient is engaged in a therapeutic relationship, the key is to help him or her develop motivation to comply with treatment, and to change behaviours such as drug use that impact negatively on treatment. Techniques of motivational interviewing are the mainstay of treatment in this phase (see chapter 5).
- Active treatment: Treating both the drug-use problems and the mental health symptoms is the focus of this phase. Medication and cognitive behavioural strategies are the most common approaches, and usually allow effective integration of treatment.
- Relapse prevention: Once significant changes in health status have been achieved, the main aim is to prevent relapse, be it in the drug use or in the mental health disorder. Cognitive behavioural relapse prevention strategies are particularly useful in this context.

The key principles of treatment are:
- safety
- stabilisation
- comprehensive assessment and treatment planning
- clinical case management
- treatment integration.

Key processes to consider

In addition to the key principles mentioned above, there are several other processes that should be attended to.

Conceptual frameworks

The complexity of the problems that people with coexisting mental health and drug use disorders present with means that a range of treatment approaches are often indicated. Many of these will originate from different theoretical paradigms. Using approaches that are conceptually compatible is important in trying to put together an integrated treatment package. The following are conceptual models that fit well and are often combined in the treatment of coexisting disorders to enhance comprehensiveness and integration:
- bio-psyschosocial and disease models
- the engagement–persuasion model
- stages of change and motivational interviewing
- various cognitive–behavioural approaches, including relapse prevention.

The 12-step abstinence-focused approaches, while widely used in some countries, do not fit as neatly with the other models mentioned, and patients with coexisting disorders may have more difficulty engaging in abstinence-focused treatments. They certainly have a place, however, for those patients who are attracted to them.

Therapeutic alliance

Throughout the treatment process, consideration must be given to fostering the therapeutic alliance between patient and clinician. While dealing with issues of safety must take precedence, the therapeutic alliance provides the context within which other aspects of treatment take place.

Clinical responsibility

All people in treatment should have a clinician who is clearly designated to hold clinical responsibility. This person should be identifiable at all times.

Treatment issues for special-needs groups

There are several groups who may not engage well in treatment unless their special needs are met, and the general principles of treatment need to be elaborated upon to take this into account. Of particular importance are the following:
- cultural needs for Aboriginal Australians, New Zealand Māori, and Pacific nations peoples
- rural needs
- sexual orientation
- gender

Specific combinations of coexisting disorders

Because coexisting drug use and mental health disorders are heterogeneous, the general principles of treatment need to be informed by knowledge of the nature of specific combinations of problems.

Alcohol and mood disorders

Alcohol is commonly associated with a depressive syndrome that can be identical to a major depressive episode. In the majority of cases, these depressive symptoms abate with in a few weeks of abstinence from alcohol, and in that case the depressive symptoms are considered secondary to the alcohol use. In a minority of cases, however, the depression persists as a primary disorder, requiring specific treatment. In this case the standard treatments for depression can be easily combined with treatment for the alcohol and drug problems.

Bipolar disorder and alcohol dependence commonly coexist. There is a suggestion that alcohol may worsen treatment response and increase the speed of cycling of bipolar disorder, and that elevated mood makes relapse to drinking more likely.

Alcohol and psychosis

Alcohol-use disorder has been associated with a significant increase in the risk of hallucinations and delusions in those with psychotic disorders. Patients with schizophrenia who use alcohol are more likely to be non-compliant with medication, to experience increased psychotic symptoms, to suffer more medical problems, and to have higher rates of disruptive behaviour when unwell.

Cannabis and mood

There is little research into the effects of cannabis on mood disorders, but case series and clinical anecdote suggest that it might significantly elevate mood. As such, it possibly induces and exacerbates mania in people with bipolar disorder. It might also increase the intensity of psychotic symptoms that arise due to the mood disorder.

While a lowering of mood can occur in conjunction with cannabis intoxication, it is unlikely that cannabis use causes a depressive syndrome. There is a lack of evidence regarding the relationship between cannabis and depression, but clinical impressions lean towards the view that cannabis use may improve depressive symptoms in some people.

369

Cannabis and psychosis

Mild psychotic symptoms such as paranoia are a common part of cannabis intoxication, but cannabis can also induce a psychosis that persists for several days after intoxication. In most cases this psychosis is self-limiting if no further cannabis is used.

Cannabis probably precipitates the earlier onset of schizophrenic psychosis in those prone to develop the disorder. It is known to increase rates of hospitalisation, to increase the rate of psychotic relapse, and it probably increases the intensity of psychotic symptoms.

Opiates and mental health disorders

Opiates may induce hallucinatory experiences in some individuals, but there is little evidence that the drugs themselves induce psychiatric syndromes. Opiate dependence is important for dual diagnosis because of the very high rates of psychiatric syndromes that accompany people in treatment for opiate dependence. These especially include major depression, social phobia, and other anxiety disorders. It is likely that developmental and social factors that lead to the development of opiate dependence also increase the risk of a person developing a mental disorder, and the psychosocial circumstances associated with opiate dependence may also be a significant precipitant of psychiatric disorder in some individuals. However, many people who use opiates do not develop psychiatric illness. Rather, it seems that for those who do use opiates, the presence of a psychiatric disorder is one of the main factors in their seeking help for their opiate use.

Stimulants and mental health disorders

Stimulants such as amphetamines may be associated with a range of psychiatric symptoms as part of intoxication. The most widely described syndrome that persists beyond intoxication is amphetamine psychosis, in which a brief psychotic reaction may last for several weeks before ameliorating. In some cases, a more chronic schizophrenia-like illness may be precipitated by amphetamine use, though it is unclear if amphetamines cause this or merely precipitate an underlying psychotic illness in those with a vulnerability to it.

Anxiety disorders and drug use

High rates of drug use disorders are found in people with anxiety disorders. This is complicated by anxiety symptoms that often occur as part of an alcohol or drug withdrawal syndrome. Attempting to stop drug use before treating the anxiety disorder is optimal, but it is frequently not possible. Most anxiety treatments are effective to some degree in those whose drug use continues but is stable.

Potentially abusable medications prescribed for mental health problems

Two classes of drugs in particular, the benzodiazepines and the anticholinergics, are widely prescribed to patients with mental illnesses and are thought to have significant liability to abuse.

Benzodiazepines

Benzodiazepines are widely used in mental health settings to treat anxiety, insomnia, and agitation. The addiction potential or liability to abuse of benzodiazepines varies between individuals, and those with a predisposition to alcohol or drug dependence are more likely to have problems controlling their use of benzodiazepines prescribed for mental health purposes. It is also important to recognise that benzodiazepines differ in their abuse liability and their range of side-effects, with those with a slower onset of action such as nitrazepam or oxazepam being less likely to be abused.

The use of these drugs for short periods in a controlled environment, such as an inpatient unit, is probably safe and warranted for most patients. However, there are reasonable alternatives to benzodiazepines for most conditions for which they may be indicated, and they should therefore be used with caution in less controlled environments. This is especially pertinent for patients with a history of abusing other drugs or with a family history of alcohol or drug dependence. When a clinician decides that a benzodiazepine is indicated, consideration should be given to using those drugs with a lower abuse potential (see chapter 11).

Anticholinergics

Anticholinergic medications such as benztropine and orphenadrine are valuable adjuncts to the use of antipsychotic medication due to their ability to reduce extrapyramidal side-effects. These medications are occasionally abused for the euphoria and hallucinations they can induce, but they can also induce unwanted side-effects, including impairment of memory and cognition after long-term use, and a withdrawal syndrome. A toxic delirium may result, although it is less clear that these symptoms are always welcome (see chapter 12).

With increasing use of the newer atypical antipsychotics such as risperidone and olanzapine, the need to prescribe these medications should decrease.

Case study

You are a GP in rural community. Geoff, a 55-year-old man of European descent, comes to see you complaining that he has been feeling despondent over the last few weeks and is not enjoying life like he used to. He currently lives with his 75-year-old aunt, having separated from his wife 15 years ago. He puts his low mood down to the pressures of caring for his frail aunt and to his lack of money.

You are aware that Geoff has a history of bipolar affective disorder that began in his early teens, and that this has led to 18 acute psychiatric admissions from the age of 27 years, mostly for mania. He is currently seen approximately once a month by a mental health outreach team and is known to be compliant with medication (lithium carbonate 1250 mg at night, with a recent serum level of 0.9 mmol/L).

Assessment indicates that Geoff drinks three to five jugs of beer four times weekly when manic, and one to two jugs two to three times weekly when not manic. He has a history of moderate alcohol dependence (no withdrawals). He completed a six-week residential alcohol treatment program 10 years ago, and was abstinent for 12 months after this before relapsing during a manic episode. He occasionally attends Alcoholics Anonymous meetings when his mood is well controlled. He has four past convictions for driving under the influence of alcohol, and three for dangerous driving at excessive speed when sober but manic. He has a past history of heavy gambling, and he currently bets on horses regularly. He spends much of his sickness benefit on gambling and alcohol. His mental health outreach team are aware of the drinking and gambling problems but rarely discuss them with him.

You talk with Geoff about the pressures he is under, and, using a motivational approach, guide him to consider the interconnection between his gambling, alcohol use, mood problems, and social stresses. You specifically point out that alcohol use is likely to destabilise his mood disorder, and that when his mood disorder is destabilised it is likely to limit his ability to control his alcohol use and his gambling. You note that all three problems will increase his financial and social difficulties, and this will in turn worsen his bipolar disorder and alcohol dependence. Together, you agree that a period of abstinence from alcohol for several months would be useful, and you contact his mental health case manager to inform the outreach team of the situation.

Three weeks later you are called to see Geoff at the police station after he was arrested following a high-speed car chase. He appears intoxicated and irritable. He gives a two-week history of increasingly elevated mood, currently manic. You contact the local alcohol and drug services, but they are unwilling to get involved with Geoff on the grounds that his problems are clearly related to his mental illness. The local psychiatric services inform you that his problems seem to be related to alcohol intoxication, but eventually agree to admit him to an acute psychiatric unit to keep him safe. You try to get Geoff to accept admission willingly, but he refuses to do so. Accordingly you initiate compulsory admission on the grounds of his risk to himself and others from his poor judgment, especially behind the wheel of a motor vehicle.

Geoff presents to your surgery six weeks later. His mood has returned to normal and he has been discharged from hospital with sodium valproate added to his lithium. While he did not consume alcohol during his time in hospital, he has had one or two jugs of beer on three occasions since. He has continued to gamble in moderation without significant losses. He reports that he was told in hospital to stop drinking, but he is not receiving any help to do this.

You discuss with Geoff various options for treatment. For his alcohol problem these are attendance at Alcoholics Anonymous, since this has previously proved useful, and the use of medications such as naltrexone to control his alcohol craving, coupled with a cognitive–behavioural approach to alcohol control that would fit well with the treatment approaches for his mood disorder. For his gambling, you discuss involvement of pathological gambling specialists, and attendance at Gamblers Anonymous. You also suggest he could access consumer-based support groups for his mood disorder.

You contact Geoff's mental health case manager, and the case manager agrees to take a lead role in coordinating Geoff's overall management. As a move towards this you suggest that a meeting be convened which involves the range of agencies involved in Geoff's care. This would include the police, social services, gambling and alcohol and drug treatment agencies and his mental health outreach team. The meeting would have the aim of clarifying the role of each agency and coordinating responses, so that a single, coherent approach is shared and reinforced by all people involved. You also suggest the involvement of people involved with the care of his aunt, so that the use of support services for her could be maximised to reduce the stress on Geoff.

Case points

Geoff's case illustrates:
- the complex interactions between substance use and mental health problems
- coexisting alcohol and drug use and mental health disorders leading to multiple problems in multiple areas, and the need to involve a range of different services with differing approaches to treatment
- that coexisting disorders highlight the gaps and poor coordination between alcohol and drug and mental health services that is inherent within health systems
- that treatment can usefully be organised under five key headings:
  1 Safety
  2 Stabilisation
  3 Comprehensive assessment and management planning
  4 Clinical case management
  5 Treatment integration.

REFERENCES AND FURTHER READING

Treatment Protocol Project 1999, 'The patient with a dual diagnosis', in *Acute Psychiatric Inpatient Care: A Source Book*, World Health Organisation Collaborating Centre for Mental Health and Substance Abuse, Brown, Prior & Anderson, Burwood, New South Wales, pp. 144–55.

US Department of Health and Human Services 2000, 'Assessment and treatment of patients with coexisting mental illness and alcohol and other drug abuse', in *Treatment Improvement Protocol* (TIP), Series 9, Substance Abuse and Mental Health Services Administration, Center for Substance Abuse Treatment, Rockville MD.

21

Professional Issues

Moira Sim, Eric Khong, Gary Hulse, Rose Friend & Gavin Cape

This chapter deals with three major alcohol and drug issues confronting the medical profession.

The first issue concerns the role of the medical practitioner in relation to general patients who use alcohol and drugs. Doctors see people who use a range of drugs at varying levels. For the majority of these patients, drug use is not associated with significant harm. However, for a subsection of patients, drug-use patterns are problematic and commonly associated with psychosocial and physical harm. Many of these people fail to report, and some even to acknowledge, their drug use.

Drug use may be illicit (for example heroin, amphetamines) or licit (for example alcohol, tobacco). Within this context there are many barriers to the medical practitioner raising the issue of alcohol and other drug use. Even when the presence of drug use is known, its extent may be hidden. The medical practitioner is effective in changing alcohol and other drug-use behaviour, and can improve health even when drug use continues. It is therefore argued that a duty of care exists to raise alcohol and other drug issues with patients to improve health outcomes.

The second issue concerns the patient who seeks psychoactive drugs from the doctor. Such a patient confronts the practitioner with difficult decisions about prescribing. This chapter examines strategies to help the doctor find a healthy balance between the two extremes of becoming over-involved and being uncaring.

The third issue is that drug abuse and dependency occurs within the medical fraternity, as in other parts of the population. This chapter identifies risk factors and signals of problem alcohol and other drug use, and suggests how to deal with these. It is highlighted that medical practitioners have a professional duty to ensure that prompt intervention is provided to all colleagues who develop these problems, and that there are potential medico-legal consequences to non-reporting of impairment. Medical Boards and the Medical Council have developed supportive mechanisms for medical practitioners in this situation.

GENERAL BARRIERS IN RAISING ALCOHOL AND OTHER DRUG ISSUES

There are a number of commonly recognised barriers to medical practitioners raising alcohol and other drug issues with patients. These need to be acknowledged and overcome.

Is this the role of the medical practitioner?

Medical practitioners sometimes fear that asking about alcohol and other drug use might be an intrusion. However, patients see this as a valid role of the medical profession. Doctors (especially general practitioners) see the majority of the population every year. Furthermore, alcohol and tobacco use causes substantial morbidity, and medical practitioners are effective in changing drug-use behaviour. This gives the medical community an unparalleled opportunity to influence health outcomes.

375

> Medical practitioners have a duty to influence drug-using behaviour in the community.

The less glamorous side of medicine

Medical practitioners often consider patients with alcohol and other drug problems to be disruptive to their practice, and choose not to encourage service delivery to them. In addition, with relatively few medical practitioners sympathetic to drug users, those who are sympathetic tend to attract other patients with similar problems. This further discourages practitioner involvement with this group. The reality is, however, that there is no such thing as a drug- and alcohol-free medical practice. All practices have patients who use licit and illicit drugs. These patients simply conceal drug use, particularly if they believe this will prejudice the medical practitioner against them. However, without such crucial information, diagnoses may be incorrect, and unnecessary investigations and ineffective treatments offered.

> Most people who use illicit drugs are only too grateful to find a medical practitioner who understands their ambivalence to drugs and the effects they have on their lives.

Many medical practitioners view all patients who use drugs (particularly illicit drugs) as being desperate and deceitful. However, those who work with illicit drug users know how rewarding this work can be. Many illicit drug users feel judged by others, and are appreciative of the relationship with a practitioner with whom they can be open. When difficult gains are made, for example gradual reduction from a heavy consumption of benzodiazepines, the personal reward as a health professional is greater. Sometimes merely continuing to engage a poorly compliant patient with complex problems can be a huge achievement in itself. Over time (usually years), other gains follow. In addition, skills learned in the management of the problem drug-use patient (for example motivational interviewing, limit setting) are invaluable for other areas of medicine.

Practitioner experience

The traditional culture of undergraduate medical education insists that students must always appear to know everything. Medical graduates learn not to raise issues, such as illicit drugs, that might display their ignorance. However, the admission of ignorance creates the opportunity to learn from patients and gives time to seek answers.

On the other hand, medical practitioners, like other people in the population, may smoke tobacco or cannabis and drink alcohol. It is easy to minimise the importance of these behaviours in patients if they parallel one's own behaviour. However, medical practitioners should always take every opportunity to promote health in all patients.

Organisation of medical care

When caring for people with chronic complex problems, professional isolation can lead to a sense of being overwhelmed. Developing systems to share care can reduce the load and lead to more effective care.

In a practice setting, it is important to agree on a common approach to patients to prevent the process of 'splitting', where a patient's behaviour with each individual practitioner leads to conflicts and inconsistencies in practice between practitioners. Discussion between colleagues, and clear documentation of advice to patients and treatment plans, can mitigate this.

Overcoming barriers

Recognising these barriers and placing them in a more balanced perspective will assist the practitioner to transcend these issues. While there are barriers to working with patients with alcohol and other drug-related problems, it is rewarding work that can reap long-term health outcomes.

WORKING WITH PATIENTS: COMMONLY ENCOUNTERED ISSUES

A number of special issues are frequently encountered when managing patients with complex problems, including those with alcohol and other drug problems. It is useful to consider these and develop strategies to deal with them.

Patient groups

Patients use alcohol and other drugs and acknowledge harm related to this use at varying levels. One can consider patients in four groups. The corresponding actions to take in each case are outlined in table 21.1.

Table 21.1   Using the opportunity to deal with drug issues

Patient category	*Opportunity for action*
Presenting complaint unrelated to alcohol and other drug use.	To identify hazardous drug use and to encourage behaviour change early (for example reduce tobacco use or binge drinking on weekends), and to reduce harm if drug cessation is not likely (for example discourage driving under the influence of alcohol).
Presenting complaint related to alcohol and other drug use, but patient unaware of this connection.	To link symptom or problem with alcohol or other drug use (that is, personalise the effect of drug), and offer help.
Presenting complaint clearly related.	To emphasise link between the symptom or problem and the alcohol or other drug use, and offer help.
Drug seeking (for example seeking opioids or benzodiazepines).	To engage the patient in a therapeutic relationship, to offer a controlled safer drug regime, and to offer harm reduction until drug cessation is practical.

377

Window of opportunity

Brief advice from medical practitioners can be highly effective, especially when offered prior to the development of severe pathology. When the presenting complaint is related to alcohol and other drug use, this opportunity should not be missed. Advice linked to the personal effects of a drug can be a strong stimulus for change (see chapter 5). For example, a 50-year-old man whose doctor explains that alcohol worsens his blood pressure and diabetes control is more likely to heed medical advice to reduce his alcohol intake than to respond to a public advertisement against excessive alcohol use outside that context.

Boundaries

People who use drugs in a way that is considered unacceptable to society often have concerns about confidentiality. When they do disclose information to a medical practitioner, there may be complex matters revealed, and problems may be difficult to solve. Medical practitioners may find themselves in the dilemma of wanting to help and do as patients ask, but having medico-legal responsibilities that prevent certain actions. Being aware of responsibilities and limits of confidentiality, as well as developing good boundaries and support mechanisms, is essential for healthy practice.

Confidentiality

Patients may want to keep issues such as alcohol and other drug use concealed from others (including family). There may be shame about the extent of licit drug use or fear of the legal implications (for example custody of children). In general, without consent medical practitioners may not disclose information obtained in a professional capacity to a third party. Confidentiality promotes trust and honesty, and is essential to the therapeutic relationship. Medical practitioners must explain the limits of confidentiality (that is, situations in which this cannot be maintained, such as high risk of harm to self or others).

Developing good boundaries

Medical practitioners graduate with an expectation of being able to help people, but are rarely taught to set limits and to let patients take responsibility for their own problems. Mastering these skills will extend the ability to practise in a healthy manner.

Medical practitioners who treat people with problem drug use often develop a strong rapport, since these patients often feel marginalised and value this relationship. They require advocacy and long-term care. The medical practitioner is often viewed as a unique and sympathetic person colluding against the general health system (which is often percieved as judgmental and authoritarian severe). In this context, it is easy to see why medical practitioners easily begin to feel special and indispensable. But where is the line between being a good caring medical practitioner and involvement that is inappropriate and unprofessional? If a medical practitioner can answer 'yes' to the following questions it may be time to reflect, to talk with colleagues, or, in some cases, seek professional help.

Questions to ask yourself about your boundaries with patients

- Do you tell your patients details about your own personal life?
- Do you think frequently about particular patients and their management, including on days off?
- Do you feel that you are the only one who can effectively treat your patients?
- Do you think that other medical practitioners do not understand your patients, and feel the need to advocate for them constantly?
- Do you find yourself rescuing patients (for example, patients keep attending in crisis unannounced despite being asked to make appointments, but you continue to squeeze them in)?
- Do you find yourself saying one thing and doing another (for example, telling your patient that you will not prescribe, and then doing so)?
- Do you socialise with patients? Sometimes this is unavoidable (for example, in rural or remote practice), but where it cannot be avoided can you separate the times when you are a medical practitioner and when you are a friend? Socialising with patients is a major problem if you feel that your behaviour as a medical practitioner is compromised, for example if for reasons of friendship and not professional judgment you prescribe a drug you would rather not prescribe.

When one is directly involved in a consultation process it can be difficult to step back and observe the process. A colleague or professional supervisor may be able to see when an alternative solution is more appropriate as in the following case.

Case study 1

Phil is a 35-year-old male doctor who prescribes benzodiazepines to a female friend who has had a recent traumatic separation. When requests to do late-night home visits and prescribe benzodiazepines increase, he feels increasingly uncomfortable but unable to extricate himself from the situation. Discussion with a colleague enables him to set some clear boundaries and to arrange a transfer of her care to another medical professional.

379

Feeling cheated

Medical practitioners often feel cheated when patients with alcohol or drug problems do not tell them the truth, for example when patients hide the fact that a relapse has occurred. Yet the same medical practitioners react differently when they discover that their diabetic patients have lied about their diet or exercise. However, the situations are not dissimilar.

Patients may hide the truth for fear of a punitive outcome (for example cessation of a drug on which they are dependent), or from a desire to please the practitioner. The person who uses alcohol and other drugs usually feels guilty and expects to be punished following a relapse. Tell patients from the outset that relapse is common, and that if it occurs you will continue working with them. Focus on what the patient views as progress while leaving your personal feelings out of the interaction. For example, 'How do you feel about the past week?' is better than 'I'm really proud of you for not drinking for a whole week!'

Missed appointments

Many medical practitioners assume that patients with problematic drug use will miss appointments. While a degree of flexibility is always needed, patients usually respond well to clear explanations of expectations and follow through of consequences. While medical practitioners may be sympathetic to the problems experienced, not setting clear limits can result in the medical practitioner feeling devalued and used.

The dilemma

People who use drugs in a harmful manner are at risk of overdose and other complications. When caring for them, the doctor has to make judgments about the potential for causing harm by prescribing, versus the risk of continued drug use and alienation from the helping profession.

Table 21.2   The dangers of prescribing

Patient level	*Practice level*	*Societal level*
Avoidance	**Easy target**	**Violence**
May help to avoid other treatment options (for example managing depression, detoxification)	Increases the likelihood of other drug-seeking patients presenting to the practice since prescribers who are easy targets become well known to subgroups of drug users.	May increase the potential for violence
Drug dependence		**Illicit supplies**
May facilitate drug dependence		May increase supplies of licit drugs in illicit markets.
Overdose		
May increase the risk of overdose death, particularly in combination with alcohol and other illicit drugs. While strategies such as daily dispensing can reduce the risk of overdose, there remains a high risk of abuse and harm.		

The risks of prescribing

Before prescribing psychoactive drugs it is useful to consider the impact at a number of levels, as illustrated in table 21.2.

There are safer methods of prescribing and these are described below in the discussion of drug-seeking behaviour.

The regulatory dilemma

The doctor is placed in an invidious position of being both helper and 'police officer' because of notification requirements. While offering help, the doctor is frequently required to notify the local authorities of suspected drug addicts. There is a duty of care both to the patient and to the public enshrined in legislation, and this can be a barrier to disclosure, particularly of illicit drug use.

The need for notification can, however, be helpful in stabilising behaviour. For example, when a patient on long-term opioids for chronic pain is suspected of seeking extra opioid supplies, the doctor may explain that attempts to seek additional opioids elsewhere will result in notification of dependence. This allows the doctor and patient to establish a plan for improved treatment of chronic pain while addressing the development of dependence.

Intoxication

From time to time patients may present intoxicated. Where consciousness is impaired, refer the patient immediately to a hospital for neurological monitoring. All doctors should ensure that they are skilled in the management of overdose. Remember that an intoxicated patient cannot give legal consent to treatment. When a patient is unable to consent to treatment (for example where consciousness is impaired by drugs or alcohol), and the treatment proposed is not urgent, wait until the patient has regained the capacity to consent. All episodes of intoxication should be documented.

Criminal activities

As medical practitioners we may become aware of criminal activities that our drug dependent patients become involved in to support their drug habits. Patients should be informed of limits to confidentiality. Medical records are not immune to warrants, and medical practitioners can be subpoenaed to give information. In general it is best to avoid discussing criminal activities, since these are largely peripheral to the medical practitioner's role in patient care. However, if, during the course of work, information comes to light that might help to prevent harm to the public, medical practitioners have a duty to report this (for example knowledge of intention to commit a crime that may put others at risk of harm). If unsure of the appropriate action in such situations, contact your medical defence organisation promptly.

Drug-seeking behaviour

Drug-seeking behaviour has been described as 'the presentation of people falsely reporting symptoms in order to obtain a prescription or requesting a drug in order to maintain an abuse or dependence pattern of drug use'. However, this is just one end of a continuum, and many patients who seek drugs of dependence may have genuine distress for which they seek help.

Recognising drug seeking

Doctor shopping is an extreme form of drug-seeking behaviour in which an individual obtains large quantities of prescribed psychoactive drugs. Doctor shoppers are people who attend multiple doctors in search of drugs of abuse (also see chapter 14). A high index of suspicion should be held when benzodiazepines or opiates are requested, particularly by patients who are new to the practice. See 'Strategies for assessment and management of drug seekers' on page 384.

Right to refuse to see or prescribe for a patient

Prescribing to a patient who may be doctor shopping is risky, as outlined above under the risks of prescribing. A doctor can refuse to offer treatment to a patient as long as the situation is not life-threatening and there is access to other practitioners. However, engaging a patient in dialogue and offering further care without necessarily prescribing any drugs of dependence, can be a positive step. When the drug seeker realises that the doctor will not prescribe but is still interested in caring for him/her, an opportunity to address general health concerns becomes possible.

Understanding drug-seeking behaviour

Drug-seeking behaviour may be the most successful means a person has found to relieve the experience of genuine distress. Drug use may be used to dull emotional or physical pain and to fill a void.

> ➡ Compassion and understanding are key characteristics expected of health professionals. But compassionate insight alone leaves the doctor at risk of collusion, 'at-risk' prescribing, becoming the 'soother' and enabler of drug dependence, perpetuating a dependent relationship, and in danger of professional misconduct.

The management of the drug seeker

In managing a drug-seeking person, the two extremes of over-involvement (poor boundaries) and over-distancing (not caring) are easy pitfalls and can be managed by setting clear boundaries (see 'Developing good boundaries' above). Remember that long-term decisions do not have to be made immediately. When feeling under pressure to prescribe, saying 'no' and inviting the patient back for review can be a good technique.

Some useful statements to use when saying 'no' are:

- 'I'm sorry, I don't think that is a reasonable treatment. However I do recommend ...'
- 'I believe using such a medication in this situation will cause more problems. I don't prescribe it. What I can offer is ... (for example medication) or ... (for example referral). It is your choice.'
- 'In this situation I suggest a team approach. I would like you to see ...'
- 'If you had these previously, I will need to find out more from the doctor who used to prescribe it before I can do the same. In the meantime ...'
- 'Before I start to prescribe such medications I need authorisation from the health authorities. Unfortunately, there are people who go to different doctors looking for medication like these and I have been warned not to start these without first checking.'

> When saying 'no', offer alternatives. If patients choose not to follow through with alternative advice or options, it is their prerogative. You do not have to offer alternatives that you are uncomfortable with, and you do not have to take responsibility for their decisions not to take what you offer them.

If you feel the need to prescribe on the day, a small amount (for example 5 × 5 mg diazepam) is unlikely to result in an overdose or a reputation as an easy target. An appointment can be scheduled the next day so that a further assessment and discussion can take place. People who are drug seeking but not keen to engage in a therapeutic dialogue are unlikely to return the next day. For safer prescribing, consider the strategies for assessment and management of drug seekers outlined below.

Engage the patient—use common sense, courtesy, and the appropriate level of neutrality needed to establish effective relationships with patients. Don't pretend to know what you do not know. Refer on if you feel unable to manage the situation.

Managing patients with chronic pain

The continuum of pain and dependence

Among patients who present to medical practitioners seeking analgesia there is a continuum from the patient who is clearly drug seeking and for whom opiates are inappropriate, to the patient who genuinely requires potent analgesia. To complicate matters, patients who fit criteria for abuse or dependence may suffer genuine pain and require opiate analgesia. This is a controversial area where over- and under-prescribing is common and associated with significant morbidity. Seek help from a pain specialist if unsure.

The use of opiates for chronic pain

The decision to use opiates in the treatment of chronic pain should only be made after a full assessment of the cause of the pain, exploration of non–pharmacological treatment and minor analgesia, and consultation with a pain specialist. In general, avoid opiate treatment outside hospital for anyone with a history of previous or continuing drug dependence except in acute emergencies prior to hospital transfer, for example an apparent fracture. Opiates should also be avoided in the psychologically unstable, in young people, and in those with obscure pathology or a complex compensatable problem (for example compensation for injury).

Managing chronic pain in suspected opiate dependence

In managing pain for a known or suspected opiate dependent person:

- Establish an honest and supportive relationship (accept the patient's experience of pain).
- Learn about and explain the pain syndrome.
- Be clear and consistent.
- Define specific goals and expectations, as well as the consequences of not achieving these (for example review of current prescribing arrangements and establishment of an alternative, such as a supervised methadone maintenance program that is more appropriate for the treatment of dependence).
- Take time to make significant decisions such as whether to use opiates for chronic pain. Pain may be experienced as severe, but an inappropriate decision to commencing opiate treatment may result in greater pain later. The patient has managed to survive up till that point without your urgent intervention. There are other options. Do not let yourself be pressured into a decision without having the necessary information and specialist support. If there is urgent need, a hospital admission may be more appropriate.
- Arrange an assessment at a chronic pain clinic (preferably multidisciplinary).
- Diagnose and manage other mental and physical problems.
- Use physiotherapy, counselling, cognitive-behavioural therapy, psychotherapy, relaxation, meditation, self-expression techniques, hypnosis and other therapies, in addition to pharmacotherapy.
- Decide on the roles of each practitioner involved, define a primary practitioner, and establish good communication between practitioners who share care.
- Monitor treatment progress, compliance, and symptoms regularly.

Strategies for assessment and management of drug seekers

Assessment

Identity

- Establish the identity. People who seek psychoactive drugs from multiple doctors may use false identities. Be cautious if you do not know the patient.

Diagnosis

- Establish the diagnosis. It is illegal to prescribe solely to maintain dependence, except in specific programs such as methadone maintenance programs. What other issues need to be dealt with?
- Are there warning signs? Are the story or symptoms inconsistent? Has the person recently moved into the area with an accompanying letter from a specialist (who cannot be contacted) endorsing opioid use? Has the patient presented late in the day or on a weekend? Does the patient request a specific drug and reject other options? Does the patient claim to need prescribed drugs to stay off illicit drugs? Does the patient claim to have lost or been robbed of a script or medication? Does the patient threaten suicide or harm to someone if he/she does not get what he/she wants?
- Do you feel uneasy? Treat the patient with respect, but listen to your intuition and feelings of suspicion, and delay decisions to another appointment to give time to find out more information.

Management

Immediate management of drug-seeking behaviour

- Is there a clear contraindication to prescribing immediately? Is the person intoxicated? Does intoxication need to be dealt with further?
- Is it helpful to get more information immediately? Can you call the health authorities that have information on doctor shoppers or registered addicts? Checking this information with the patient in the consulting room with you lets the patient know that you are able to access health authorities and information easily. On the other hand, calling with the patient outside the room gives more freedom to speak without being heard. Either can be useful.
- Is there any reason that drugs need to be prescribed immediately? Does the patient appear to be in withdrawal? Are the withdrawals from a drug that has the potential to cause complications? Is an alternative plan required (for example admission into a detoxification unit)?
- If prescribing is required immediately, how can you increase safety? Use small amounts where possible (for example limit the amount prescribed or dispensed).
- If prescribing is not needed, learn to say 'no' firmly but compassionately. Offer alternatives to drug treatment. Offer referral to a drug clinic.

Long-term plan for drug-seeking behaviour

- Establish the primary problem that needs to be dealt with. If the issue is dependence, discuss treatment options (see chapter 5).
- If the issue is pain, establish a pain management plan, using a multidisciplinary pain management team where possible.
- If the patient is a recreational drug user who is unwilling to reduce or cease this use, then use this as an opportunity to practise harm reduction (see chapter 5) and to establish a relationship.

Other issues that need addressing
- Are there other health issues that need to be addressed? Is drug use a method of managing depression or anxiety?

Caution

Prevent theft
- Prescription pads and stationery with letterheads are useful in obtaining licit drugs illicitly. Make sure that you do not turn your head or leave the room with the patient present.

Always document
- the reasons for prescribing in the history and examination
- the management decisions, doses, and amounts of addictive drugs prescribed
- any intoxication
- advice given about the risk of overdose (including the increased risk with poly-drug use).

Personal or staff safety
- Although violence does not generally take place, all practices should be prepared for this. If threatening behaviour occurs, explain that this is not acceptable. If he/she persists, stand up and calmly ask the patient to leave. If he/she does not, warn that the police will be called, and follow through with this if he/she does not comply. If personal or staff safety is at risk because of refusal to prescribe, it is better to prescribe and to call the police afterwards. Plan ahead, have a practice policy in place, and train staff to ensure that they know what to do in a threatening situation.

Case study 2

Andrew is a 55-year-old GP in a small rural town where he has been the Jones' family doctor for 25 years. He has delivered all their children, and their families often share Sunday evening dinners and picnics. Stephanie, the youngest Jones, suffers a serious motor vehicle accident in the city and returns home to recuperate from a fractured femur and pelvis on slow-release morphine tablets. Andrew encounters difficulty controlling Stephanie's pain, and is called out with increasing frequency at night to administer intramuscular opiate injections.

Scenario 1
Andrew is unable to control Stephanie's pain despite increasing her opiates and the frequency of home visits. The family becomes more concerned and frustrated by Stephanie's suffering. Andrew feels obliged to look after Stephanie

and feeling guilty about the poor pain control acquiesces to her demands for increasing analgesia. Mr and Mrs Jones decide to take their daughter to another GP for a second opinion, and are referred to a pain specialist in the city. Andrew finds out and is upset that the Jones have lost faith in him. They cease to have any relationship from that point.

Scenario 2

Andrew finds that he is unable to control Stephanie's pain adequately. He supplements her analgesia with NSAIDs and paracetamol, which help only temporarily. Andrew discusses a referral to the pain management clinic at the hospital, and this is accepted. After a few weeks in the hospital and completion of a pain management course, Stephanie is successfully established on a new analgesia regime. From time to time, Andrew is still called to review her regime, but he does this in conjunction with the pain specialist. He finds setting limits easier this way. The Jones still continue to see him at a professional and social level.

ALCOHOL AND OTHER DRUG USE BY DOCTORS

Like other people in society, medical practitioners use and can develop problems related to alcohol and other drugs. However, there are special issues for the medical practitioner in this situation, and these can prevent the practitioner seeking help. Early recognition and intervention of such problems in oneself and in colleagues is likely to result in better outcome for the medical practitioner and for society.

Patterns of alcohol and other drug use

Prevalence

The prevalence of alcohol and illicit drug use in medical practitioners has been shown in several British and US studies to be at least as high as that in the general population. The American Medical Association has estimated lifetime prevalence of alcohol and drug dependence among medical practitioners to be 6–8% and 1–2% respectively. The lifetime prevalence of substance abuse among medical practitioners in Australia has been estimated to be about 7.7% (Wijesinghe & Dunne 1999). Using this latter figure, one could expect that a staggering 4000 out of the 50 000 medical practitioners in Australia and 800 out of the 10 000 in New Zealand would at some point in their lives develop a substance abuse disorder. Substance misuse is the major reason that medical practitioners in Australia and New Zealand come before the disciplinary section of Medical Boards or the Medical Council.

Risk factors

There are high rates of suicide, marital disturbance, and physical and emotional problems in the medical profession. The stresses associated with medical practice, such as long hours of work, fatigue, pressure on time and resources, the demands of the job and patients, fear of failure, fear of litigation, as well as ambivalence to and disillusionment with medicine, have a large part to play in the aetiology. Coupled with ready access to drugs, these can lead to inappropriate drug use. Risk factors for increased vulnerability are discussed in the section 'Early signs of impairment in the medical practitioner' on page 389. Statistically, male medical practitioners, particularly general practitioners, anaesthetists, and emergency physicians, are at higher risk.

Professional responsibility

Impediments to seeking help

Denial is part of the picture of developing drug dependence, and is reinforced by the culture of medical training. High expectations are conferred on the new medical graduate, who is welcomed into a noble profession. The great sense of responsibility to live up to expectations work against early admission of the need for help. The practitioner who begins to acknowledge a problem usually fears the public implications of disclosure. This is compounded by the conspiracy of silence among family, friends, and colleagues, leaving the practitioner isolated. Unfortunately, many cases are detected at later stages when intervention involves penalties that range from temporary withdrawal from work, with its concomitant stigmatisation, to de-registration.

Duty of care to the public

When a medical practitioner is not functioning well, there are enormous implications for public safety. A medical practitioner has a duty to ensure that he/she practises only when fit to do so. Seeking help early results in the best personal outcome and public good.

Taking care and responsibility for oneself as a medical practitioner

The doctor's own drug use

Most people consume some form of psychoactive drug (for example caffeine, alcohol, tobacco). The medical community is not immune to the negative effects of these drugs, but medical practitioners with drug dependency are often capable of working undetected for many years before a crisis occurs. By the time drug dependence has an impact on work performance, the problem is severe.

Warning signs

There are a number of warning signs of problematic alcohol and other drug use, long before any effects at the workplace become apparent. These are outlined below.

The aim of early intervention is to deal with underlying issues before effects on the workplace occur. Medical Boards or the Medical Council usually regard the doctor as impaired, and deal with the matter as an illness rather than an offence.

Early signs of impairment in the medical practitioner

The following list is adapted from Centrella (1994), and Weir (2000).

Risk factors
- unresolved psychological issues
- family history of alcohol or other drug dependence, or depression/suicide
- pattern of high achievement, habitual overwork
- lack of pursuits or relaxation time outside of medicine
- expectation of always coping.

Personal
- feelings of depression, anxiety, and guilt
- fatigue and physical symptoms
- self-prescribing of psychoactive drug
- daily drug use★
- the use of the drug begins to take precedence over other activities, changes in social preferences, social withdrawal★
- driving under the influence of drugs, accidents★
- public intoxication★
  ★ These signs generally occur later and suggest that urgent help is required.

Family/social
- domestic disputes, extramarital affairs, frequent absences

Work
- ambivalence about career choice
- professional isolation
- stressful work conditions
- feeling of indispensability at work
- not being able to say 'no' when this is the preferred option.

Self care

It is tempting to self-diagnose and to self-treat when one has access to knowledge and therapies. It also seems much easier and practical to seek corridor consultations and refer oneself to various specialists when needed. However, this delays proper

389

diagnosis and treatment of illnesses. Medical practitioners deserve to give themselves the same standard of care available to the general population.

There are several basic tenets for the safe practice of medicine.

- Every medical practitioner and his/her family should have his/her own general practitioner.
- Avoid self-medication.
- Be aware of your own fallibilities.
- Be aware of your own consumption of alcohol and other drugs, and avoid using these to relieve stress.
- Balance your work life with your social life.
- Maintain an emphasis on healthy living and learn ways to manage your own stress.
- Know the effects of alcohol and drugs and be able to spot the early warning signs of misuse (see above).
- Find regular opportunities to reflect on personal and professional conduct and well-being.

Under no circumstances should one ever self-prescribe psychoactive drugs. It is unethical and dangerous to self-prescribe and self-administer a controlled substance.

COLLEAGUES WHO ARE IMPAIRED BY ALCOHOL AND OTHER DRUG USE

When colleagues develop problems related to drug and alcohol use, medical practitioners have a duty to intervene to protect the colleague and the public.

Barriers to involvement

Medical practitioners may hold stereotypes of drug users that conflict with the picture of a peer developing drug dependence. Raising the issue of drug use in a colleague can be difficult, and medical practitioners may collude to protect a colleague from the negative consequences of revelation of drug dependence. This establishes a conspiracy of silence that denies early intervention.

Responsibility to colleagues and to the public

Regardless of a medical practitioner's wish to protect a colleague, the first responsibility of a medical practitioner is to first do no harm to patients, *primum non nocere*. It is therefore never reasonable to wait passively for the impaired practitioner to acknowledge the presence of a problem or for severe incapacity to develop. There are potential medico-legal consequences for medical practitioners who do not report suspicions of impairment in practising colleagues. In some jurisdictions mandatory reporting is legislated, and this is an increasing international trend.

Warning signs

Signs of drug dependence at the workplace usually occur late. Friends and family are more likely to notice early behaviour changes (see the early signs of impairment above). Changes at work can be summarised as follows.

Late changes in the impaired medical practitioner

History
- recurrent job changes, especially from one community to another
- intervals between employment
- acceptance of jobs that are inappropriate or for which he/she is overqualified.

Appearance
- physical deterioration; fatigue
- signs of intoxication or withdrawal, for example smell of alcohol, sedation, slurring of speech, loss of coordination.

Mental state
- erratic mood and personality
- poor memory.

Behaviour
- frequent personal medical complaints
- persistent overwork
- absences from work
- loss of reliability, lateness
- indecision and errors
- accidents
- inappropriate prescribing and over-prescribing
- seen to be taking pills or alcohol at work
- 'locked bathroom' syndrome
- increasing isolation professionally and socially.

Staff
- staff concerns.

Patient
- patient complaints.

391

Why get involved?

The prognosis for medical practitioners with drug dependence is generally good, especially if early intervention can be offered. Protecting a colleague is more likely to result in a loss of respect and confidence, not only in the colleague but also in the whole profession.

> ➡ Professional self-regulation is preferable to external regulation but relies on effective use of established mechanisms by the profession.

Tackling drug issues in a colleague

When a problem is suspected, early action is likely to improve the outcome. Resources and strategies are outlined below.

Resources

If you become alerted to problematic alcohol or other drug use in a colleague, there are a number of resources available to both you and your colleague.

Local Medical Boards or the Medical Council

All Medical Boards (in Australia) and the Medical Council (in New Zealand) have developed mechanisms for dealing with confidential enquiries about one's own or a colleague's suspected impairment. Procedures are aimed towards restoring ability to work and public confidence. Doctors are a scarce resource, and all efforts are made to rehabilitate, support and monitor so that public safety can be assured.

Where the problem is acknowledged by the practitioner, and treatment and monitoring is accepted, public disclosure may be avoided. A voluntary decision to take leave (if deemed to be required) is preferable to involuntary suspension. De-registration and disciplinary proceedings are not taken lightly, and generally only occur after serious offences (for example supply of drugs to the illicit market) or after multiple opportunities to demonstrate improvement have been unsuccessful.

Medical Boards and the Medical Council:
- are mandated to protect the public
- may establish a plan to assess, treat, and support the impaired medical practitioner
- aim to return the doctor to work where possible
- impose disciplinary procedures as a last resort.

Doctors' Health Advisory Service

Within Australia and New Zealand, organisations listed as the Doctors' Health Advisory Service facilitate independent expert advice, assessment, and treatment of suspected impaired practitioners. These focus on assistance, and are not directly aligned with the disciplinary arms of Medical Boards or the Medical Council.

The Doctors' Health Advisory Service:
- focuses on assistance—advice, assessment, and treatment
- is not directly aligned with the disciplinary arms of Medical Boards and the Medical Council
- can be contacted anonymously by the impaired doctor or a concerned other.

Medical defence organisations
Medical defence organisations can advise about the medico-legal implications of not reporting suspected impairment or errors in patient management.

Preparing the ground

When signs of drug dependence are suspected, it is essential to document the events (for example late attendance, episodes of intoxication, mistakes made) objectively, clearly, and as soon as possible.

Raising the issue with a colleague

Early intervention
Colleagues and friends may note early warning signs of problematic drug use (see page 389). At this point gentle confrontation may be a sufficient stimulus for the practioner concerned to seek help. If there is no reason to suspect any form of impairment in the workplace, it may be enough for the friend or colleague to take a supportive role, encouraging and facilitating engagement in treatment.

Case study 3

Anne is a dedicated 20-year-old medical student who starts her clinical rotations in her third year. She feels stressed by the demands of hospital work and out of place as a medical student in the clinical hierarchy. She feels incompetent with clinical procedures, and makes mistakes. Anne feels tired all the time, and when one of her friends on the campus gave her some amphetamine pills she found that she felt confident on the wards and able to study better. She starts using amphetamines prior to major ward rounds.

Scenario 1

Over time Anne finds that while the effect of the amphetamines is helpful, she gets moody and tired on the days that she doesn't use them. Feeling increasingly stressed by her medical studies, she feels incapable, and starts questioning her career choice. She uses more amphetamines to help her study, loses weight, becomes irritable, and often feels ill. Anne starts injecting amphetamines and is very careful, using clean injecting equipment from the wards, but occasionally shares equipment with her boyfriend. She contracts Hepatitis C that eventually comes to the attention of the faculty, and they suggest she terminate her medical studies.

Scenario 2

Anne continues to be stressed by her medical studies and uses more ampheta-mines to help her cope. Her registrar notices her lack of clinical skills and poor performance, and they have a meeting. He is sympathetic to her prob-lems and offers her extra help. Anne is quite frightened to realise that her drug use may have come to the attention of others. She resolves to seek counselling through the university clinic. Over time she gains confidence and ceases amphetamine use.

Case study 4

Paul is a 38-year-old GP whose wife has recently left him and taken his two young children interstate. He works long hours in a large and very busy seven-day practice in a low socioeconomic area where doctor shoppers are common. Paul has in recent years taken an interest in helping drug-depen-dent people. As another doctor at the practice, you hear from patients about how badly Paul's wife has treated him and about how she prevents him from seeing the children. Paul always appears tired. He tends to prescribe larger amounts of benzodiazepines and opioids, and this creates resentment among his colleagues.

Scenario 1

Paul works increasingly longer hours, attending almost every day to see his patients on Sundays and public holidays. He becomes isolated from others at the practice who blame him for making the practice a target for doctor shoppers. You become aware from patients that they are obtaining prescrip-tions from him late at night at his home. His self-care appears to have deteriorated. His documentation in the notes becomes more erratic, so that often patients are apparently prescribed opioids with no record of this in the notes. One day Paul is found to be clearly intoxicated at work. He insists that he is just tired, but this is obviously not enough to account for his appear-ance. Practice staff express concerns, and the practice partners send him home and contact the Medical Council. The surgery undergoes major disruption, as all of Paul's patients have to be rebooked with other doctors. It then becomes clear that some unethical prescribing has occurred, with some opioids being apparently prescribed for patients who are unaware of this. Paul is suspended from working for six months. He is allowed to return to work with supervision from the practice principals and ongoing urine screens. Although an option for Paul was return to the same surgery, he chooses to work in a government agency and avoids contact with people from the previous surgery.

Scenario 2

Two of the practice partners who knew Paul prior to his working at the surgery ask to see him after work one day. They express concern about some rumour spread by patients about his private life, and ask how he is coping with the separation. It is apparent that Paul has been very depressed, and has been using benzodiazepines to sleep and to reduce anxiety during the day. He has also been self-prescribing antidepressants. He feels that work has become the only thing that keeps him sane. He realises that he shouldn't really talk about his private life to patients, but finds it a relief to talk when patients ask, and then feels guilty for having done so. Paul agrees to see a psychiatrist, and the two partners ensure that they regularly check in with Paul every week. Paul is invited to take part in some of their social activities, some of which he attends. Over time Paul seems to be more able to set limits with patients in relation to his prescribing.

Intervention at the point of crisis

Impairment is usually noted following a crisis at work (for example if an anaesthetist is found to be intoxicated prior to a scheduled operation). A crisis can be viewed as a positive point of intervention. When impairment has been identified, colleagues must ensure that an assessment takes place, help is offered, and patients are protected. If there is reason to suspect that patient safety might be compromised, it is unacceptable to allow the medical practitioner to remain at work. Sick leave should be taken until full assessment and an acceptable treatment, support, and monitoring plan is put into place under the auspices of the local Medical Boards or the Medical Council.

When tackling the issue of impairment at work, consider the approaches set out below. If the impaired doctor refuses to cooperate with these approaches, colleagues must report this to the Medical Board or the Medical Council, which is authorised to act on this.

Tackling impairment in a colleague

Who

It is usually better to have more than one person present to raise the issue, since this helps to reinforce the gravity of the situation and may be useful should disputes occur about what is discussed. This needs to be done sensitively, as the impaired doctor is likely to feel defensive. It is, however, better for the impaired doctor to know that the issue is in the open, and that colleagues are united in their wish to tackle the issue and to help.

When

This should be done when the impaired doctor is not intoxicated, and as soon as practicable after the event that has led to the suspicion of impairment.

Where

This should be done in a quiet and private place.

How

The issue should be raised non-judgmentally.

What

- State the facts (for example what happened, when, who was involved).
- Express concern about the doctor as well as about patient safety.
- Anticipate denial, alternative explanations, and expressions of competence.
- Listen to explanations and look at options, but do not waver from a need to ensure patient safety.

Result

- Agree on temporary cessation of work if patient safety cannot be ensured.
- Agree on immediate assessment by a psychiatrist or other relevant health professional.
- Agree on report to the Medical Board or the Medical Council.
- Document the above and obtain consent to forward this to the Medical Board or Medical Council.

Helpful factors

Medical practitioners, like other people, are more likely to do well when adequately supported by family, friends, and colleagues. Support groups can be very important in the recovery of medical practitioners from drug dependence. These resources should be harnessed where possible, since this is likely to improve prognosis.

> The risk of depression and suicide is significant and special vigilance is required since medical practitioners who choose to suicide are likely to be successful.

Early intervention and likely outcome

If intervention can be offered early, for example when drug use is infrequent, disruption at work may be avoided. Remember that while temporary job cessation might be required, most medical practitioners will return to work with monitoring and support. Waiting for hard evidence can have disastrous consequences.

In general the prognosis is excellent for medical practitioners with substance misuse. However, the longer the problems have existed the more entrenched and resistant to treatment they become. For this reason all medical practitioners should take responsibility for maintaining high professional standards. This includes being vigilant and willing to act early for the best outcome for colleagues who are impaired by drug use, and for the best outcome for the health of the community.

REFERENCES AND FURTHER READING

Brandon, S. 1997, 'Persuading the sick or impaired doctor to seek treatment', *Advances In Psychiatric Treatment*, vol. 3, pp. 305–11.

Brook, D. 1997, 'Impairment in the medical and legal professions', *Journal of Psychoactive Research*, vol. 43, pp. 27–34.

Centrella, M. 1994, 'Physician addiction and impairment—current thinking: a review', *Journal of Addictive Diseases*, vol 13, pp. 91–105.

Doctor Shopping Project, Professional Review Division, Pharmaceutical Benefits Scheme, Health Insurance Commission 2001 http://www.hic.gov.au/

Graziotti, P.J. & Goucke, C.R. 1997, 'The use of oral opioids in patients with chronic non-cancer pain. Management strategies', *Medical Journal of Australia*, vol. 167, pp. 30–4.

Parran, T. Jr 1997, 'Prescription drug abuse. a question of balance', *Medical Clinics of North America*, vol. 81, pp. 967–78.

Weir, E. 2000, 'Substance abuse among physicians', *Canadian Medical Association Journal*, vol. 162, p. 1730.

White, J. & Taverner, D. 1997, 'Drug-seeking behaviour', *Australian Prescriber*, vol. 20, pp. 68–70.

Wijesinghe, C.P. & Dunne, F. 1999, 'Impaired practitioners notified to the Medical Practitioners Board of Victoria from 1983 to 1997', *Medical Journal of Australia*, vol. 171, pp. 414–17.

Index